Pharmaceutical Compounding and Dispensing

John F Marriott

Senior Lecturer, Pharmacy Practice
Aston University School of Pharmacy, UK

Keith A Wilson

Head of School
Aston University School of Pharmacy, UK

Christopher A Langley

Lecturer in Pharmacy Practice
Aston University School of Pharmacy, UK

and

Dawn Belcher

Teaching Fellow, Pharmacy Practice
Aston University School of Pharmacy, UK

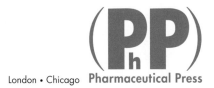

London • Chicago   Pharmaceutical Press

Published by the Pharmaceutical Press

An imprint of RPS Publishing

1 Lambeth High Street, London SE1 7JN, UK
100 South Atkinson Road, Suite 206, Grayslake, IL 60030-7820, USA

© Pharmaceutical Press 2006

 is a trade mark of RPS Publishing

RPS Publishing is the publishing organisation of the
Royal Pharmaceutical Society of Great Britain

First published 2006

Typeset by Type Study, Scarborough, North Yorkshire
Printed in Great Britain by Cambridge University Press, Cambridge

ISBN-10 0 85369 575 X
ISBN-13 978 0 85369 575 2

A catalogue record for this book is available from the British Library

Contents

List of figures

List of tables

Contents of CD-ROM

Still images

The following is a list of the images contained on the accompanying CD-ROM and an indication of where the image is referenced in the text.

Chapter 2

Chapter 4

Chapter 5

Chapter 8

Chapter 12

Additional still images on CD-ROM

Video images

The following is a list of the videos contained on the accompanying CD-ROM.

About the authors

John F Marriott

John Marriott is a pharmacist, registered in the UK for the last 25 years. He practised in both community and hospital sectors, holding a variety of positions, latterly as Chief Pharmacist at the Royal Wolverhampton Hospitals NHS Trust, before joining the academic pharmacy department at Aston University, where he took over as the Head of the Pharmacy School in 2005.

He has a proactive role in teaching in the department and is working on the development of electronic methodologies to support pharmacy learning and teaching. In addition he has wide, active research interests, principally in the areas of clinical pharmacy/pharmacology and medicines management. Current project themes revolve around the PK/PD of paediatric drug use and formulation, control of antibiotic prescribing and medicines wastage.

Keith A Wilson

Keith A Wilson graduated in pharmacy from Aston University in 1971. He is now Professor of Pharmacy at Aston University with research interests in the practice of pharmacy and particularly in public policy and pharmacy services and pharmacy education. He has over 30 years' experience in teaching on pharmacy undergraduate and postgraduate programmes and is a subject reviewer for the QAA in pharmacy and pharmacology and a member of the RPSGB accreditation panel since 1999.

Christopher A Langley

Chris Langley is a qualified pharmacist who graduated from Aston University in 1996 and then undertook his pre-registration training at St Peter's Hospital in Chertsey. Upon registration, he returned to Aston University to undertake a PhD within the Medicinal Chemistry Research Group before moving over full time to pharmacy practice. He is currently employed as a Lecturer in Pharmacy Practice, specialising in teaching the professional and legal aspects of the degree programme.

His research interests predominantly surround pharmacy education but he is also involved in research examining the role of the pharmacist in both primary and secondary care. This includes examining the pharmacist's role in public health and the reasons behind and possible solutions to the generation of waste medication.

Dawn Belcher

Dawn Belcher is a qualified pharmacist who graduated from the Welsh School of Pharmacy in 1977 and then undertook her pre-registration training with Boots the Chemist at their Wolverhampton store. After registration she worked as a relief manager and later as a pharmacy manager for Boots the Chemist until 1984. While raising a family she undertook locum duties for Boots the Chemist and in 1986 became an independent locum working for a small chain of pharmacies in the West Midlands while also working for Lloyds Chemist. In 1989 she began sessional teaching with the pharmacy practice group at Aston University which continued until she took a permanent post in 2001. She now enjoys teaching practical aspects of pharmacy practice while still keeping an association with Lloydspharmacy, where she is employed as a relief manager.

Preface

Pharmacists or their pharmaceutical equivalents have been responsible for compounding medicines for centuries. Recently this role has been challenged in the pharmaceutical literature with suggestions and recommendations that it is inappropriate for the pharmaceutical practitioner to compound medicines in a local pharmacy environment. Notwithstanding this valid debate, it is clear that a vast array of skills and knowledge with regard to medicines compounding has been accrued and refined, certainly over the last two centuries. In the present environment it is possible that this knowledge and skill base might be dispersed and ultimately lost. However, it is not beyond the bounds of imagination to conceive that there will be times, albeit possibly in the face of some form of environmental, cultural or local emergency, that pharmacists might be called upon to extemporaneously compound medicines when conventional supply chains are either unavailable or have broken down.

This text has been designed with a number of functions in mind. First, it is important to be aware of some of the historical pathways that have led to the present technological position of pharmacists. In addition, unless many of the antiquated measuring systems, methodologies and formulations are not preserved in some reference work, they might be lost forever, or at least be totally unavailable except to the dogged historian. Primarily, however, this work is intended as a reference-based tutorial to the methods employed in medicines compounding. The text has been designed to allow students and practitioners to be able to examine either all or part of the subsequent chapters in order to familiarise themselves with the compounding techniques necessary to produce products of appropriate quality and efficacy. In addition, the text is supported by moving images in order to augment the necessary techniques and expertise.

The text also has a role when considering the design and implementation of standard operating procedures (SOPs) pertinent to certain sectors of professional practice today. Although we do not expect all practitioners of pharmacy to be compounding medicines on a daily basis, we hope that should the need arise this text will effectively support any work of this nature that might be encountered.

John F Marriott
Keith A Wilson
Christopher A Langley
Dawn Belcher
Birmingham, United Kingdom
May 2005

Acknowledgements

The authors are grateful to everyone who assisted them during the preparation of this book.

Special thanks are given to Edward Belcher for offering his advice and extensive pharmaceutical compounding knowledge during the preparation of Part 2 of the book.

In addition, the authors are also grateful to Mike Turner who offered advice and the use of his equipment during the preparation of the video images on the accompanying CD-ROM.

Finally, the authors are also very grateful to the Museum of the Royal Pharmaceutical Society of Great Britain for allowing access to various museum pieces during the assembly of the still images on the accompanying CD-ROM and for the assistance offered by Briony Hudson (Keeper of the Museum Collections) and Peter Homan (Honorary Secretary of the British Society for the History of Pharmacy) during the collection of the images.

Museum of the Royal Pharmaceutical Society

The Royal Pharmaceutical Society has had a museum collection since 1842. The 45 000 items collected since then cover all aspects of British pharmacy history, from traditional dispensing equipment to 'Lambeth delftware' drug storage jars, and from proprietary medicines to medical caricatures.

In addition to displays in the Society's headquarters building, the Museum offers historical research services based on its collections, and also research of pharmacists' family histories and the history of premises. The Museum has a large photographic archive and can supply images for reproduction. Books, postcards, greetings cards and other merchandise based on the Museum's collections are available directly from the Society and by mail order.

Museum of the Royal Pharmaceutical Society, 1 Lambeth High Street, London SE1 7JN, UK. Tel: +44(0)20 7572 2210.
museum@rpsgb.org
www.rpsgb.org/museum

British Society for the History of Pharmacy

The British Society for the History of Pharmacy was formed in 1967, having originated from a committee of the Royal Pharmaceutical Society. It seeks to act as a focus for the development of all areas of the history of pharmacy, from the works of the ancient apothecary to today's ever changing role of the community, wholesale or industrial pharmacist.

For further details about membership and events, contact: The British Society for the History of Pharmacy, 840 Melton Road, Thurmaston, Leicester LE4 8BN, UK. Tel: +44(0)116 2640083.
bshp@associationhq.org.uk

Part 1

History of compounding

1

Historical perspective

1.1 The origins of the pharmacy profession

It is impossible to determine when humans first began to mix substances and concoct preparations that produced either perceived or real therapeutic effects, but it is known that the compounding of medicinal preparations from materia medica of animal, vegetable and mineral sources has been practised in a sophisticated form by a range of ancient civilisations. The societies of ancient Egypt, Greece, Rome and the Arabian cultures, for example, all developed complex levels of medical knowledge, integrating various aspects of pharmacy and medicines compounding.

The ancient Egyptian cultures exerted an influence upon social and scientific development throughout the period extending from approximately 3000 BC to 1200 BC. Clearly, throughout this period of diverse cultural development, Egyptian society was supported by specialist medical and pharmaceutical practice. Archaeological research shows widespread evidence of medicines compounding being central to the therapeutics practised by the ancient Egyptians. Examples of medicines chests containing dried drugs and the tools associated with compounding have been found. Written works on papyrus have also been discovered that describe contemporary materia medica, formulae, remedies and the weights and measures used. Many of the vegetable-based drugs, animal products and minerals described are recognisable today, and indeed some remain in current use.

Prepared drugs were also a feature of the various Mesopotamian civilisations that existed in parallel with the Egyptian cultures. Again, some of the drugs used by the Assyrians, such as opium, myrrh and liquorice, are still used today.

The ancient Greek civilisations made known contributions to medicine and pharmacy principally between approximately 1250 BC and 285 BC. It would appear that the ancient Greek medical practice used fewer drug-based therapies than the Egyptian and Mesopotamian cultures. Despite this, around 400 drugs are described by Hippocrates, writing around 425 BC. Interestingly, Hippocrates also emphasised the importance of pure water in medicine and the necessity for absolute cleanliness in surgery, features which are still causing problems in the treatment of patients today.

After the disintegration of the ancient Greek civilisation around 220 BC, many Greek physicians moved to either Rome or other parts of the Roman Empire. Prior to this period Roman medical and pharmaceutical practice had revolved around religious and superstitious ritual, principally conducted by the lower sections of society such as slaves (*servi medici*) and wise-women (*sagae*). Drugs and prepared medicines were used by the Romans, but compounding again appeared to be chiefly carried out by less prominent sections of society, with herb-gatherers (*rhizotomi*), drug pedlars (*pharmacopoloe*) and those trading in salves (*unguentarii*) being in evidence.

By around 30 BC, under the influence of imported Greek practice, the status of some of those practising medicine had risen, and until the fall of the Roman Empire a substantial number of influential practitioners were in evidence, including Celsus, Dioscorides and Galen. Each of these great practitioners left written works containing information on drugs, medicines and compounding, which formed the basis of therapeutics well into the seventeenth century.

As the Roman Empire disintegrated, the West entered the Dark Ages and medical and pharmaceutical practice was transformed into a 'monastic'-driven system. During this time, although some Graeco-Roman therapeutic principles were preserved, practice was largely based upon religious and superstitious beliefs. By contrast, in the Eastern Byzantine area of the Roman Empire, centred on Constantinople, which remained until 1453, much of the classical literature on therapeutics and drug trading links was retained. An additional eastern repository and incubator of medical knowledge developed in Arabia during the Dark Ages. Traditional Graeco-Roman medical texts were translated into Arabic and compiled with other works collected from the Far East. The Arabs of this period also derived information from their studies on alchemy.

Many important texts containing information on drugs and compounding were compiled by the great Arab physicians of the seventh to thirteenth centuries, including those by John Mesuë Senior (d. 857), Abu Mansur (*c.* 970), Ibn Sina (Avicenna, *c.* 980–1036) and Ibn al Baitar of Malaga (1197–1248). Typical of the texts of the period and area is the *Corpus of Simples*, compiled by Ibn al Baitar of Malaga, which largely contains information on drugs and compounding originating from older classical works. There is, however, some evidence to show that at least 300 previously unused medicinal agents were described by the key Arabic texts dealing with pharmaceutical preparation. Many of these new agents appear to have arisen from introductions by the Arabs from the Far East, and include cloves, betel nut, rhubarb, nux vomica and the widespread use of cane sugar as a component of formulations.

By the eleventh century, Europe was beginning to emerge from the post-Roman Dark Ages. New concepts in medical and pharmaceutical practice were developed and disseminated along Graeco-Arabian lines of communication, which spread from areas around the Mediterranean, where close contact had been established with Arabian invaders.

In centres of learning throughout Europe, traditional medical works were resurrected and refinement of these principles was begun by employing a more scientific approach to medicine.

In the thirteenth-century German court of Frederick II, apothecaries translated many of the earlier Arabic pharmaceutical works into Latin. As a result of these activities, around 1240, Frederick II issued an edict that defined the role of pharmacists as an entity distinct from other professions.

In England, the origins of the pharmaceutical profession arose principally from trading arrangements that had begun in Roman times and continued throughout the Dark and Middle

Ages. Close links had been formed with continental Europe, particularly France following the Norman invasion and the subsequent Crusades.

The dealing in medicines and materia medica fell under the trades of 'mercery' and 'spicery', the latter being traded by spicers and pepperers. These merchant bodies were amongst those who formed Guilds during the medieval period and the spicers began to evolve into a body concentrating upon the manipulation and compounding of medicines. It is from this group that the specialist apothecary arose.

By the fifteenth century the apothecaries were highly specialised in the art and practice of pharmacy, and it was during this period that the long-standing disagreements with the physicians began to emerge. This conflict arose primarily because apothecaries were not only compounding and dispensing medicines, they were also involved with providing medical advice. Physicians protected their status by petitioning the crown and Henry VIII issued a regulation that restricted the practice of medicine to physicians by stipulating that practitioners had to be examined and ratified by the Bishop of London or the Dean of Saint Paul's.

1.2 Foundation of the Royal Pharmaceutical Society of Great Britain

For centuries disputes had occurred between physicians, apothecaries and chemists and druggists in relation to their respective rights to practise pharmacy and to provide medical advice. These disputes led to the introduction of a number of keynote elements of legislation which placed controls upon medical and pharmaceutical practitioners.

During the eighteenth and early nineteenth centuries the number of Members of the Royal College of Physicians was relatively small (around 100) and they generally concentrated on the treatment of wealthy patients, with some *pro bono* work amongst the poor. However, at this time a large middle class existed who were able to pay for consultations and treatments. This group most often sought advice and help from apothe-

caries and surgeon-apothecaries. The Society of Apothecaries had been founded in 1617 and subsequently ratified an extensive apprenticeship system for members.

In 1703 a long-standing dispute between the College of Physicians and the Apothecaries regarding the authority to prescribe medicines erupted in the 'Rose case', in which apothecary William Rose was prosecuted by the College for allegedly practising medicine without a licence. This case progressed through the courts, culminating in an appeal in the House of Lords. The final outcome resulted in the finding that apothecaries could give advice to patients and prescribe medication in addition to compounding and selling medicines, though they could only seek remuneration for any activity involving the supply of medicines.

Despite the controlled existence of the College of Physicians and the Society of Apothecaries, by the nineteenth century there were such large numbers of either unqualified or poorly qualified individuals practising that it became apparent that legal reform of the education and registration procedures was necessary. Eventually the Apothecaries Act was passed in 1815, under which the Society of Apothecaries was made responsible for education and registration of apothecaries. A subsequent court decision made in 1829 ruled that apothecaries could make charges for their professional advice, a reversal of the previous situation.

The Apothecaries Act (1815) also clarified the status of chemists and druggists, stating that their activities in procuring, compounding and selling drugs would be unaffected by the legislation. Thus, the Apothecaries Act (1815) effectively enabled chemists and druggists to practise pharmacy without imposing any educational or performance requirements on their activities. The ability of the chemists and druggists to secure such an important concession in the Apothecaries Act was due, in part, to the concerted lobby presented by this group, which had previously formed an Association of Chemist and Druggists in 1802. The Association of Chemists and Druggists was reconfigured and expanded to form the General Association of Chemists and Druggists in 1829. This was soon disbanded, however, following the achievement of one of the aims of the group, notably the removal of duty levied on certain compounded medicines.

In 1841 a Bill was introduced to the Commons by Mr Benjamin Hawes to amend the laws relating to the medical profession of Great Britain and Ireland. This Bill intended to effect a drastic reorganisation of the way medicine was practised. The impact of the proposed legislation on chemists and druggists would have been to require them to be regulated by examination before practising, since any activities involving patients, such as recommending therapies or treating minor ailments, would have been regarded as practising medicine.

Chemists and druggists, particularly from London, began to form an opposition strategy to the proposed Bill. Some of these established practitioners were cognisant, however, that many of their body were poorly educated and that they had been fortuitous under the terms of the Apothecaries Act (1815) in being able to practise effectively without regulation. Meetings were held in February 1841 at which the main wholesalers were greatly in evidence, including representatives from Allen, Hanburys and Barry, Savory, Moore and Co and John Bell and Co. The outcome of this meeting was that vociferous representations were made to Parliament opposing the Hawes Bill, supported by a written petition sporting over 600 signatures from chemists and druggists all opposed to any moves to remove their right to prescribe and recommend medicines. Through these efforts and those of other professionals the Hawes Bill was withdrawn.

The campaign to enable the education and registration of chemists and druggists was not forgotten, however. Jacob Bell believed that the solution to this problem resided in the formation of a unified society formed from the chemists and druggists practising in Great Britain. The proposed society was intended to serve a number of functions, principally to present a unified front in promoting and protecting the interests of pharmacists, developing the education of the membership and ultimately enhancing the status and prestige of pharmacists.

The initial meeting to promote this concept was held at Bell's house and has been referred to subsequently as 'the pharmaceutical tea-party'. There were sufficient numbers of chemists and druggists motivated by the recent dealings of the Hawes Bill to warrant further meetings to develop the formation of the proposed new society. A subsequent meeting, chaired by William Allen FRS, was held in the Crown and Anchor Tavern in the Strand on 15 April 1841. During this meeting a resolution was adopted to form an association of chemists and druggists called 'The Pharmaceutical Society of Great Britain' and a formal report was then sent to over 5000 prospective members.

At the inaugural meeting of the new Society, held on 1 June 1841, rules were drafted and approved and a temporary committee agreed until the general meeting planned for May 1842. By the end of 1841 around 800 members had joined the Society and in 1842 the membership had increased to 2000. In November of that year the Society petitioned for a Royal Charter, which was granted on 18 February 1843.

1.3 Pharmacy legislation

It is useful to consider the historical development of relevant legislation that has influenced the manner in which pharmaceutical compounding has been conducted in the UK. Before the 1850s, medicinal products could be sold by any individual, who was at liberty to use the title 'pharmaceutical chemist'. Moreover, there were no formal controls on the premises from which such individuals operated the business of selling medicines, with obvious outcomes in terms of the quality and uniformity of products available.

1.3.1 Important legislation since 1850

The Pharmacy Act 1852

This Act provided the legislative framework underpinning the original aims embodied by the formation of the Pharmaceutical Society. Under this legislation the Pharmaceutical Society was empowered to examine the proficiency of prospective pharmacists and to issue membership certificates, thereby restricting the title 'pharmaceutical chemist', although it did not restrict the use of 'chemist' or 'druggist' as titles.

The Pharmacy Act 1868

This extended the scope of the 1852 Act to require the Registrar of the Pharmaceutical Society to keep registers of pharmaceutical chemists, chemists and druggists and apprentices or students. The titles 'chemist' and 'druggist' were restricted under this Act. It also introduced restrictions on the sale of poisons by developing a 'Poisons List'. Items from this list could only be sold by pharmaceutical chemists and by chemists and druggists. Naturally these restrictions had a major impact upon the nature of products that could be legally compounded and sold.

Poisons and Pharmacy Act 1908

The control of poisons was further extended in aspects of the Pharmacy Act 1908, in that the list of poisons was expanded. In addition, this Act laid out the terms under which a body corporate could conduct the business of a chemist and druggist, thus further controlling the compounding process.

National Insurance Act 1911

The pharmaceutical profession has been intimately involved with the movements to establish a welfare state. The National Insurance Act of 1911 was passed at the time that the Secretary of the Pharmaceutical Society of Great Britain, William Glyn-Jones, was a Member of Parliament. The influence of the Society, through Glyn-Jones, ensured that pharmacists were the principal dispensers and compounders of medicines for those patients prescribed medication in accordance with this Act. Accordingly this established the beginning of the process whereby pharmaceutical professionals could develop the dispensing element of their businesses. Not surprisingly, this legislation also led to the pharmacist contractors being requested to 'discount' their activities when it became apparent that original estimates of costs were not viable.

Venereal Disease Act 1917

For a number of years both the medical and pharmaceutical professions had called for controls to be placed upon the unsubstantiated advertisement of 'patent' medicines. In 1917 the Venereal Diseases Act made the advertising of remedies for venereal diseases illegal in the same way that the later Cancer Act (1939) prohibited the advertising of treatment for neoplastic disease. These Acts were the precursors of the advent of evidence-based pharmacotherapy.

Ministry of Health Act 1919

This Act created the Ministry of Health and transferred responsibilities for health from other bodies which were further developed in later legislation.

Therapeutic Substances Act 1925

This Act controlled the licence to manufacture a stated list of products that could not be tested by chemical methods. This list contained agents such as vaccines and sera and was extended later, notably when greater numbers of antibiotics were introduced.

Pharmacy and Poisons Act 1933

Under this legislation the Pharmaceutical Society was charged with ensuring compliance with the Act, leading to the development of both the Statutory Committee as a disciplinary body and the pharmaceutical inspectorate. All pharmacy premises were registered under this Act, which also dictated that all registered pharmacists must be members of the Pharmaceutical Society. These measures clearly had great bearing upon the pharmaceutical environments in which compounding operations were being conducted. The Pharmacy and Poisons Act (1933) also established the Poisons Board, which was created to advise the Secretary of State with respect to the composition of the Poisons List.

Pharmacy and Medicines Act 1941

This Act further defined the nature of premises in which medicines could be sold, restricting such sales to shops rather than temporary structures such as stalls and barrows. The need to indicate the composition of proprietary medicines was also established, reversing the situation that existed under the Medicine Stamp Act (1812), which exempted the need to show the composition of these medicines if an appropriate duty had been paid.

National Health Services Act 1946

This legislation led to the development of an all-embracing Health Service, including the availability of pharmaceutical services which extended to the whole population. One of the outcomes of this Act was that pharmacist contractors became the almost exclusive compounders and dispensers for prescriptions under the legislation, with few exceptions such as emergencies and in very remote areas.

National Insurance Act 1946

The Health Ministries in the UK became responsible for the general practitioner and pharmaceutical services, hospitals, mental health and local authority services, together with aspects of public health (water supplies, sewage).

Pharmacy Acts 1953 and 1954

Under this legislation the register of chemists and druggists was abandoned and a new register of pharmaceutical chemists was established. All those listed in the abolished registers were incorporated into the new version.

Therapeutic Substances Act 1956

Previous legislation was rationalised under this Act and control of both the manufacture and the sale and supply of agents listed as therapeutic substances was combined in this single piece of legislation.

1.4 Development of the pharmacopoeias

Formularies and pharmacopoeias have been in use for almost as long as medicines have been compounded, but most of the early pharmaceutical texts only exerted a local influence on medicines usage.

One of the earliest, formally developed and widely accepted compilations of medicines compounding was the *Antidotarium Nicolai* of Nicolaus Salernitanus (from *c.* 1100), which contained 139 complex prescriptions in alphabetical order in conjunction with monographs and references to simples (drugs) and pharmaceutical preparations (electuaries). Nicolaus Salernitanus was the superintendent of the Medical School of Salerno, which was particularly active following the conquest of Salerno by the Normans in 1076 to around 1224 when it began to decline in influence. This period equates to the peak influence of Arabian medicine in both the East and the West. The *Antidotarium Nicolai* was compiled at this institution and became probably the most widely accepted pharmacopoeia of the Middle Ages. Many elements from it were in use long after the thirteenth century. Indeed, it was made the official pharmacopoeia in Naples and Sicily by Ferdinand II in the early sixteenth century and a number of preparations current in the twentieth century can be traced to it.

Uptake and official recognition of pharmaceutical texts was generally an ad hoc affair until the early part of the sixteenth century. At this time throughout Europe a number of city-based or municipal pharmacopoeias were developed, which were intended to be implemented in certain specified towns and districts. Inevitably, some of these works became more widely recognised.

Two particular examples of sixteenth-century pharmaceutical texts applied widely across Europe were *Chirurgerye* by John Vigon, which appeared in England in a translation by Bartholomew Traheron (1543), and the *Most Excellent Homish Apothecary* by Jerome Brunschweig, which was produced in an English translation (1561). The former work listed simples according to their qualities, and specific formulae were given for 'oyntmentes, cerates, pilaysters, oyles, pilles and confections'. The latter text contained many remedies, including confections, spices, spiced fruits and pills.

1.4.1 The first recognised pharmacopoeia?

Perhaps the first widely recognized pharmacopoeia was the *Dispensatorium* of Valerius Cordus (1515–1544) (first edition 1546). This contained many old formulae derived from traditional sources, including Galen, Avicenna, Mesuë and Rhazes, but also contained a number of unique references to medicines, including the first accurate description of nux vomica and many preparations of essential oils. The *Dispensatorium* of Valerius Cordus was adopted by the Senate of Nuremberg, which gave rise to the work being known later as the 'Nuremberg Pharmacopoeia'. It was well known in England in the sixteenth century, along with other similar works such as *The Grete Herball*, an English translation of *Le Grant Herbier en Francoys* (1516–1520), which was itself sourced from the first herbal compiled in French, *Arbolayre* (c. 1485).

In the *Dispensatorium* the herbs, minerals and other crude drugs were arranged in alphabetical order and information was given about their identification, sources, preparation and uses, together with some detail of pathology and therapeutics.

1.4.2 The first London Pharmacopoeia (*Pharmacopoeia Londinensis*) 1618

Within a few years of its foundation in 1518, the College of Physicians indicated that it would be beneficial to develop some form of national formulary or pharmacopoeia that would act as a standard reference source for physicians and apothecaries in England. This concept presumably arose from positive experiences of the early College founders with texts such as the *Recettario fiorentino* (which was established in Florence in 1498 and then used widely throughout Italy) itself based upon the *Antidotarium* of Nicolaus Myrepsius, which was a thirteenth-century work. In June 1585 the concept of a standard pharma-

copoeia was debated by the College, but it was not until 1589 that it was decided formally to develop a text under the stewardship of 24 illustrious physicians. These physicians were charged with detailing the preparations to be included. Notably, no pharmaceutical personnel were involved directly, though it was indicated that appropriate advice from pharmacists should be sought when compiling any details of the methods of preparation and dosages to be recommended.

The manuscript was ready for publication in 1617 following a lengthy period of examination by expert physicians. The Pharmacopoeia was finally published on 7 May 1618 following a Royal proclamation issued in April 1618 directing all apothecaries to use this text in their practice. Strangely, this first edition of the Pharmacopoeia was replaced in December of the same year by the first 'official' edition, which was a substantially revised and expanded version of that published in May. Since the 'official' December 1618 Pharmacopoeia contained a greater number of pages and the number of simples included had been expanded from 680 to 1190, as were the number of complex preparations, it can only be assumed that disagreement within the College of Physicians had led to the re-evaluation of the list of recommended products.

The Pharmacopoeia contained a large number of simples, of which over half were of plant origin (roots, herbs, leaves and seeds). The compound preparations were collected under headings that are largely recognised today. Syrups, decoctions, oils, waters, liniments, unguents, plasters, powders, conserves, salts, chemicals and metals all appeared. Other less well-recognised groups of medicaments were also included (e.g. Tragematae, which refer to sugar and spice mixtures). Significant quantities of materia medica of animal, vegetable and mineral origin were also included. Most of these were included as compound preparations requiring expert technical manipulation in an apothecary's premises for their production. For example, the 1618 'Official' Pharmacopoeia contained around 178 simple waters, many of which would require distillation (or evaporation) in their production.

Many of the compound preparations in the Pharmacopoeia contained a huge number of ingredients. It was common to find preparations with between 10 and 30 components, and certain products took the compound formulation approach to the extreme. For example Confectio de Hyacinthi contained in excess of 50 ingredients and the Great Antidote of Matthiolus, which was used against poison and plague, was made up of over 130 components.

It is clear that a high level of pharmaceutical expertise was required to compound these treatments, but paradoxically many of the preparations would be of little therapeutic value. The Pharmacopoeia contained a large number of items and preparations that had been derived from older and even ancient texts, including various materia medica of animal origin, including dessicated whole animals and excrements. Neverthless, newer chemical therapies were also included, for example various mineral acids, Mercurius Dulcis (calomel) and some iron preparations, which would be expected to produce positive therapeutic outcomes if used in appropriate conditions. The introduction of these newer therapies appears to be the result of the actions of the King's physician, Sir Theodore de Mayerne, who had a particular interest in experimental pharmacy.

1.4.3 Subsequent London Pharmacopoeias

The 1618 London Pharmacopoeia was revised in subsequent versions in 1621, 1632 and 1639.

The 1650 edition of the London Pharmacopoeia (second edition)

This edition was a 212-page, indexed document, published under the auspices of the Commonwealth and was obviously intended to have wider influence than previous editions, which only applied to England. The 1650 Pharmacopoeia was also arranged under headings of simples and a range of compound preparations, the form of which would be readily recognisable today. Waters, spirits, tinctures, vinegars, syrups, decoctions, conserves, powders, pills, lozenges, oils, ointments, plasters and salts were all represented, together with a larger number of chemical entities (Medicamenta Chymicae Praeparata), such as the mercury salts. Significantly, a six-page section still included a miscellany of bizarre substances clearly thought to be of pharmaceutical use, including prepared worms and millipedes, lard and powdered lead.

The London Pharmacopoeia 1677 (*Pharmacopoeia Collegii Regalis Londini*) (third edition)

This edition was dedicated to Charles II and contained most of the simples and therapeutic preparations, both compound, animal and herbal, included in the previous edition. The 1677 edition began to address the need to categorise the increasing number of inorganic chemical entities used therapeutically. Categories for metals (e.g. gold, silver), *metallis affinia* (e.g. mercury, cinnabar) and *recrement metallica nativa* (e.g. cobalt, bismuth) were included. This edition also gave specific details concerning weights and measures.

The London Pharmacopoeia 1721 (fourth edition)

Contributors to this work included Sir Hans Sloane (1660–1753), who donated land for the Chelsea Physic Garden. It is not surprising, therefore, that this edition included accurate botanical descriptions of plants in addition to even more chemical entities.

The London Pharmacopoeia 1746 (fifth edition)

This edition contained many important revisions and a large number of obsolete preparations were removed. Despite the obvious attempts to modernise this edition, the text was still written largely in Latin.

However, the details outlined in this Pharmacopoeia indicated that contemporary physicians, despite working only with observational evidence, were striving to change their therapeutic practice towards treatment with less intricate, efficacious products geared to containing only active ingredients. Thus, there was an active movement away from the older, elaborate complex preparations. This edition was said to excel in Galenic pharmacy.

With a few exceptions, the classes of preparations included in the 1746 edition would have been recognisable and in common use in the early twentieth century. The relative importance of each product grouping can be derived by looking at the contents list and noting the number of pages devoted to each section. The contents, with first section page number, were as follows: Pondera et Mensurae 1, Materia Medica 3, Praeparationes Simpliciores 22, Conservae 27, Condita 29, Succi 30, Extracta et Resina 31, Olea per Expressionem 35, Olea per Distillationem 36, Sales et Salina 40, Resinosa et Sulphurea 53, Metallica 55, Aquae Stillatitiae Simplices 65, Aquae Stillatitiae Spiritosae et Spiritus 69, Decocta et Infusa 75, Vina 82, Tincturae Spirituosae 86, Mixturae 96, Syrupi 98, Mella et Oxymelita 105, Pulveres 108, Trochisci et Tabellae 115, Pilulae 118, Electaria 122, Aquae Medicamentosae 132, Olea per Infusionem et Decoctionem 134, Emplastra 136, Unguenta et Linimenta 142, Cerata 150, Epithemata 152.

Apothecaries' recommended books (Henry Pemberton 1746)

Despite the development and promotion of official pharmaceutical works, it is clear that from the sixteenth to the eighteenth centuries, those involved with compounding relied in their professional lives upon a range of texts that detailed therapies arising from both traditional, classical pharmaceutical sources and those originating from more modern trends and discoveries. This premise can be exemplified by the following list of texts for the practising apothecary recommended in the mid eighteenth century by Dr Henry Pemberton, the Gresham Professor of Physic.

Pemberton indicated that two classical works on simples by Avicenna (AD 980–1037) and Serapion (200–150 BC) should be consulted, together with *De synonymis* and *Quid pro quo* on substitutes (Simon Januensis, thirteenth century). Also recommended was *Liber Servitoris* of Bulchasim (Ben Aberazerin, 936–1013), which examined the preparation of minerals, plants and animal materials, the *Antidotarium* of Johannes Damascenus (or Mesuë, d. 857), which was arranged in classes rather like the sections detailing

galenicals in current pharmacopoeias, the *Dispensatory (De compositione)* of Dessen – Bernardus Dessenius Chronenburgius (Lyon, 1555) and the *Antidotarium* of Nicolaus de Salerno (twelfth century), which presented galenical compounds arranged alphabetically. Two editions of the latter work were referred to: the first *Nicolaus Parvus* (common edition) and *Nicolaus Magnus*, which was an expanded version containing more preparations.

The London Pharmacopoeia 1788 (sixth edition)

This edition of the London Pharmacopoeia signalled the movement from the recommendation and use of ancient multicomponent preparations to the wider adoption of chemical medicines. A number of Torbern Bergmann's names for chemical salts were used and a range of new drugs, including several examples of alkaloids, was introduced. (Bergmann was an eighteenth-century chemist who produced the definitive table for chemical affinities in 1775.)

There was also a physical difference between this edition of the London Pharmacopoeia and its predecessors, in that the pages were substantially smaller (approx 8 cm × 13 cm). It was also recognised that many practitioners were less proficient in Latin, as the foreword indicated that a translation of the 1788 Pharmacopoeia would be available soon.

In addition, there was further evidence that a more rigorous scientific approach had been adopted with regard to the selection of information provided in this edition. The binomial system of plant nomenclature was adopted, as were details of temperatures using the newly developed Fahrenheit mercury thermometer, and a more rational naming system for compounds was used, rejecting some of the more traditional nomenclature (e.g. Ferrum Ammoniacale rather than Flores Martiales).

The London Pharmacopoeia 1809 (seventh edition)

This edition was produced on a larger page size than the previous 1788 edition and the practice of publishing a Latin-to-English translation was continued. The 1809 edition was republished with corrections in 1815, reputedly because of serious criticisms made by a London chemist and druggist, Richard Phillips FRS (1777–1851). In this and subsequent editions, the need to follow directions and weighing and measuring instructions in the Pharmacopoeia was stressed. The trend to review and replace older nomenclature was also continued (e.g. Acidum Sulphuricum replaced the rather ancient term Acidum Vitriolicum).

The London Pharmacopoeia 1824 (eighth edition)

This edition was dedicated to George IV and continued the trend to include the fruits of contemporary experimental research. The temperatures in Fahrenheit of both sand and water baths were defined and a number of specific weights were included in the monographs for a range of compounds. For example, it was stated that alcohol prepared by distillation on a water bath from rectified spirit treated with potassium subcarbonate should have a specific weight of 0.815.

The table of contents for the 1824 edition contained 223 articles, of which 175 were of vegetable origin, together with a further 320 compounds and preparations which were arranged in product groupings that are clearly recognisable today (with the proviso that they were still in Latin). Very few of the ancient and often bizarre materia medica, based on animal (including human) material, so much the mainstay of the older Pharmacopoeias, survived in the 1824 edition. However, some intriguing examples remained, such as lard, Cornu Ustum (animal charcoal from burnt ivory), suet, Spongia Usta (burnt sponge, which was rich in iodine for thyroid conditions) and Testae Preparatae (oyster shells used as an antacid).

The London Pharmacopoeia 1836 (ninth edition)

The 1836 edition differed substantially from those published earlier as it was in alphabetical order. It was produced following the appointment of a Pharmacopoeia Revision Committee by Richard Phillips FRS and colleagues.

Many new alkaloids (morphine, quinine and strychnine) and the halogens iodine and bromine, together with a number of potent agents (e.g. hydrocyanic acid and ergot), were included. The increase in the number of new drug entities included reflected the efforts directed at experimental research being actively conducted around this time. This increased research effort was also reflected in this edition of the Pharmacopoeia in terms of advances in chemical analysis and identification. Indeed, the 1836 edition has been said to herald the advent of drug standardisation, as details were included concerning the determination of substance purity.

The last London Pharmacopoeia 1851 (tenth edition)

This was the last edition of the London Pharmacopoeia for which the College of Physicians was entirely responsible. As might be expected, many new medicaments appeared, including cod liver oil, morphine salts, atropine, ferrous iodide syrup and chloroform, which had only recently been first used as an anaesthetic agent.

1.4.4 The Edinburgh Pharmacopoeias

The *Pharmacopoeia Collegii Regii Medicorum Edinburgensium* was first produced in 1699. It is possible that this small first edition of 1699 was modelled upon the London Pharmacopoeia, as it closely resembled the early English volumes.

The 1699 Edinburgh edition contained details of simples, compound preparations and a variety of chemicals used in therapeutics. Despite the inclusion of the latter more advanced preparations, this Pharmacopoeia was largely based upon ancient traditional remedies and materia medica.

The pharmacopoeias produced in Scotland were revised regularly, and by 1774 the sixth edition had been reached. By this time much of the older materia medica had been excluded.

The 1783 edition of the Edinburgh Pharmacopoeia stipulated that the measurement of quantities of both solids and liquids should be made by weight in a similar manner to the pharmaceutical customs practised in France at this time. In this edition there is also an interesting example of eighteenth-century evidence-based practice. Digitalis was re-introduced into the 1783 edition following the ground-breaking work performed by William Withering in 1775, despite having been removed from earlier editions presumably because of the perception that this agent was therapeutically ineffective.

Further changes in later editions of the Edinburgh Pharmacopoeia mirrored those adopted in London. In 1839, English was adopted as the pharmaceutical language rather than Latin, and this edition also began to give instructions on how the purity of drug substances could be determined.

In 1841 the last edition of the Edinburgh Pharmacopoeia was published, and this remained in use until the first British Pharmacopoeia was issued in 1864 (see Section 1.4.7). This final edition reversed the weighing recommendations of 1839 and the Imperial weights and measures system was introduced.

1.4.5 The Dublin Pharmacopoeia (*Pharmacopoeia Collegii Medicorum Regis et Reginae in Hibernia*)

The Royal College of Physicians in Ireland also produced its own Pharmacopoeia. Editions were produced in 1793 and 1805 for exclusive use by College members. However, in 1807 an edition was produced and endorsed by the College for general issue. This contained a descriptive list of drugs approved for use together with preparation and compounding details and advice concerning equipment and official weights and measures. However, no dosage recommendations were given in this edition.

Further editions were issued in 1826 and 1850. It is interesting that although the Dublin Pharmacopoeia was clearly based in principle on elements of its counterparts from London and Edinburgh, in some respects the Irish Pharmacopoeia was more advanced and forward thinking. The 1851 edition had largely excluded any ancient, ineffective preparations, and avoirdupois weights replaced the troy system previously used. In addition, chloroform appeared only three years after its first use as an anaesthetic in 1847. Moreover, the final edition stipulated that poisons must be dispensed in bottles of distinctive shape.

1.4.6 Unofficial reference works

Clearly, prior to the publication of the first London Pharmacopoeia in 1618 all pharmaceutical texts and reference works were technically 'unofficial'. The production of the first official Pharmacopoeia, however, did not prevent the development of other unofficial reference works: indeed, the production of official texts in Latin in some ways promoted the need for translations, which often then contained additions by the author.

In 1649 Nicholas Culpeper (1616–1654) published *A Physicall Directory*, which was effectively an unauthorised translation of the 1618 London Pharmacopoeia with additional comments on the therapeutic uses of the substances included. This work was produced in many subsequent editions.

A *New London Dispensatory* was published by William Salmon (1644–1713) in 1676. This work was continually developed to include information on pharmaceutical practice and was produced in a total of eight editions up to 1716.

The trend to produce translations and interpretations of the official London Pharmacopoeia continued throughout the eighteenth and early nineteenth centuries and many of these texts served to support the need for improved teaching and learning experiences in pharmaceutical practice and therapeutics. Examples of these supplementary pharmaceutical texts include *Pharm Universalis* (1747) by Robert James, *The London Dispensatory* (1811) by A.T. Thomson, *The Pupil's Pharmacopoeia* (1824) by William Maugham, the *Supplement to the Pharmacopoeia* (1828) by S.F. Gray and the *New London Manual of Medical Chemistry* (1831) by William Maugham.

1.4.7 The British Pharmacopoeia (BP)

The Medical Act (1858) led directly to the production of the first British Pharmacopoeia in 1864. Under this Act the General Medical

Council for Medical Education and Registration was set up and given responsibility to publish a book listing medicines and compounds, their method of preparation together with weights and measures necessary for preparation and mixing. The name of the work was specified as *The British Pharmacopoeia*, and the need to alter, amend and republish in response to scientific developments was recognised and empowered.

The Medical Council Act (1862) further stipulated that the British Pharmacopoeia would be the official reference for the British Isles, superseding the London, Edinburgh and Dublin Pharmacopoeias.

Significantly, at the first meeting of the General Medical Council in November 1858 a decision was made to ensure involvement of the Pharmaceutical Society in the preparation of the British Pharmacopoeia and to appoint paid pharmaceutical experts to assist with appropriate chemical and pharmaceutical research. Four Pharmacopoeia committees were established, one each for England, Scotland, Ireland and the Pharmaceutical Society, in order to assist with Pharmacopoeial development, and in December 1858 a Pharmaceutical Society representative was also appointed to the London subcommittee of the British Pharmacopoeia.

The result was the 1864 British Pharmacopoeia, which in many ways resembled other contemporaneous pharmaceutical texts, being of a similar page size. It was published in English and consisted of two parts, both in alphabetical order. Part I (161 pages long) listed monographs for the therapeutic agents, giving details of material sources, characteristics, relevant preparations containing the substance in question and chemical tests. Part II (233 pages long) listed preparations and compounds considered to be of therapeutic importance. Collected appendices contained details of information required in the practice of pharmacy, including symbols, weights and measures and substances and equipment used in medicines preparations and analysis.

Subsequent editions and addenda

Mr Peter Squire, the Pharmaceutical Society's representative for British Pharmacopoeia development, produced *A Companion to the British Pharmacopoeia* soon after publication of the first edition of the British Pharmacopoeia. This book was widely consulted within the profession and after numerous editions was incorporated in *Martindale's Extra Pharmacopoeia*.

The second edition of the British Pharmacopoeia appeared in 1867, since the first edition apparently received an unfavourable reception in the professional community. An addendum was published in 1874, a third edition in 1885, followed by an addendum in 1890 and a fourth edition in 1898.

The 1898 fourth edition differed from the pattern set in the 1864 first edition in that the distinct parts (Part I Materia Medica and Part II Preparations) were amalgamated. It was clear from the monographs in this edition that most of the manufacture of chemical substances had been taken over by wholesale manufacturers rather than being encompassed as part of the general pharmacy-based activity. Also, by 1898 examples of enzymes (pepsin, glycerin of pepsin), hormones (pancreatic solution, dry thyroid, thyroid solution) and vitamins (lemon juice) had been included in the British Pharmacopoeia. As might be expected given the impetus for research into medicines at the time, a wide range of agents with therapeutic value were added to the 1898 edition. Many resulted from the fruits of the extensive overseas exploration undertaken by the Victorians and included crude drugs such as quillaia, coca, cascara and strophanthus, together with chemical substances of botanical origin such as aloin, codeine phosphate, physostigmine sulphate and strychnine hydrochloride. The active research undertaken at this time also yielded a range of other organic chemicals, such as apomorphine hydrochloride, liquid paraffin and saccharin, in addition to many inorganic chemicals and minerals, including bismuth salicylate and kaolin.

In the next edition of the British Pharmacopoeia, published in 1914, doses were expressed using both metric and imperial units. A statement was included that qualified this action, expressing the expectation that 'in the near future the (metric) system will be adopted by British prescribers'. In reality it was to be well over 50 years until this happened, the Government only in 1965 announcing support for the metrification of the UK 'within 10 years'.

It was a further 18 years before the appearance of the next revised edition of the British Pharmacopoeia, in 1932. Such a long interval arose in part through the obvious disturbances to political and social structures caused by World War I and partly because times of serious conflict tend to accelerate developments in both the medical and pharmaceutical fields: the consideration, evaluation and assimilation into the British Pharmacopoeia of the significant therapeutic and practice advances made during and following World War I took time to effect.

The preparatory work to produce the 1932 British Pharmacopoeia began in 1928 when a Pharmacopoeia Commission of six members was convened. The full-time Secretary of the Commission was Dr CH Hampshire, who had previously been the Chief Pharmacist at University College Hospital, London. Naturally the 1932 British Pharmacopoeia contained many developments, particularly with regard to the biological and serological agents that had had a significant impact in World War I with vaccination against typhoid and tetanus. Certain categories of preparation, such as wines and pills, were reduced in number and details of standards and tests associated with the determination of therapeutic substances, such as insulin and antitoxins as defined by the Therapeutic Substances Act (1925), were added. This edition continued to use both imperial and metric measurements and firmly established the principle of 'solids by weight and liquids by measure'.

Seven addenda to the 1932 edition of the British Pharmacopoeia were produced between 1936 and 1945, some of which were compiled to address the need for alternatives to official BP medicinal products in response to the failure of supply lines for some pharmaceuticals during World War II.

The seventh edition of the British Pharmacopoeia was finally produced in 1948 after major revisions of the previous version, necessitated by the significant technical and scientific advances made before and during the war period. A number of monographs were included to address new drug discoveries and developments, including certain of the sex hormones and, notably,

penicillin. The General Medical Council (GMC) actually described the production of the seventh edition as 'a more complex and laborious task than any of its predecessors, not excluding the original British Pharmacopoeia of 1864', which reflects the degree of work required to update the previous edition. Reflecting on the workload imposed by the rapid expansion of pharmaceutical discoveries, the GMC also indicated that new editions of the British Pharmacopoeia should appear every five rather than 10 years. The Medical Act (1950) extended this principle further to enable the date of implementation of future British Pharmacopoeias and addenda to be determined in advance, principally to allow those involved in drug manufacture to have studied and prepared for new standards.

In accordance with the new five-year implementation interval, the eighth edition of the British Pharmacopoeia was issued in 1953 after only one addendum to the previous edition in 1951. English replaced Latin in the titles used in the 1953 edition, although in some cases an abbreviated Latin synonym was retained. As might be expected, developments in analysis were reflected by the inclusion of an increased number of assays, and capsules, both hard and soft, were introduced as a new dosage form.

Again only one addendum to the 1953 edition was produced in 1955, which contained new disintegration tests for tablets, before the implementation of the ninth edition in 1958.

The 1958 edition continued the trend to add monographs referring to the products of pharmaceutical research and development and to actively remove preparations of little or no value. At this time, there was a significant increase in the appearance of psychoactive agents, notably those considered to be sedatives or tranquillisers. A number of radioactive isotopes also appeared. Naturally, there was an appropriate extension and modification of assay details and procedures to embrace these new pharmaceutical developments.

An addendum to the 1958 edition in 1960 included a number of monographs describing important extensions to the range of antibiotics and immunological agents, such as a parenteral poliomyelitis vaccine.

It is clear, though, that by the late 1950s, the British Pharmacopoeia was no longer considered to be a reference text useful in the daily common practice of pharmacy other than by those involved in quality assurance or large-scale manufacture of pharmaceuticals, and other texts were more often utilised.

The British Pharmacopoeia is still published on the recommendation of the Medicines Commission in accordance with section 99(6) of the Medicines Act 1968 (see Part 2, Section 2.5.1).

1.4.8 The British Pharmaceutical Codex (BPC)

By the end of the nineteenth century leading practitioners of pharmacy were highlighting some perceived inadequacies of official texts such as the British Pharmacopoeia. These critics cited issues such as the failure to embrace medicines used elsewhere in the world, particularly in other parts of the Empire, the exclusion of medicines thought to be valuable but not yet established, and agents excluded despite being in common use. It was recognised that many non-official texts had attempted to provide information about such agents but none had robust professional backing. In 1903 the Council of the Pharmaceutical Society decided that an appropriate single-volume work should be developed in order to provide accurate information about medicines commonly used throughout the British Empire and those officially recognised in France, Germany and the USA in addition to the UK.

The response was the publication by the Pharmaceutical Society in 1907 of the first British Pharmaceutical Codex (BPC), which was described as 'An Imperial Dispensatory for the use of Medical Practitioners and Pharmacists'. The 1907 British Pharmaceutical Codex contained monographs on medicinal substances of chemical, vegetable and animal origin. Details of these substances, including sources, histology

and chemical composition, details for tests, information on mechanisms of action and uses, formulae for preparations and information to facilitate prescribing and dispensing, were included. The text was arranged with substances in alphabetical order and contained some innovations, for example the 'ml' was used rather than the 'cc'. The content was largely based upon the British Pharmacopoeia together with information from various respected hospital formularies and reference works from the USA and Australia.

Further editions of the British Pharmaceutical Codex were produced in 1911, 1923 and 1934. In the latter edition, surgical dressings were included as a separate section. This trend was extended in the 1940 BPC supplement, which specifically referred to 'standard dressings' that had been accepted in accordance with the Drug Tariff as part of the National Health Insurance Acts.

Subsequent editions were issued in 1949, 1954, 1959, 1963, 1968 and 1973 and the content was continually refined to reflect current therapeutic practice.

1.4.9 The International Pharmacopoeia (World Health Organization)

The first volume of the International Pharmacopoeia was produced in 1951 in Latin with English and French translations. This volume consisted of a collection of monographs on drugs and chemicals with appendices dealing with reagents, tests and biological assays. The second volume followed in 1955 and contained details and formulae for preparations involving the agents specified in the 1951 volume. The range of agents and information was extended in a Supplement issued in 1959, which also detailed International Biological Standards.

2

Obsolete dosage forms, equipment and methods of preparation

The activities of an apothecary or pharmacist in compounding a medicine using traditional methods was often referred to using the term *secundum artem*, literally meaning 'to make favourably with skill'. This embraces both the high level of technical ability used and the appropriate knowledge base required to successfully undertake compounding procedures that result in a medicine acceptable to patients.

The following sections are devoted to descriptions of the nature, preparation, equipment and technology associated with the compounding of some traditional drug forms, compounds and formulations, most of which have become defunct during the twentieth century. They are presented here in part to satisfy historical interest and partly as a repository of methods and skills that would otherwise be lost completely to the general pharmaceutical world.

The preparations, forms and formulations that may still be encountered in current practice, albeit in specialised situations, are considered in Part 2 of this book.

2.1 Obsolete pharmaceutical preparations and preparative methods

2.1.1 Galenicals

Most of the active constituents of traditional extemporaneously prepared products originated from plant or animal sources. Although it was likely that the therapeutic effects of these preparations could be attributed to one active ingredient, isolation of discrete active constituents was either technologically impossible or prohibitively expensive. In addition, it was commonly believed by early practitioners that under certain circumstances, extraneous constituents present in impure forms of medicines could exert beneficial actions on the therapeutic ingredients. This is why various galenicals, which evolved before the ability to separate active ingredients accurately, became commonplace in pharmaceutical compounding.

Today, 'galenicals' is a term that is applied loosely, and often incorrectly, to name any type of preparation (elixirs, solutions, waters etc.) irrespective of whether it is an extract of a crude drug or a solution of chemicals. Historically, however, true galenicals were pharmaceutical preparations obtained by macerating or percolating crude drugs with alcohol of an appropriate strength or some other solvent (menstruum), which was carefully selected to remove as completely as possible only the desired active components, leaving the inert and other undesirable constituents of the plant in the solid phase (marc).

The ancient Greek physician Galen (Claudius Galenus of Pergamum, AD 131–201) was the first to devise solutions of the active constituents of plants, hence the term galenicals. Since that time, pharmacists have tried to improve upon Galen's techniques and prepare galenicals that are stable, free from inert material and therapeutically efficacious as well as concentrated, for ease of handling. Examples of true galenicals include decoctions, extracts, infusions, tinctures, vinegars and oxymels. Aromatic waters, although not true galenicals, will also be outlined in the following sections.

Some examples of galenicals have been retained in practice today and are obtained from alkaloid-bearing plants, e.g. Belladonna Tincture BP (see Example 2.19, page 28).

2.1.2 Bougies

Bougies are solid preparations that are designed to be inserted into the urethra, nose or ear in order to exert a local or systemic effect in a similar manner to the modern suppository.

The urethral bougie was generally formulated in glycerinated gelatin and was designed to be pencil shaped, with a point at one end. Generally a glyco-gelatin 2 g bougie was approximately 7 cm in length, whereas, a 4 g version was 14 cm long. If a bougie was compounded using Theobroma Oil as a base, then its weight was approximately half that of an equivalent-sized bougie formulated in a gelatin base. The gelatin versions were better than those moulded in oil as they were more flexible, which aided insertion into the urethra. If a firmer consistency of the bougie was required then acacia mucilage could be substituted for either glycerin or water in the formulation.

Henry Wellcome devised a version of the urethral bougie with an elongated bulb near the tip that reputedly reduced the likelihood of involuntary expulsion on insertion.

The mould for the urethral bougie had to be warmed before pouring the mass in order to facilitate complete filling. Finished bougies were then often rolled in lycopodium powder after removal from the mould in order to stop them sticking to surfaces. Glyco-gelatin bougies had to be protected from excessively dry or moist air by storing in a tightly closed container in a cool place in order to maintain their integrity.

Nasal bougies were similar to urethral bougies, although they were shorter, approximately 2.5 cm in length, and weighed approximately 1.5 g. They were usually prepared using a glyco-gelatin base as this was more suitable for the medicaments that were to be incorporated into the product.

Aural bougies, also called ear cones, were conical in shape, usually about 1.25 cm in length and weighed between 250 and 400 mg. References disagree on the common base used for aural bougies. The British Pharmaceutical Codex 1949 stated that unless otherwise directed, they should be made with Theobroma Oil BP base, but most pharmaceutics textbooks of the period (e.g. Cooper and Gunn, 1950) suggest the use of glyco-gelatin bases.

 See Picture 1

2.1.3 Cachets (capulae amylaceae, oblata)

Cachets were developed from the early practice of masking the taste of unpleasant bitter or nau-seating drug powders by encapsulating the offending substance in bread and jam. Develop-ments from this practice involved the production of thin wafer sheets from flour and water which could be dried and stored. In order to administer a powder the dry wafer was floated on water. When it had softened, a tablespoon was passed underneath the wafer and it was lifted out. The powder was then placed into the spoon-shaped depression and the corners of the wafer folded over to enclose it. Water was then poured onto the spoon and the packet swallowed.

In its most well-developed form a cachet com-prised two lenticular or spoon-shaped flanged discs made from rice paper. The drug substance was placed within the saucer-shaped depression in one half of the cachet and was sealed in by placing the second half on top. A cachet could be sealed by moistening the flanges, usually by quickly passing them over a piece of wet felt, and then sticking them together (wet-type seal). Sophisticated sets of apparatus were devised for the filling and sealing of larger numbers of cachets. These included pourers to avoid powder contaminating the flange of the cachet and specialised holding and sealing devices.

A dry-seal type of cachet was also developed that consisted of a body to hold the powder con-tents and a cap that interlocked over the body to form a seal.

Cachets had to be moistened before swallow-ing in order to render them soft, elastic and slippery, though there was a certain 'knack' to this procedure.

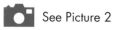 See Picture 2

2.1.4 Collodions

These are liquid preparations, intended for external use, containing highly volatile solvents (usually a base solution of pyroxylin (soluble gun-cotton) in a mixture of ether and alcohol) that evaporate to leave either a mechanical or a therapeutic film. Col-lodions had to be applied to the skin using a soft brush. Although almost obsolete, Flexible Collo-dian BP and Salicylic Acid Collodian BP are still listed in the modern British Pharmacopoeia (2004).

2.1.5 Confections

Confections (older terms: conserves, electuaries) were thick, sweet, soft, solid preparations into which one or more drug substances were incorpor-ated. They were designed to provide an agreeable method of administration for bitter or nauseating drugs, while offering a convenient method of preservation (e.g. Confection of Senna BP).

2.1.6 Decoctions (decocta)

A decoction differs from an infusion in that one or more crude drug bases, either whole or suitably prepared, were boiled with water for a specified time, usually 10 minutes or until a given volume was obtained. The preparation was then strained and, if necessary after cooling, made up to volume with more distilled water, which was passed through the original filter to ensure that as much extract as possible had been removed from the marc. This process left an aqueous prep-aration similar to 'clear soup'. If decoction was followed by evaporation, then a solid or semi-solid extract was produced.

Where a number of ingredients were to be included in the decoction then they were added at different times during the process. Hard ligneous drugs were added first, with the addition of aro-matics and volatile oils near the end of the process in order to minimise loss of active principles.

The object of a decoction was to produce an aqueous solution containing soluble active drug principles that were not degraded by heat. Clearly few drugs were suited to preparation in this manner.

Example 2.1 Decoction of Chondrus BPC (Decoctum Chondri) (BPC 1949, page 1091)

Formula:

Chondrus   25 g
Water   to 1000 mL

Method: Wash the chondrus in cold water to remove impurities and boil with 1200 mL of water for 15 minutes. Strain while hot and, if necessary, pour sufficient water over the contents of the strainer to produce the required volume when cool. It should be Freshly Prepared.

Dose: 30–120 mL, or more.

Use: As a demulcent in the treatment of irritating coughs.

 Example 2.2 Extract of Cannabis BPC (Extractum Cannabis) (BPC 1949, page 1118)

Formula:

Cannabis, in coarse powder   10 oz
Alcohol (90%)   a sufficient quantity

Method: Exhaust the cannabis by percolation with the alcohol (90%) and evaporate to the consistency of a soft extract.

Dose: ¼–1 gr.

Because decoctions are aqueous products they are very susceptible to decomposition and therefore they should be freshly prepared (see Section 6.8.2).

Decoctions fell from use in the early 1950s and the last official examples of formulae appeared in the BPC 1949.

2.1.7 Extracts (extracta)

Extracts are produced by the action of various solvents (aqueous, alcoholic, ethereal, acetic or ammoniated), using a variety of processes (expression, maceration, decoction, percolation), which may be followed by evaporation with or without vacuum assistance to produce liquid, semi-solid or solid products. Where the juices of fresh plants were obtained by expression and evaporation, the resultant extracts were frequently termed *succi spissati* (inspissated juices).

Extracts were intended to contain the active principles of crude drugs while minimising the amount of inert matter present. In general, extracts contained a higher proportion of active drug principles than equivalent infusions, decoctions or tinctures. The most common extracts encountered were either solid or liquid extracts.

Solid extracts varied in consistency depending on their degree of concentration. They were termed either soft extracts, with a consistency between that of a pill mass and a paste, or dry extracts. Soft extracts were semi-sticky masses formed by concentration from a liquid extract. They have fallen from current use because it was difficult to standardise the degree of 'softness' and therefore their consistency with any degree of accuracy. In addition, soft extracts often hardened on storage, producing a tough mass that was difficult to handle. This also means that the strength of a soft extract could vary significantly depending on preparation and storage.

Dry extracts replaced soft extracts as the solid extract of choice as these could be standardised, they varied less in strength and were generally easier to handle. Storage was less likely to cause significant problems, although granular dried extracts were preferred to those that were powders, as powdered varieties were more likely to absorb moisture from the air and become a solid block.

Liquid extracts are still commonly used in extemporaneous compounding, the main example being Liquid Liquorice Extract BP. Liquid extracts are usually prepared by the 'reserve percolate process' (see Section 2.1.10).

2.1.8 Eye discs (lamellae)

Lamellae were small discs of a glyco-gelatin base that were intended to be placed onto the cornea of the eye, where they would be allowed to

Example 2.3 Liquid Extract of Hamamelis BPC (Extractum Hamamelis Liquidum) (BPC 1973, page 682)

Formula:

Hamamelis, in moderately coarse powder	1000 g
Alcohol (45%)	to 1000 mL

Method: Exhaust the hamamelis with the alcohol by percolation, reserving the first 850 mL of percolate; evaporate the subsequent percolate to the consistency of a soft extract, dissolve it in the reserved portion, add sufficient alcohol to produce 1000 mL, allow to stand for not less than 12 hours and filter.

Use: Because of its astringent properties, hamamelis and its preparations are used in the treatment of haemorrhoids. It is also used in toiletry preparations.

Example 2.4 Liquid Extract of Liquorice BP (Extractum Glycyrrhizae Liquidum) (BP 1963, page 449)

Formula:

Liquorice, unpeeled, in coarse powder	1000 g
Chloroform water	a sufficient quantity
Alcohol (90%)	a sufficient quantity

Method: Exhaust the liquorice with chloroform water by percolation. Boil the percolate for 5 minutes and set aside for not less than 12 hours. Decant the clear liquid, filter the remainder, mix the two liquids and evaporate until the weight per millilitre of the liquid extract is 1.198 g. Add to this liquid, when cold, one-fourth of its volume of alcohol (90%). Allow to stand for not less than four weeks; filter.

Dose: 2–5 mL.

Use: Used in cough mixtures and to disguise the taste of nauseous medicines.

Example 2.5 Glycerite of Tar (Glyceritum Picis Liquidae) (Remington, 1905, page 1351)

Formula:

Tar	65 g
Magnesium carbonate	125 g
Glycerin	250 mL
Alcohol	125 mL
Water	to 1000 mL

dissolve in the lachrymal secretions. The active ingredient, which was often an alkaloid, would be released for a local effect.

2.1.9 Glycerins (glycerita or glycerites)

These were produced by dissolving or incorporating substances in glycerin (or glycerin solutions). The principal use of glycerins was to provide a simple and rapid method of producing an aqueous solution of a drug that was not otherwise readily soluble. Many of the glycerins were made in a concentrated form that could be easily diluted with water or alcohol without precipitation.

2.1.10 Infusions (infusa)

Infusions are dilute solutions containing the water-soluble extracts of vegetable drugs. They were prepared by macerating drugs in water for short periods of time, varying from 15 minutes to 2 hours. The volume of the product depends on the quantity of menstruum retained by the marc, which should not be pressed. The degree of comminution of the drug, the temperature used for the preparation of the infusion and the length of maceration chosen depended upon the nature of the drug and the constituents to be extracted.

Infusions were usually prepared in earthenware vessels (latterly glass was used). The drug was added to the vessel usually suspended in some way or enclosed in muslin (like a modern teabag) so as to be just below the surface of the water. If the drug sank to the bottom of the vessel the mixture would need occasional stirring. If hot water was added to prepare the infusion it would be weighed into a previously tared and warmed vessel to prevent cracking of the measure. Often a layer of cloth was wrapped around the infusion container in order to reduce heat loss and hence aid the extraction process. When the specified infusion time had elapsed, the product was strained and the marc removed as quickly as possible so as to allow the preparation to cool before use. The supernatant formed the infusion, which was generally unstable and needed to be Freshly Prepared (see Section 6.8.2). Infusions containing a drug that was freely soluble or those containing a high proportion of starch were prepared with cold water. Fresh infusions should be dispensed within 12 hours. Sometimes highly concentrated forms of infusions were prepared.

A number of types of special infusion apparatus were developed (e.g. Alsop's Infusion Jar, Squire's Infusion Mug). These had in-built supports for the crude drug substance positioned at an appropriate level in the container and also featured specially designed pouring spouts. Infusion devices were often made by customising tea or coffee pots.

 See Picture 3

The BP and BPC recommend the use of concentrated infusions from which infusions can be prepared by diluting one volume of concentrated infusion to 10 volumes with water. This applies to all formulae for concentrated infusions since reformulation in 1968; any formula that predates 1968 will be required to be diluted to eight volumes with water.

Two different methods of producing a concentrated infusion have been used in the following examples. The Orange Peel Infusion Concentrated BPC (Example 2.10) and Concentrated Compound Gentian Infusion BP (Example

---

 Example 2.7 Infusion of Catechu BP (Infusum Catechu) (BP 1885, page 205)

Formula:

Catechu, in coarse powder	160 gr
Cinnamon bark, bruised	30 gr
Distilled water, boiling	10 fl oz

Method: Infuse in a covered vessel for half an hour and strain.

Dose: 1–2 fl oz.

Use: An astringent used in internal mixtures to treat diarrhoea.

 Example 2.8 Compound infusion of horseradish (Infusum Armoraciae Compositum) (Pharmaceutical Journal Formulary, 1904, page 22)

Formula:

Fresh horseradish root, sliced	1 oz
Black mustard seed	1 oz
Compound spirit of horseradish	1 oz
Distilled water, at 150–180 °F	20 fl oz

Method: Macerate the seed and root for 2 hours with the water; then strain and add the spirit.

Dose: 1–2 fl oz as a warm stimulant.

Use: Used as a counterirritant and vesicant for external application and as a carminative in small amounts.

 Example 2.6 Infusion of Valerian BPC (Infusum Valerianae) (BPC 1911, page 1224)

Formula:

Valerian rhizome, bruised	½ oz
Distilled water, boiling	1 pt

Method: Infuse in a covered vessel for 15 minutes and strain.

Dose: ½–1 fl oz.

Use: To treat hysteria as it is said to depress the nervous system. Also used as a carminative.

Example 2.9 Fresh Acid Infusion of Rose BPC (Infusum Rosae Acidum Recens) (BPC 1949, page 1156)

Formula:

Red rose petal, dried and broken	¼ oz
Dilute sulphuric acid	60 m
Water, boiling	10 oz

Method: Mix the red rose petal with the boiling water in a covered vessel, add the dilute sulphuric acid, infuse for 15 minutes, and strain.

Dose: ½–1 fl oz.

Use: As a vehicle for gargles containing alum or tannin.

Example 2.10 Orange Peel Infusion Concentrated BPC (Infusum Aurantii Concentratum) (BPC 1973, page 704)

Formula:

Dried bitter orange peel, cut small	500 g
Alcohol (25%)	1350 mL

Method: Macerate the dried bitter orange peel in 1000 mL of alcohol in covered vessel for 48 hours and press out the liquid. To the marc add the remainder of the alcohol, macerate for 24 hours, press out the liquid, and add it to the product of the first pressing. Allow the mixed liquids to stand for not less than 14 days and then filter.

Dose: 2.5–5 mL.

Use: Flavouring and as a bitter with carminative properties.

Example 2.11 Concentrated Compound Gentian Infusion BP (Infusum Gentianae Compositum Concentratum) (BP 1973, page 217)

Formula:

Gentian, cut small and bruised	125 g
Dried bitter orange peel, cut small	125 g
Dried lemon peel, cut small	125 g
Alcohol (25%)	1200 mL

Method: Macerate the gentian, the dried bitter orange peel and the dried lemon peel in a covered vessel for 48 hours with 1000 mL of the alcohol (25%); press out the liquid. To the pressed marc, add 200 mL of the alcohol (25%), macerate for 24 hours, press, and add the liquid to the product of the first pressing. Allow to stand for not less than 14 days and then filter.

Dose: 1.5–4 mL.

Use: A bitter to stimulate gastric secretion and stimulate appetite.

potential loss of volatile constituents. The dried bitter orange is cut into small pieces in order to expose the oil glands embedded in the peel.

Alcohol 25% is used for the menstruum because volatile oils are more soluble in alcohol than in water. Alcohol also acts as a preservative, discouraging the development of moulds and preventing fermentation.

In double maceration, the first maceration process extracts most of the soluble matter but leaves an amount of liquid that is inseparable from the marc; this is likely to contain a significant amount of soluble matter. The second maceration process is intended to achieve a better extraction through addition of menstruum to the marc. The resultant liquids from both macerations are combined and allowed to stand for 14 days. The expression process expels mucilaginous and albuminous matter, which slowly precipitates on standing. On completion of the precipitation process the liquid is filtered, after which it remains clear and bright.

By contrast, the Senega Infusion Concentrated

2.11) are prepared by double maceration, where the filtrate is the finished product and no evaporation process is used. This is because both the preparations contain volatile constituents that would be dissipated by evaporation, and also because in the percolation process the active ingredients must be ground more finely and in the comminution process there would be further

Example 2.12 Senega Infusion Concentrated BPC (Infusum Senegae Concentratum) (BPC 1973, page 704)

Formula:

Senega, in coarse powder	500 g
Dilute ammonia solution	a sufficient quantity
Alcohol (25%)	to 1000 mL

Method: Extract the senega with the alcohol by percolation, reserving the first 750 mL of percolate. Continue percolation until a further 1000 mL has been collected, evaporate to a syrupy consistence, dissolve the residue in the reserved portion, gradually add dilute ammonia solution until the product is faintly alkaline, add sufficient of the alcohol to produce the required volume, and mix. Allow to stand for not less than 14 days and filter.

Dose: 2.5–5 mL.

Use: To irritate the gastric mucosa and give rise to a reflex secretion of mucus in the bronchioles. It is used with other expectorants in the treatment of bronchitis.

Box 2.1 Reserve percolation

When a crude drug is extracted by the percolation process, only 70–80% of the active constituents are obtained. This high concentration is achieved mainly by the 24-hour maceration process when the first quantity of menstruum is added. Subsequent percolates become less and less concentrated and the final percolate may be very weak, containing a very low concentration of active ingredient.

When a concentrated preparation is required, such as in the case of some concentrated infusions and liquid extracts, the first strong percolate is reserved. The subsequent weaker percolates are then collected and evaporated to produce a soft mass or syrupy liquid, which is then added to the strong percolate. This method avoids subjecting the whole percolate to heat, which may have a detrimental effect on the active constituents.

BPC described above (Example 2.12) is made by the 'reserve percolation' process (Box 2.1), which is generally restricted to the production of a concentrated infusion where the original drug is a hard drug and therefore more difficult to extract. With senega, a tough, woody drug, there are no volatile constituents to be lost and therefore a method employing heat is suitable.

2.1.11 Juices (succi)

Juices were prepared by expression from fresh natural products (e.g. belladonna, hemlock, henbane, lemon, broom, dandelion).

2.1.12 Lozenges (trochisci, troches)

Lozenges were solid dose forms designed to dissolve slowly and disintegrate in the mouth. They were used principally for drugs exerting a local action in the mouth and throat. They were prepared by mixing the active substance with one of four bases (the lozenge mass), which generally contained sugar and mucilage. Base one comprised sugar and gums in a blackcurrant paste; base two comprised sugar and gums with rosewater; base three was a simple base of sugar acacia and water; base four comprised sugar, acacia, tolu tincture and water.

The lozenge mass was rolled into a flat sheet of appropriate thickness on a lozenge board using a cylindrical roller, and shaped lozenges were cut from this using a metal cutter. Finished lozenges were then weight checked and dried. The lozenge weight was determined by the thickness of the flat sheet of mass for a given cutter size.

2.1.13 Mucilages (mucilagines)

Mucilages are thick, viscous, adhesive aqueous solutions or extractions of gums. There are two official mucilages: Mucilage of Acacia BP (BP 1953, page 854) and Mucilage of Tragacanth BPC (BPC 1949, page 924) that are used as thickening agents in medicines for internal use. Mucilages were traditionally used as suspending agents for insoluble substances in mixtures. They have also been used to thicken the continuous phase of an oil-in-water emulsion system. A mucilage of starch has been used for its emollient effects on the skin and other mucilages have been used as water-miscible bases for dermatological preparations and as lubricating agents for catheters and some surgical instruments.

Since mucilages are prone to decomposition they should not be made in quantities greater than required.

2.1.14 Oxymels (acid honeys)

Oxymel is the term applied to purified honey (Mel Depuratum) to which acetic acid has been added. There are many examples of oxymels formulated with active ingredients.

2.1.15 Pills (pilulae)

Pills were small, solid, oral dose forms of a globular, ovoid or lenticular shape. They were the most common oral dose form in the nineteenth century for drugs with smaller volume doses. They were perceived to be relatively easy to make and compact in quantity, masked unpleasant tastes and odours, were stable for long periods and were easy to administer. It was only during the twentieth century that the poor bioavailability characteristics of pills as a dose form were

discovered: pills were as likely to pass through the gastrointestinal tract unaltered as to disintegrate and deliver active ingredients, particularly when used in a coated form.

In order to compound pills by hand, a pill base or mass was constructed from which the prescriber often directed that a given weight of mass should be made into a specified number of pills.

The pill mass consisted of two parts: the active ingredients and the excipient, which gave the mass the appropriate consistency of adhesiveness, firmness and plasticity. A generic pill excipient would probably contain glucose, glycerin, powdered acacia and benzoic acid. The latter was often used as a preservative and might be omitted if only a small batch of pill mass was being compounded. This excipient formed a colourless, very adhesive liquid that was usually prepared in advance of compounding the pills.

The active ingredients and excipient were triturated in a mortar with a special pill pestle and kneaded into an homogeneous mass that could be divided into the desired weight.

The required weight of mass was then rolled into an elongated cylinder on a pill tile, which often incorporated a measuring scale to aid

---

Example 2.14 Squill Oxymel BPC (BPC 1973, page 765)

Formula:

Squill, bruised	50 g
Acetic acid	90 mL or sufficient quantity
Purified water, freshly boiled and cooled	250 mL
Purified honey	a sufficient quantity

Method: Macerate the squill with the acetic acid and water for seven days. Strain the liquid and press the marc. Mix the drained and expressed liquids and heat to boiling to coagulate expressed cell contents and then filter whilst hot. To every 3 volumes of this solution add 7 volumes of honey and mix thoroughly.

Dose: 2.5–5 mL.

Use: Mild expectorant in cough mixtures.

Example 2.13 Oxymel BPC (BPC 1973, page 764)

Formula:

Acetic acid	150 mL
Purified water, freshly boiled and cooled	150 mL
Purified honey	to 1000 mL

Method: Mix thoroughly.

Dose: 2.5–10 mL.

Use: Demulcent and sweetening agent.

cutting and division. Small quantities of mass were rolled using a pill spatula that had very little 'spring' and featured a broad end or a flat impervious board. The cylindrical pill mass was then cut either by hand or using a pill divider (a grooved roller) and then rolled into the final shape using a pill roller (resembling interlocking jar lids) or between the fingers.

Larger quantities of pills were generally made using a special pill machine. This consisted of two hardwood boards on which were mounted brass plates indented with hemispherical grooves (cutters). A cylindrical 'pipe' of pill mass would be laid across the grooves of the lower board. The upper and lower boards could be interfaced so that the grooves corresponded, and the upper board had handles which allowed the compounder to cut the mass into uniform pieces. Different sized pills could be cut by using different sized cutting plates.

Pills were prevented from sticking to either the tile or the machine by use of a dusting powder such as rice flour.

Pills were often coated with a variety of substances such as gold or silver leaf, gelatin or varnish (by treating with a solution of sandarac in ether and alcohol, which was allowed to evaporate), chocolate or keratin. The coating of pills effectively disguised unpleasant tastes and odours, rendered the pill more attractive and, in the case of precious metals, added to their therapeutic efficacy. Commercially produced pills were often given a sugar or pearl (using finely powdered talcum or French chalk) coating which was difficult to accomplish on a small scale.

Pills were usually dispensed in a flat, circular or square box which was preferably made so shallow that the pills could not lie on top of one another. A light coating of dusting powder was included in the pill box to prevent freshly made pills adhering to each other.

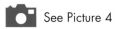 See Picture 4

2.1.16 Plasters (emplastra)

In this context, a plaster was an adhesive substance that required the aid of heat to spread it and was intended for external application to the skin. A plaster mass (often containing plant mucilages) was melted, then spread using a hot plaster iron on plaster leather (sheepskin), chamois, linen or calico cut to a specific size and/or shape as ordered by the prescriber. It should be noted that the term 'plaster' would describe both the adhesive mass itself and the completed spread plaster.

The plaster was firm at room temperature but spread easily when heated, remaining soft and pliable without melting when in contact with the skin.

Hand spreading was largely replaced by a mechanised process in the very early twentieth century.

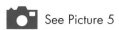 See Picture 5

2.1.17 Poultices

Poultices were preparations of a thick, semi-solid base, which were often heated and applied to a body part or area on a cloth in order to draw infection.

2.1.18 Resins

Resins are solid preparations consisting of the resinous constituents of vegetable matter. They are soluble in alcohol and in most organic solvents but insoluble in water. To manufacture resins the vegetable matter is subjected to an extraction process using 90% alcohol (or in some instances a weaker alcohol solution). In order to isolate the resin the alcoholic extract is concentrated and poured into water. This results in the precipitation of the resin, which can be subsequently washed with water, dried and powdered. An example of a resin produced in this manner is Podophyllum Resin BPC.

Oleo resins are combinations of volatile oils and naturally occurring resins and are generally found by cutting into the trunks of trees in which they occur. The best-known natural oleo resin is turpentine resin, which is found in 80–90 species of *Pinus* and is used to produce Turpentine Oil BPC.

Prepared oleo resins are concentrated liquid

preparations produced by percolating drugs containing both a volatile oil and a resin with an appropriate solvent (e.g. acetone or alcohol) and then concentrating the percolate until the solvent has all evaporated. Capsicum Oleoresin BPC is an example of a prepared oleo resin.

Gum resins are natural exudates of plants that are a mixture of gum and resin. An example is Myrrh Resin BP, which is concentrated from the stem of *Commiphora molmol* (Engler).

2.1.19 Snuffs

A snuff is a prepared powdered drug that is sniffed vigorously up the nose for a local and/or systemic action.

2.1.20 Syrups

Syrups are concentrated solutions of sucrose or other sugars at a concentration of at least 45% m/m. Flavoured syrups provide a sweet vehicle to mask the taste of nauseous medicaments. Syrups were particularly popular in older formulations as high concentrations of sucrose prevented the decomposition of matter extracted from vegetable drugs. The syrup exerted an osmotic pressure such that the growth of bacteria, fungi and moulds was inhibited. Sucrose also retards oxidation because it is partly hydrolysed into the reducing sugars glucose and fructose.

Medicated syrups are made of ingredients used in extemporaneous dispensing and thus form a stock solution of certain drugs (e.g. Tolu Syrup BP).

Flavoured syrups contain aromatic or pleasantly flavoured substances and are designed to be used as flavourings or vehicles for extemporaneous preparations, for example Blackcurrant Syrup BP, Lemon Syrup BP and Orange Syrup BP.

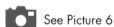 See Picture 6

2.1.21 Tinctures (tincturae)

Tinctures are alcoholic solutions of drugs prepared by adding alcohol (or occasionally ether) to a substance using maceration or percolation.

Tinctures are particularly useful intermediates as they can, in most cases, be kept for long periods without deterioration or loss of potency. This is because of the preservative properties of the alcohol that is used in their preparation. Generally they are prepared by a process of maceration, where the ingredients are placed in an enclosed container with the whole amount of the solvent and are allowed to stand for seven days with occasional stirring. The resulting mixture is then strained, the marc is pressed, and the two liquids are combined. The resultant tincture is clarified by filtration or by allowing to stand and decanting off the clear solution.

Tinctures can also be produced by a percolation process. In this process the solid ingredients are moistened evenly by sufficient solvent and left in an enclosed container for 4 hours. This damp mass is then packed into a percolator, sufficient additional solvent is added and the top of the percolator is closed. When the liquid is about to drip, the lower outlet of the percolator is closed, sufficient solvent is added to give a shallow layer above the mass, and the mixture is allowed to macerate in the closed percolator for 24 hours. The percolation process is then allowed to proceed slowly until the percolate measures about three-quarters of the required volume of the finished tincture. The marc is pressed, the expressed liquid is added to the percolate and sufficient solvent is added to prepare the required volume. Once again the combined liquids are clarified by filtration or by allowing to stand and decanting the clear solution.

 Example 2.15 Quillaia Tincture BP (Tinctura Quillaiae) (BP 1988, page 1022)

Formula:

| Quillaia liquid extract | 50 mL |
| Ethanol (45%) | to 1000 mL |

Method: Mix, allow to stand for not less than 12 hours and filter.

Dose: 2.5–5 mL.

Use: An emulsifying agent.

Example 2.16 Aromatic Cardamom Tincture BP (Tinctura Carminative) (BP 1988, page 1019)

Formula:

Cardamom oil	3 mL
Caraway oil	10 mL
Cinnamon oil	10 mL
Clove oil	10 mL
Strong ginger tincture	60 mL
Ethanol (90%)	to 1000 mL

Method: Mix all ingredients together.

Dose: 0.12–0.6 mL.

Use: Carminative and flavouring agent.

Example 2.17 Compound Cardamom Tincture BP (Tinctura Cardamomi Composite) (BP 1963, page 140)

Formula:

Cardamom seed, freshly removed from the fruit, immediately reduced to a moderately coarse powder, and used at once	14 g
Caraway, in moderately coarse powder	14 g
Cinnamon, in moderately coarse powder	28 g
Cochineal, in moderately coarse powder	7 g
Glycerol	50 mL
Alcohol (60%)	sufficient to produce 1000 mL

Method: Moisten the mixed powders with a sufficient quantity of alcohol (60%), and prepare 900 mL of tincture by percolation. Add the glycerol and sufficient alcohol (60%) to produce 1000 mL. Filter if necessary.

Dose: 2–5 mL.

Use: Carminative and flavouring agent.

Example 2.18 Compound Gentian Tincture BP (Tinctura Gentianae Composite) (BP 1963, page 341)

Formula:

Gentian, cut small and bruised	100 g
Cardamom seed, freshly removed from the fruit, immediately bruised and used at once	12.5 g
Dried bitter orange peel, cut small	37.5 g
Alcohol (45%)	1000 mL

Method: Prepare by maceration.

Dose: 2–5 mL.

Use: A bitter used to stimulate appetite.

Example 2.19 Belladonna Tincture BP (Tinctura Belladonnae) (BP 1988, page 1018)

Formula:

Belladonna Herb, in moderately coarse powder	100 g
Ethanol (70%)	a sufficient quantity

Method: Prepare about 900 mL of a tincture by percolation.

Dose: 0.5–2 mL.

Use: Antispasmodic.

 See Picture 7

2.1.22 Vinegars (aceta)

The use of vinegars has now declined but they are worthy of mention as their use as a menstruum for medicinal preparations dates back to ancient times. Vinegar itself was used as an antiseptic during outbreaks of plague, and vinegars were particularly popular in France, many

Example 2.20 Squill Vinegar BPC (Acetum Scillae) (BPC 1973, page 823)

Formula:

Squill, bruised	100 g
Dilute acetic acid	to 1000 mL

Method: Macerate the squill with the dilute acetic acid in a closed container for seven days, shaking occasionally, strain, press the marc and heat the combined liquids to boiling to coagulate expressed cell contents; allow to stand for not less than seven days and filter.

Dose: 0.6–2 mL.

Use: A mild expectorant ingredient in cough mixtures.

different formulae being quoted in the French Codex.

Medicated vinegars were solutions of drugs in dilute acetic acid, which is a good solvent and possesses antiseptic properties. Wine and cider vinegar were abandoned as a base because of the variations in composition and quality encountered.

In the UK there is only one official vinegar remaining (Squill Vinegar BPC).

It is worth noting that vinegar (acetic acid) is being used currently in burns units to treat *Pseudomonas aeruginosa* infections in wounds.

2.1.23 Waters (aquae)

Waters are simply an aqueous solution of a volatile substance and are prepared by aqueous distillation and hot or cold solution. The volatile substance can be either solid, liquid or gaseous.

Aromatic waters are saturated solutions of volatile oils or other aromatic substances in water. The main purpose of a water is to serve as a pleasant flavouring; however, some do have a mild therapeutic action, usually carminative. Nowadays aromatic waters are usually prepared from their equivalent concentrated water. The concentrated water is diluted with 39 times its volume of freshly boiled and cooled purified water.

Chloroform water

Chloroform is an anaesthetic when inhaled. When taken by mouth, it has a pleasant taste and causes a sensation of warmth. Orally it is used as a carminative, a flavouring agent and a preservative. In products made extemporaneously, it is added either as Chloroform Water BP (also referred to as Single Strength Chloroform Water BP), Double Strength Chloroform Water BP or as Chloroform Spirit BP.

Chloroform Water BP or Double Strength Chloroform Water BP is often added to oral dosage forms as a simple preservative. Originally, Chloroform Water BP and Double Strength Chloroform Water BP were both prepared using Chloroform BP and freshly boiled and cooled purified water.

Chloroform Water BP (BP 1988, page 1022)

Chloroform BP	2.5 mL
Freshly boiled and cooled purified water	to 1000 mL

Double Strength Chloroform Water BP (BP 1988, page 1022)

Chloroform BP	5 mL
Freshly boiled and cooled purified water	to 1000 mL

Both of these products were prepared by adding the Chloroform BP to a bottle containing the water and shaking until the chloroform dissolved in the water. Double Strength Chloroform Water BP was more difficult to prepare as the amount of chloroform present was near to the limit of solubility (chloroform is soluble 1 in 200 parts of water).

In 1959 Concentrated Chloroform Water BPC was developed.

Concentrated Chloroform Water BPC 1959 (BPC 1959, page 1161)

Chloroform BP	100 mL
Alcohol (90%) BP	600 mL
Water	to 1000 mL

The chloroform was dissolved in the alcohol and the water added gradually with shaking to produce the required volume.

Nowadays, in community pharmacies, Chloroform Water BP and Double Strength Chloroform Water BP are always made using a concentrate.

Chloroform Water BP (Single Strength Chloroform Water BP) is prepared using a 1 in 40 dilution of Concentrated Chloroform Water BPC 1959:

Concentrated Chloroform   2.5 mL
Water BPC 1959

Freshly boiled and cooled   to 100 mL
purified water

Double Strength Chloroform Water BP is prepared using a 1 in 20 dilution of Concentrated Chloroform Water BPC 1959 (see Key Skill 2.1):

Concentrated Chloroform   5 mL
Water BPC 1959

Freshly boiled and cooled   to 100 mL
purified water

A similar method to that outlined in Key Skill 2.1 would be employed in the preparation of Chloroform Water BP (Single Strength Chloroform Water BP).

It is worth noting that chloroform preparations made using Concentrated Chloroform Water BPC 1959 will contain a residual ethanol concentration of about 1.5% v/v. This is due to the presence of alcohol in the Concentrated Chloroform Water BPC 1959 (see Example 2.21). The ethanol would not be present if the preparation was made from Chloroform BP and freshly boiled and cooled purified water alone. This means that although officially the product produced is not a BP formula, it is widely accepted to be the equivalent available in pharmacy today. Although this should not normally cause a problem, it should be borne in mind that for certain patients (e.g. neonates and children, patients on certain types of medication and patients who cannot consume alcohol for religious reasons), this may not be a suitable preparation to use.

 Key Skill 2.1 Method for preparation of Double Strength Chloroform Water BP

1. Measure approximately 85–90 mL of freshly boiled and cooled purified water in a 100 mL conical measure.
2. Measure 5 mL of Concentrated Chloroform Water BPC 1959 in a 10 mL conical measure and add to the water. Stir vigorously.
3. Make up to volume (100 mL) with more freshly boiled and cooled purified water and stir.

Note: This is one of the few times that it is acceptable to dissolve in a conical measure rather than a glass beaker (see Section 6.2.3).

 Example 2.21 Concentrated Chloroform Water BPC 1959 (Aqua Chloroformi Concentrata) (BPC 1959, page 1161)

Formula:

Chloroform   100 mL
Alcohol (90%)   600 mL
Purified water, freshly boiled   to 1000 mL
and cooled

Method: Dissolve the chloroform in the alcohol and add sufficient water in successive small quantities to produce the required volume, shaking vigorously after each addition.

Dose: 0.4–0.8 mL.

Use: Flavouring and preservative.

Other concentrated waters

Example 2.22 Concentrated Anise Water BP (Aqua Anisi Concentrata) (BP 1988, page 1022)

Formula:

Anise oil	20 mL
Alcohol (90%)	700 mL
Purified water, freshly boiled and cooled	to 1000 mL

Method: Dissolve the anise oil in the alcohol and add sufficient water in successive small quantities to produce the required volume shaking vigorously after each addition. Add 50 g of purified talc and shake; allow to stand for a few hours then filter. The talc is added to adsorb any precipitates thereby enabling the production of a bright clear solution.

Dose: 0.3–1 mL.

Use: Flavouring, carminative and mild expectorant.

Example 2.23 Concentrated Camphor Water BP (Aqua Camphorae Concentrata) (BP 1988, page 1022)

Formula:

Camphor	40 g
Alcohol (90%)	600 mL
Purified water, freshly boiled and cooled	to 1000 mL

Method: Dissolve the camphor in the alcohol and add sufficient water in successive small quantities to produce the required volume shaking vigorously after each addition. Add 50 g of purified talc and shake; allow to stand for a few hours then filter.

Dose: 0.3–1 mL.

Use: A mild analgesic and rubefacient for external application in liniments and lotions.

2.1.24 Wines (vina)

Wines may be either medicated or unmedicated (e.g. Vinum Xericum or sherry) and closely resemble tinctures, with the only difference being the menstruum.

The presence of alcohol in medicated wines makes them more stable than decoctions or infusions.

2.2 Old pharmaceutical equipment

Until the advent of the large-scale manufacture of proprietary medicines in the twentieth century, a typical pharmacist required premises that were suitable both for the retail of crude drugs and compounded products and as a laboratory or preparative area which could be used for compounding activities. The latter needed to be equipped with suitable apparatus for weighing, comminution, mixing, expression, filtration, heating and condensing.

Before the modern era, most of the equipment used to establish compounding laboratories was not designed specifically for pharmaceutical purposes but originated from other domestic or professional situations, such as cooking, farming, milling, brewing and distilling. Some of the development and refinement of basic laboratory equipment and techniques for more specific pharmaceutical purposes was achieved through involvement with alchemy. In addition, the fruits of new scientific discoveries were also applied to medicines compounding processes as they were refined. For example, thermometers allowed more precise control over processes involving heating.

Many images exist that show typical interiors of pharmaceutical premises used for compounding, for example the 1747 engraving of 'The Chemical Lab' in the Wellcome Museum for the History of Medicine. Possibly one of the most famous pharmaceutical interiors is depicted in the print of John Bell's Oxford Street Pharmacy from 1842 (again from the Wellcome Museum for the History of Medicine). These examples clearly depict the wide range and complexity of specialist apparatus used in compounding before the modern era.

2.2.1 Weighing and measuring

The accurate weighing and measuring of ingredients is a fundamental element of the compounding process and has been recognised as being of importance since the earliest times.

Weighing

It is likely that the development of accurate weighing techniques with the attendant equipment and technology originally arose in cultures that found the need to quantify amounts of precious metals accurately. The ancient Egyptians, Assyrians and Babylonians all used weights and scales in different forms.

The portable steelyard, which had a movable balance weight, and the beam balance suspended on a central pillar were both used by the Etruscans, who introduced their use to Western Europe before the time of Christ. These weighing methods were adopted by the Romans, and many variants of these simple systems were introduced throughout Europe. Scales of both of these types were commonly used by those compounding drugs up to the fifteenth century, when in London the single-pan (*lanx*) steelyard beam was abandoned for the two-pan (*bi-lanx*, hence balance) pivoted fixed beam type. A balance of this type mounted in a glass case is depicted in a woodcut showing the interior of an alchemist's laboratory in *Alkimy the Ordinall* by Thomas Norton (1477). Compounders of medicines of this period would also have used larger balances with fixed roof mountings for weighing more substantial amounts, as well as folding hand-held types when portability was necessary.

The use of troy weights in England was formalised by legislation in 1497, whereas the avoirdupois weight system was not formally recognised until 1532 (see Section 3.1.1). These weights were not, however, of a uniform size or shape and examples are known to be round, square and cylindrical. The problems associated with non-uniformity of weights was clearly recognised, and in 1745 the College of Physicians commented upon the differences between the troy weights used by silversmiths (ounces divided into penny-weights) and apothecaries' (ounces divided into drachms and scruples) and avoirdupois weights generally used by druggists and grocers. In response, all of the formulae in the 1746 Pharmacopoeia were presented in a common troy system.

In 1824 the pound in weight was standardised to be 5760 grains (troy) with one pound avoirdupois being equivalent to 7000 grains troy. The Weights and Measures Act (1878) further standardised weights by only recognising the pound avoirdupois, but paradoxically drugs were allowed to be sold in weights measured by the troy or apothecaries' ounce (480 gr). This system continued until metrication (see Chapter 3).

 See Picture 8

Measuring

The measurement of liquids presented another problem to those involved in medicines compounding. A number of archaeological finds indicate that measures made of metal, pottery, animal horn and glass were used by those practising pharmacy certainly in the Roman and Arabic worlds. No uniform standard volume was accepted, although use of the Roman gallon was widespread. Indeed, the College of Physicians adopted subdivisions of the Roman gallon as the units of liquid measure for the first London Pharmacopoeia of 1618.

Producing effective, accurate liquid measures from opaque materials such as pewter presented problems, as the inscription of graduations inside a measure was difficult to achieve and would be grossly inaccurate and difficult to use. Thus although some early graduated measures were constructed from translucent horn, until the introduction of graduated glass measures, first used widely in the eighteenth century, most liquid components would have been weighed.

By 1830 graduated glass measures with a lip were commonly available, being marked with minims, ounces or tablespoons.

 See Picture 9

2.2.2 Comminution

The action of grinding and breaking down substances has been practised for millennia. From the time that cereals were discovered to be a useful foodstuff, humans have developed increasingly sophisticated methods of rendering large particles to a powder. Simple querns, basically two abrasive stones moved against each other to provide a grinding action, were an early feature of human development. The simple quern was refined and became the concave mortar and convex pestle, familiar as a universal symbol of pharmacy today. The ancient Egyptians and Romans both used the pestle and mortar and many examples in a wide variety of materials are known, including marble, basalt, iron and bronze.

The use of the pestle and mortar has been central to compounding activities in the British Isles from Anglo Saxon times and intact examples exist from as early as the beginning of the fourteenth century. The pestle and mortar combination appeared in a variety of sizes, formed from a wide range of materials. Smaller versions were naturally intended to be used on a bench and were generally made from marble, limestone, glass or wood. The latter were generally constructed from lignum vitae and were chiefly used to grind spices and aromatic substances. The advantages and disadvantages of different materials and the need to reserve different types of pestle and mortar for certain drug substances was well known by the seventeenth century. In a text from this period it was described how poisons should not be ground in a mortar for general use and that a glass mortar was most appropriate for substances to be combined with syrups (*A detection of some faults in unskilful physitians, etc.* Recorde, R, *The urinal of Physic*, London, 1651).

Larger pestles and mortars were generally made from iron or bronze and were used in larger scale operations for powdering fibrous vegetable drugs and caked chemicals. Some mortars could be very large by today's standards and needed to be mounted upon their own wooden support with the corresponding pestle suspended from an overhead beam. Often mortars were of such a size that they were cast by bell founders using the same techniques as employed to make bells.

Problems encountered with these early examples of pestles and mortars included the shedding of particles following pulverisation of drugs in a metal mortar and the dissolution of limestone and other stone mortars under the action of acids. The great ceramic technologist Josiah Wedgwood solved these problems by developing 'biscuit porcelain' in the 1770s, which was ideal for forming both pestles and mortars. The use of this material was widespread by the nineteenth century and pestles and mortars from this period are often referred to as 'Wedgwood mortars'.

 See Picture 10

2.2.3 Equipment for the manipulation of formulations

Spatulas used to manipulate formulations have been made in a variety of forms for centuries. They come in wood, horn, bone, bronze, iron and steel in a variety of sizes, shapes and degrees of flexibility, and examples exist from all eras since the Roman period.

 See Picture 11

2.2.4 Other old pharmaceutical equipment

Descriptions of many other types of old pharmaceutical equipment can be found elsewhere in this chapter. Some examples are:

- Bougie moulds (Section 2.1.2)
- Cachet sealing equipment (Section 2.1.3)
- Decoction apparatus (Section 2.1.6)
- Infusion pots and mugs (Section 2.1.10)
- Lozenge containers, lozenge board, rollers and cutters (Section 2.1.12)
- Pill mortar, pill pestle, pill roller, pill rounder, tile with graduated scale, pill container, pill spatula, pill cutter, pill machine and pill counter (Section 2.1.15)
- Plaster iron (Section 2.1.16)
- Tincture bottles and tincture press (Section 2.1.21).

2.3 Old pharmaceutical containers

A major concern of the compounders of medicines was to find a suitable container in which to present the finished product to the patient in a form that could be easily handled, while retaining pharmaceutical efficacy. There is a wide range of stock containers with specific functions for compounding ingredients which are now rarely seen.

2.3.1 Glass phials

The glass phial has certainly been used since Roman times as a method to present liquid preparations to patients. The unit dose round phial was probably the most common method of presenting compounded medicines during the sixteenth and seventeenth centuries, and the practice continued well into the nineteenth century. The pharmacist prepared sufficient phials for the required number of doses and directions were written on a label tied to the neck of the phial.

Phials were made in shapes, sizes and colours characteristic of the period in which they were produced. These have been catalogued by WA Thorpe in his book *English Glassware in the 17th Century, Catalogue of Old English Glass* (Churchill, London, 1937). In the early fifteenth century phials were generally between 5 and 12.5 cm tall and had a wide base tapering in a steeple shape to a narrow neck. Those from the sixteenth century were generally made of dark green glass up to 12.5 cm with a slight taper. Variants in the sixteenth and seventeenth centuries were cylindrical but still of dark green glass. In the seventeenth century and beyond the phial began to be produced in thinner glass of a lighter colour in an oval or globular shape. These were superseded in the later seventeenth and eighteenth centuries by lighter coloured, mould-blown cylinders around 7.5 cm high or pear-shaped bottles between 5 and 7.5 cm tall. In the middle of the eighteenth century white glass phials were introduced.

2.3.2 Medicine bottles and containers

Medicine bottles for oral and external liquids only came into common use in the early part of the nineteenth century. When first produced, these were hand-made and individually blown

into a flat iron mould. By the start of the twentieth century semi-automated production of glass medicines bottles had begun, with fully automated production commencing in the 1920s. These later, machine-produced bottles often had dosage graduations indicated by moulded protrusions on the side of the bottle. Naturally, bottles from these periods were generally sealed with a cork stopper.

Special poisons bottles were introduced from around 1859 when the idea for the sharply contoured hexagonal or octagonal bottle with vertical or diagonal fluting discernible by feel was patented by John Savory and RW Barker. The Pharmacy Act of 1868 secured the future for this type of container by effectively empowering the Pharmaceutical Society to regulate the keeping, dispensing and selling of poisons in a bottle rendered distinguishable by touch.

During the sixteenth and seventeenth centuries, solid and semi-solid preparations were traditionally supplied in pottery jars between 2.5 and 7.5 cm tall. This type of jar was generally glazed and sealed with either a metal lid or a cover made of parchment tied at the neck of the jar. More affluent patients received their medications in decorated Delft pottery jars.

Glazed jars made of porcelain, stoneware or earthenware with lids were mass produced from the middle of the nineteenth century.

An alternative container for topical preparations and some solid unit dose oral forms used since the fifteenth century was the 'chip box', which was generally a round or oval box constructed from hand-cut shavings of wood. These came in a variety of sizes for different purposes. The chip box was produced on a mass scale by the 1840s, but was superseded by cardboard boxes lined with impervious greaseproof paper.

 See Picture 12

2.3.3 Bulk liquid containers

Specially designed glass stock bottles with specific functions were commonplace in the nineteenth century.

Emulsion and viscous liquid bottles

Wide-mouthed glass containers were used to store and supply viscous liquids and particularly emulsions.

Oil bottles

Oil bottles had a funnel-shaped neck which flared out from the shoulder of the bottle. The close-fitting ground glass stopper was grooved on one side, which allowed excess oil to drain from the stopper back down into the stock bottle. The whole neck and stopper assembly was further protected by a removable glass dome dust cover, which prevented debris sticking to the top of the bottle while in storage.

Syrup bottles

Bottles designed to contain stock syrups were also made with a flared neck. In this case the stopper was designed to fit only loosely in the neck of the bottle, resting on a flange around the stopper. Thus, although dust and debris was excluded and the fit of the flanged top to the neck was sufficiently good to prevent evaporation, the stopper was not tight enough to allow drying sugar crusts to cause the stopper to become stuck.

 See Picture 6

Bulk liquid containers

Two commonplace standard stock bottles for bulk liquids were the Winchester quart bottle, which was of 80 oz capacity, and the Corbyn quart bottle of 40 oz capacity. The latter was probably introduced by Corbyn, Stacy and Co. of London.

The demijohn, and more notably the carboy, are other examples of large-volume containers principally constructed from glass. The swan-necked carboy has probably gained greater recognition latterly as a decorative item, and is instantly recognisable as a symbol representing pharmacy and pharmaceutical compounding.

 See Picture 13

3

Historical weights and measures

Although all modern pharmaceutical formulae are expressed in grams and litres, these are not the only systems that have been used historically. It is important that compounders are aware of older weighing systems as, although most formulae encountered will be expressed using the metric system, it is not inconceivable that some old formulae may still be encountered today. These old systems of measuring and weighing were called the 'apothecaries' system' and the 'imperial system'.

In accordance with current weights and measures regulations it is illegal to use the apothecaries' or imperial systems when dispensing prescriptions. Unfortunately, a number of older formulae were never updated and anyone looking at old extemporaneous dispensing formulae, whether from official texts or as a result of examining old prescription books, will need at least a rudimentary understanding of the process of metrication.

3.1 Metrication

3.1.1 Weights

Apothecaries' weights

Historically, grains (gr) were the standard unit of weight (originally based on the weight of one grain of barley) and formed the base unit of the apothecaries' system. Scruples, drachms (pronounced 'drams') and apothecaries' (troy) ounces were all multiples thereof (see Table 3.1).

Imperial weights (avoirdupois)

The imperial system (also called the avoirdupois system) was introduced for bulk counter sales and was based on an imperial pound of 7000 grains. Further units of avoirdupois ounces were also used. The relationship between these units and grains is shown in Table 3.2.

Table 3.1 Relationship between grains, scruples and apothecaries' (troy) ounces

Grains	Scruples	Drachms	Apothecaries' or troy ounces
20	1		
60	3	1	
480	24	8	1

Table 3.2 Relationship between grains, avoirdupois ounces and avoirdupois pounds

Grains	Avoirdupois ounces	Avoirdupois pounds
437.5	1	
7000	16	1

Table 3.3 Relationship between minims, fluid drachms, fluid ounces and pints

Minims	Fluid drachms	Fluid ounces	Pints
60	1		
480	8	1	
9600	160	20	1

3.1.2 Volumes

Within the imperial system, minims (m) were the standard unit of volume. Fluid drachm (fl dr), fluid ounces (fl oz) and pints (pt) were all multiples thereof (see Table 3.3).

3.1.3 The relationship between weights and volumes

- 1 fluid ounce of water weighs 1 ounce (avoirdupois).
- 110 minims of water weigh approximately 100 grains.

The different abbreviations and symbols historically used in pharmacy and their meanings are summarised Tables 3.4 and 3.5. When symbols were used, the figures were written in Roman numerals after the symbol. For example:

ʒ i = 1 drachm
ʒ iii = 3 drachms

ʒ iv = 4 apothecaries' ounces

Unit one could also be expressed as 'j' (e.g. ʒ j = ʒ i), but where two or more units were expressed together, only the final one was expressed by 'j' (e.g. ʒ iij = ʒ iii).

'Half' was expressed either by ss or fs. For example:

ʒ ss = ʒ fs = ½ dr or ½ fl dr
ʒ̄ ss = ʒ̄ fs = ½ fl oz
ʒ iss = ʒ ifs = 1½ dr or 1½ fl dr

Conversion between apothecaries'/imperial and metric systems

As exact scientific equivalents of the weights and measures in the systems are readily available, it would appear that simple calculation should result in the desired conversion. However, the numerical answers prove to be unwieldy to calculate and difficult, if not impossible, to handle. For example, 1 grain becomes 0.06479 grams. A more rational method of metrication was adopted when it was introduced to dispensing. It was considered more sensible to adopt a system of metrication in which well-judged 'rounding off' would result in convenient quantities without prejudice to the patient's treatment.

In addition, when the compounding process was metricated it was considered to be the ideal opportunity to improve the system of dose measurement used by the patient. Imperial doses

Table 3.4 Historical weighing and measuring units and symbols used in pharmacy

Symbol	Meaning	Example	
gr	Grain	e.g. 10 gr	= 10 grains
		or gr x	= 10 grains
m or min	Minim	e.g. 10 m	= 10 minims
dr	Drachm	e.g. 2 dr	= 2 drachms
fl dr	Fluid drachm	e.g. 2 fl dr	= 2 fluid drachms
fl oz	Fluid ounce	e.g. 2 fl oz	= 2 fluid ounces
oz (apoth)	Ounce (apothecaries')	e.g. 2 oz (apoth)	= 2 ounces (apothecaries')
			= 960 grains
oz	Ounce (avoirdupois)	e.g. 2 oz	= 2 ounces (avoirdupois)
lb	Pound (imperial)	e.g. 2 lb	= 2 pounds (imperial)
pt	Pint	e.g. 2 pt	= 2 pints

Table 3.5 The meaning of different historical symbols used in pharmacy

Symbol	Meaning	
ʒ	Drachm (dr) by weight	
	Fluid drachm (fl dr) by volume	
	60 minims (60 min, 60 m)	= ʒ i
	⅛ fluid ounce (⅛ fl oz)	= ʒ i
	Teaspoonful, metricated to a 5 mL dose	= ʒ i
℥	Apothecaries' (troy) ounce	
	Fluid ounce (fl oz)	
	480 grains	= ℥ i
	480 minims	= ℥ i
℈	Scruple	

of oral liquid medicines were measured using ordinary domestic spoons, i.e. a teaspoonful (1 fluid drachm), a dessertspoonful (2 fluid drachms) and a tablespoonful (½ fluid ounce). Owing to considerable variation in the design of spoons, this was a serious cause of error which could be further exacerbated when fractions of spoonfuls were used, a practice quite common in the treatment of infants.

In order to minimise this problem, it was decided that doses should be measured using a standard 5 mL spoon and that whole spoonfuls were to be used. In addition, it was decided to standardise on two dose volumes. A 5 mL dose for children (about one and a half teaspoons) and a 10 mL dose for adults (midway between a dessertspoonful and a tablespoonful). Any existing formulae were thus converted to these new dose volumes.

For these reasons the metrication process adopted by law (Weights and Measures Act 1970) was designed not to be scientifically exact, but to achieve the necessary adjustments and compromises. It must be emphasised that this is the only metrication process which may be used legally when compounding.

External preparations

The activity of pharmaceutical preparations is governed by the concentration of active ingredients. Therefore, for external preparations a simple method of metrication could be adopted, i.e. formulae are metricated on the basis that:

$$
\left\{
\begin{array}{c}
10 \text{ grains} \\
\text{or} \\
10 \text{ minims}
\end{array}
\right\}
\text{ in }
\left\{
\begin{array}{c}
1 \text{ fluid ounce} \\
\text{or 1 ounce} \\
\text{(apothecaries')} \\
\text{or 1 ounce} \\
\text{(avoirdupois)}
\end{array}
\right\}
\begin{array}{c}
\text{shall be} \\
\text{equivalent} \\
\text{to 2\%}
\end{array}
$$

Therefore a formula for imperial quantities is metricated by converting each quantity into a percentage concentration using the above approximation. Bulk quantities are adjusted to suitable metric equivalents (see Table 3.6).

Oral preparations

In oral preparations activity is governed by the amount of active ingredient per dose. In the metrication procedure the formula must be adjusted to show the composition of each dose. The quantity of each ingredient per dose is then metricated using the information in Table 3.6.

The metric dose volume to be adopted is decided upon and the number of doses originally prescribed is calculated. The number of metric doses and hence the quantity of preparation to be dispensed is also determined by reference to Table 3.6.

Example 3.1 Prepare the following preparation

Simple Linctus BP
Mitte ℥ vi
Sig ʒ i tid

Answer: The quantity order is in fluid ounces but the dose is expressed in fluid drachms. Convert the dose to fluid ounces:

1 fl dr = ⅛ fl oz

Calculate the number of doses ordered, i.e. 6/(⅛) = 48 doses. The metric equivalent of ʒ i is 5 mL, therefore refer to Table 3.6A and supply 40 × 5 mL = 200 mL. If the dose is expressed in terms of ℥ fs (10 mL dose) Table 3.6B is used.

Table 3.6   Dose and quantities table. Where doses and total quantities are ordered in apothecaries'/imperial/avoirdupois systems, the number of doses and the total quantities in the metric system in column 2 shall be dispensed

(A) Paediatric mixtures, elixirs, linctuses, etc. Dose volume 5 mL (obsolete dose volume 60 m)

Prescribed 1		To be dispensed 2	
Number of doses	Imperial volume fl oz	Number of doses	Metric volume mL
4	½	5	25
8	1	10	50
12	1½		
16	2	20	100
24	3		
32	4	30	150
40	5	40	200
48	6		
64	8	60	300
80	10		
96[a]	12	100	500

[a]Above 96 doses dispense 500 mL plus the metric volume opposite the balance of doses.

(B) Mixture, elixirs, linctuses, etc. Dose volume 10 mL (obsolete dose volume ½ fl oz)

Prescribed 1		To be dispensed 2	
Number of doses	Imperial volume fl oz	Number of doses	Metric volume mL
1	½	1	10
2	1	2	20
4	2	5	50
6	3		
8	4	10	100
12	6		
16	8	20	200
20	10		
24	12		
32	16	30	300
40	20		
48[b]	24	50	500

[b]Above 48 doses, dispense 500 mL plus the metric volume opposite the balance of doses.

Table 3.6   Continued

(C) External and bulk oral preparations solids/liquids

Prescribed 1 Wt/vol (av/imp) oz/fl oz	To be dispensed 2 Wt/vol (metric) g/mL
½	10
1	25
1½	50
2	
3	
4	100
5	
6	200
8	
10	300
12	
16c	500
20 fl oz	

cAbove 16 oz (1 lb) and 20 fl oz (1 pint) dispense 500 mL plus the metric volume opposite the balance of the volume.

Although in most cases metrication of oral formulae was a fairly straightforward process, emulsions provided a problem owing to their formulation. The dose for emulsions such as Liquid Paraffin Emulsion BPC was usually 1 to 4 fluid drachms (8 to 30 millilitres). It was impossible to standardise the dose to a 5 or 10 mL standard as with other oral liquid dosage forms because of the importance of the ratio of oil:water:gum in preparing a stable primary emulsion (see Sections 8.2 and 8.3.1 for further details on the preparation of a primary emulsion). Because of this anomaly, conversion of emulsions follows the directions for external and bulk oral preparations (see Table 3.6C), enabling the conversion to be based on the final volume rather than the individual dose volume.

Conversion tables for ingredients

Using the principles outlined above, it is therefore possible to produce summary conversion tables of weights and measures from imperial to metric (Tables 3.7 and 3.8). It should be borne in mind that owing to the rounding applied, these tables are to be used as a guide only.

Table 3.7 Summary conversion table for weights from grains to milligrams or grams

Grains	Milligrams	Grains	Milligrams	Grains	Grams
1/600	0.1	⅕	12.5	14–16	1
1/500, 1/480	0.125	¼	15	17–20	1.2
1/400	0.15	⅓	20	21–25	1.5
1/320, 1/300	0.2	⅖	25	26–29	1.8
1/240	0.25	½	30	30–33	2
1/200	0.3	⅗	40	34–37	2.3
1/160, 1/150	0.4	¾	50	38–43	2.5
1/130, 1/120	0.5	1	60	44–51	3
1/100	0.6	1¼	75	52–57	3.5
1/80, 1/75	0.8	1½	100	58–65	4
1/60	1	2	125	66–76	4.5
1/50	1.25	2½	150	77–84	5
1/40	1.5	3	200	85–102	6
1/30	2	3½, 4	250	103–115	7
1/25, 1/24	2.5	4½, 5	300	116–135	8
1/20	3	5½, 6	400	136–150	9
1/15	4	6½, 7½	450	151–165	10
1/12	5	8	500	166–180	11
1/10	6	9, 10	600	181–190	12
1/8	7.5	11–13	800	191–220	13
1/6	10			221–250	15
				251–275	17
				276–325	20
				326–350	22
				351–375	23
				376–400	25
				401–425	26
				426–450	28
				451–510	30

Table 3.8 Summary conversion table for volumes from minims to millilitres

Minims	Millilitres	Minims	Millilitres
1	0.06	56–64	3.5
1½	0.09	65–74	4
2	0.12	75–84	4.5
2½	0.15	85–93	5
3	0.18	94–110	6
3½	0.2	111–130	7
4–4½	0.25	131–149	8
5–5½	0.3	150–167	9
6–7½	0.4	168–185	10
8–9	0.5	186–200	11
10–11	0.6	201–220	12
12–13	0.7	221–250	14
14–16	0.9	251–275	15
17–18	1	276–300	17
19–22	1.2	301–330	18
23–27	1.5	331–370	20
28–32	1.8	371–400	22
33–37	2	401–450	25
38–46	2.5	451–500	28
47–55	3		

Part 2

Pharmaceutical forms and their preparation

4

Key formulation skills

It is necessary to master a number of key formulation skills in order to be able to produce accurate and efficacious extemporaneous preparations. This chapter outlines the key basic concepts and calculations that will be used throughout this book. All practitioners, irrespective of their own individual area of practice, must become competent in the key skills outlined in this chapter.

4.1 Weights and measures

Weighing and measuring are possibly the two most fundamental practical skills practised by a compounder. During compounding, ingredients will need to be either weighed or measured and the accuracy of the compounder's technique will have a great bearing on the accuracy and efficacy of the final product.

4.1.1 Weighing

When weighing pharmaceutical substances, the Système International d'Unités (SI) based around the gram (g), is the system that is used. Variants on the base unit are formed by 1000 times increases or divisions of the gram. Table 4.1 summarises the main units used within the pharmaceutical profession.

For weights less than 1 mg, the units of the weight are usually written in full (for example 1 nanogram rather than 1 ng, or 3.4 micrograms rather than 3.4 µg). This is because the first letter of the abbreviation (the µ or n) when written by hand may be mistaken for the letter 'm'. This could then result in dosing errors of one-thousand times plus.

Conversions between the main weighing units are essentially easy as they are all based around 1000 times multiplications or divisions of the base unit. However, care must be exercised in carrying out these calculations as errors may not be immediately obvious.

Table 4.1	Main weighing units used in pharmacy	
Unit	Abbreviation	Gram equivalent
1 kilogram	1 kg	1000 g
1 gram	1 g	1 g
1 milligram	1 mg	0.001 g
1 microgram	1 µg (or 1 mcg)	0.000001 g
1 nanogram	1 ng	0.000000001 g

Example 4.1 Convert 2.3 g into milligrams

To convert from grams to milligrams, multiply by 1000:

2.3 × 1000 = 2300 milligrams

 Example 4.2 Convert 7894 milligrams into grams

To convert from milligrams to grams, divide by 1000.

7894 ÷ 1000 = 7.894 g

4.1.2 Balances

When weighing a pharmaceutical ingredient or product, it is important to select the correct balance. Different types of balance are designed to weigh within different weight ranges to differing degrees of accuracy. For example, a balance designed to weigh 5 kg to an accuracy of

 Example 4.3 Convert 3.2 nanograms into milligrams

Using the table illustrated in Key Skill 4.1, attempt the calculation in stages. First convert from nanograms to micrograms:

3.2 ÷ 1000 = 0.0032 micrograms

Then convert from micrograms to milligrams:

0.0032 ÷ 1000 = 0.0000032 milligrams

±0.01 kg (10 g) is not going to be suitable to weigh 200 mg (0.2 g).

Broadly speaking, there are likely to be three different types of balance that will be encountered in a pharmaceutical environment. These are:

- The Class II balance or electronic equivalent
- Sensitive electronic balances
- Balances for weights greater than 50 g.

All balances have different accuracies, precisions and tolerances and it is important that the correct balance is used for a particular weighing task. In order to select the correct balance for a particular

 Key Skill 4.1 Conversion between base weight units

To convert between the base weight units, multiply or divide the figure by 1000. For conversions between more than one base unit (e.g. nanograms to grams), convert via any intermediate units (e.g. micrograms and milligrams).

Conversion from kilograms to nanograms	Conversion from nanograms to kilograms
1 kilogram	1 nanogram
× 1000	÷ 1000
1 gram	1 microgram
× 1000	÷ 1000
1 milligram	1 milligram
× 1000	÷ 1000
1 microgram	1 gram
× 1000	÷ 1000
1 nanogram	1 kilogram

weighing task, the accuracy, precision and tolerance of the balance needs to be taken into consideration. Although often misunderstood and interchanged, there are key differences between these three terms:

- **Accuracy** – is a measure of the capability of a balance to approach a true or absolute value.
- **Precision** – is the relative degree of repeatability, i.e. how closely the values within a series of replicate measurements agree.
- **Tolerance** – or 'limits of permissible errors' is the extreme value of an error permitted by specifications for a measuring instrument.

Standard dispensing balances

The balance most commonly found in pharmacies will be either a traditional 'Class II' dispensing beam balance or a modern electronic equivalent. Class II balances are similar to older Class B balances and use the same weighing techniques.

Class B balances

Class B beam balances were traditionally used in pharmacies before the introduction of Class II beam balances (and later, electronic balances). The Weights and Measures Regulations (1963) categorised weighing instruments for certain retail transactions into three different categories: Class A, Class B or Class C. The Class B balance was the balance most commonly found in pharmacies, with Class A balances being reserved for weighing amounts below the limits of a Class B balance. The weighing capabilities of the three different types of balance are summarised in Table 4.2.

Table 4.2	Traditional balance capabilities		
Balance type	Minimum weighable quantity	Increment weight	Normal maximum weighable quantity
Class A	50 mg	1 mg	1 g
Class B	100 mg (see below)	10 mg	50 g
Class C	1 g	100 mg	2 kg

 See Picture 14

As outlined in Table 4.2, Class B beam balances were designed to weigh up to 50 g in 10 mg increments. They had a nominal minimum weighable quantity of 100 mg, but in practice a higher limit was preferred for potent substances (e.g. 150 mg).

Class II balances

Class I–IV balances arose from legislation introduced in the 1980s to harmonise the laws of the European Economy Community (EEC) member states that related to non-automatic weighing instruments (Weights and Measures Act (1985)). This legislation replaced the older classification of balances under which a dispensing-type beam balance was Class B (see above). They are stamped with both a maximum and a minimum weighable quantity and so it is easier to identify whether a balance is suitable for a particular task. A traditional Class II dispensing beam balance is marked with a maximum weighable quantity of 25 g and a minimum weighable quantity of 100 mg and, as with Class B balances, Class II balances typically have a increment weight of 10 mg. As was the case with the older Class B balances, in practice many pharmacists chose to adopt a higher limit for potent substances (e.g. 150 mg).

 See Picture 15

Weighing techniques for Class B and Class II dispensing beam balances

The same weighing technique is used for both Class B and Class II dispensing beam balances. Within this section, the term 'Class II' will be used (as this is the more modern balance) but the same techniques will apply to the use of Class B dispensing beam balances.

Before use, the balance must be set up at a particular location. This should ideally be on a solid, level, firm surface. In order to ensure that the balance is exactly level, a multidirectional circular spirit level should be used, centralising a bubble contained within the level in the central circle. Once the balance has been set up at a particular location, it is important that it is not moved while in use as this will affect the accuracy of the instrument.

Next check that the scale pans are clean and that the pointer is in the centre of the scale. If the pointer is not in the centre, centralise by referring to the instructions for that particular model.

When using the balance, the weights (which are to be found in the balance drawer) are placed on the metal pan (on the left), and any ingredient being weighed is placed on the glass pan (on the right).

The following general method should be followed when using a Class II balance:

1. Obtain the ingredient to be weighed and fill in the batch number on the product worksheet (see Section 5.2, Figure 5.1).
2. Using a set of dedicated tweezers, place the correct weights on the metal scale pan (on the left-hand side). Weights should be handled as little as possible. This prevents the transfer of particles or grease from your hands onto the weights, which would alter their weight. Always use the least number of weights possible, as this will reduce error (each individual weight has its own accuracy). Note that when weights are added to the scale pan, the pointer will deflect to one side.
3. Close the weights drawer before weighing. If the drawer is left open, powder or other ingredients may fall into the drawer and adhere to the weights, altering their weight.
4. Transfer the ingredient to the glass pan using a spatula, until the pointer is central. Ensure when reading the pointer that you move to align your eye with the scale to avoid any parallax errors (see Figures 4.1 and 4.2).
5. Check the weight, the name of the ingredient, and then initial the worksheet.
6. Ask for a second, independent check of your weight from another member of staff, who will also initial the worksheet.

In some situations you may be working on your own (for example if preparing an emergency preparation outside of normal hours). On these occasions you must perform your own second check in point 6 above.

Although most Class II balances contain a graduated scale within the pointer window (usually expressed in either milligrams (mg) or grains (gr) for some Class B balances), it is best to

Example 4.4 Weighing 10 g of Zinc Oxide BP powder on a Class II dispensing beam balance

1. Check that the balance is clean and dry and that the pointer is in the centre of the scale.
2. Obtain the stock pot from the shelf and write the batch number (the number on the label after BN or LOT) in the table on the product worksheet.
3. Place a 10 g weight on the metal scale pan.
4. Using a spatula, transfer 10 g of Zinc Oxide BP onto the glass scale pan. Check that the pointer is in the centre, check the ingredient and sign your initials in the 'Dispensed by' box.
5. Ask for a second check from another member of staff. Once the check has been performed, the member of staff initials the 'Checked by' box.
6. Return the stock pot to the shelf.

Extract from the product worksheet:

Ingredient	Batch number	Quantity	Dispensed by	Checked by
Zinc Oxide BP		10 g		

weigh an ingredient using the method outlined above (i.e. by placing weights equal to the target weight on one scale pan and counterbalancing with the appropriate amount of solid or liquid until the pointer registers zero in the centre of the scale). Although useful as a guide, it is not advisable to use the scale to accurately indicate the weight of solid or liquid on a balance, as although the central point can be read easily without any parallax error, the reading of graduations at either side of the central point will be more difficult because of the angles involved.

Before weighing any ingredient, the product formula should be written out in full, in ink. If you are weighing more than one ingredient, once weighed, place each ingredient on a piece of labelled paper on the bench.

If you are weighing a greasy product, place a piece of greaseproof paper on the glass scale pan. Remember to counterbalance this piece of paper with a piece of the same weight on the other side. Check the pointer is still in the middle when the greaseproof paper is on both sides. Ensure that

Example 4.5 Weighing 10 g of Simple Ointment BP on a Class II dispensing beam balance

1. Check that the balance is clean and dry and that the pointer is in the centre of the scale.
2. Place a piece of greaseproof paper on the glass scale pan.
3. Counterbalance the greaseproof paper with a second piece on the metal pan. Check the pointer is in the centre of the scale.
4. Obtain the stock pot from the shelf and write the batch number (the number on the label after BN or LOT) in the table on the product worksheet.
5. Place a 10 g weight on the metal scale pan.
6. Using a spatula, transfer 10 g of Simple Ointment BP onto the greaseproof paper on the glass scale pan. Check that the pointer is in the centre, check the ingredient and sign your initials in the 'Dispensed by' box.
7. Ask for a second check from another member of staff. Once the check has been performed, the member of staff initials the 'Checked by' box.
8. Return the stock pot to the shelf.

Extract from product worksheet:

Ingredient	Batch number	Quantity	Dispensed by	Checked by
Simple Ointment BP		10 g		

Example 4.6 Weighing 5 g of Syrup BP on a Class II dispensing beam balance

1. Check that the balance is clean and dry and that the pointer is in the centre of the scale.
2. Place a small pot on the glass scale pan.
3. Counterbalance the pot with a second pot on the metal pan. Check the pointer is in the centre of the scale.
4. Obtain the stock pot from the shelf and write the batch number (the number on the label after BN or LOT) in the table on the product worksheet.
5. Place a 5 g weight on the metal scale pan.
6. Pour an amount of Syrup BP into a beaker to use as stock. Once an ingredient is removed from its stock container it should not be returned, to reduce the risk of contaminating the stock liquid. For this reason, avoid transferring too much as this is wasteful.
7. Transfer 5 g of Syrup BP from the beaker into the pot on the glass scale pan. Check that the pointer is in the centre, check the ingredient and sign your initials in the 'Dispensed by' box.
8. Ask for a second check from another member of staff. Once the check has been performed, the member of staff initials the 'Checked by' box.
9. Return the stock pot to the shelf.

Extract from product worksheet:

Ingredient	Batch number	Quantity	Dispensed by	Checked by
Syrup BP		5 g		

both pans can move freely and that the paper is not touching the sides of the balance or bench. If the pan's movement is hindered by the paper touching the side, the balance will not weigh accurately.

When weighing a material that can stain (e.g. Potassium Permanganate BP), remember to place a piece of paper under the weighing pan and push a large piece of paper up to (not underneath) the balance. This will catch any material that falls off the balance pan during weighing and will avoid the bench and balance becoming stained.

If the quantity of an ingredient to be incorporated into a product is quoted in grams (or other unit of weight, e.g. mg), it will be necessary to weigh the liquid ingredient rather than measuring it by volume. Any liquid can be weighed on a Class II dispensing beam balance by measuring into a small pot. Remember to counterbalance the pot first (check the pointer is in the centre).

Electronic pharmacy balances

Unlike the Class II dispensing beam balance, the scale pan on an electronic balance is usually made of metal rather than glass. This means that the ingredient to be weighed is not placed directly onto the scale pan. Solids are weighed onto a watch glass, greasy solids onto greaseproof paper and liquids into a small pot. In all three cases, tare the balance (i.e. set the electronic display back to zero) with the container for the ingredient (e.g. watch glass, greaseproof paper, etc.) on the balance beforehand. Taring the balance with the ingredient container on the balance will ensure that only the weight of the ingredient placed in the container will register on the display. By using this method, the procedure of subtracting the weight of the container from the display weight is avoided, making the weighing process easier and less susceptible to error.

Sensitive electronic balances

If the amount of substance to be weighed is less than 150 mg, it would not be appropriate to weigh the ingredient on a standard dispensing balance, such as a Class II balance, as the accuracy of the balance would make the error too large. Clearly, the smaller the amount to be weighed, the bigger the inaccuracy as a percentage of the total weight becomes. For example, measuring 200 mg on a Class II balance would result in 200 mg ± 10 mg (i.e. ±5%). When the weight to be measured is reduced to 100 mg (i.e. 100 mg ± 10 mg) this increases the percentage inaccuracy to ±10%. Further reductions in the amount to be weighed would further increase this percentage inaccuracy.

To weigh amounts below 150 mg, it is usual to use a more sensitive electronic balance. These typically have an accuracy of ±1 mg (10 times more accurate than the common pharmacy balance). The typical minimum amounts that are weighed on these balances are 50 mg for non-potent substances, increasing to 100 mg for potent substances.

In some circumstances, it will be necessary to incorporate an amount of active ingredient into a product that is less than the minimum recommended weighable quantity of a balance. In these circumstances, it is necessary to weigh a known excess of active ingredient and then dilute further during the compounding procedure. Further explanation of how this is achieved and when it is appropriate will be given within the respective product chapters.

Balances for weights greater than 50 g

The final type of balance that you are likely to find in a pharmacy are the balances designed to weigh weights over the maximum weighable weight (i.e. 25 g) of a Class II balance or electronic equivalent. These balances will be used to measure out bulk ingredients.

4.1.3 Measuring

Liquids are universally measured in litres. Although not part of the SI system of units, the litre is commonly used. A litre is defined as one cubic decimetre (0.1 m³), i.e. the volume that a cube with equal sides of 10 cm would occupy.

As described for weights in Section 4.1.1 above, there are a number of different volumes based around the litre that are in common use in pharmacy today (Table 4.3). In a similar way to weights, for volumes less than 1 mL the units of the volume are usually written in full (for example 1 microlitre rather than 1 µL). This is because the first letter of the abbreviation (the µ)

 Example 4.7 Weigh 10 g of Zinc Oxide BP on an electronic balance

1. Check that the balance is clean and dry.
2. Obtain the stock pot from the shelf and write the batch number (the number on the label after BN or LOT) in the table on the product worksheet.
3. Place a watch glass onto the balance and tare.
4. Check the display is reading zero.
5. Using a spatula, transfer 10 g of Zinc Oxide BP to the watch glass. Check the weight, check the ingredient and sign your initials in the 'Dispensed by' box.
6. Ask for a second check from a member of staff. Once the check has been performed, the member of staff will initial the 'Checked by' box.
7. Return the stock pot to the shelf.

Extract from product worksheet:

Ingredient	Batch number	Quantity	Dispensed by	Checked by
Zinc Oxide BP		10 g		

Key Skill 4.2 Determining the appropriate balance for use

It is important when weighing any ingredient that consideration is given to the accuracy of the instrument in use. All balances will have an inherent accuracy that will affect your confidence in the final product. Using the wrong balance is in some cases as bad as weighing the wrong amount. Remember that there are three main types of balance used in pharmacy and it is important to check the accuracy of each balance that you use. Typical balance ranges are detailed below, although they can vary dramatically and you must become familiar with the tolerances of the individual balance(s) that you encounter.

Type of balance	Typical minimum weight	Typical maximum weight	Typical accuracy
1. Large balance	50 g and upwards	Variable	Variable
2. Class II dispensing balance or electronic equivalent	150 mg	25 g	± 10 mg
3. Sensitive electronic balance	50 mg (non-potent) 100 mg (potent)	100–500 g	± 1 mg

Table 4.3   Main volume units used in pharmacy

Unit	Abbreviation	Litre equivalent
1 litre	1 L (or 1 litre)	1 litre
1 millilitre	1 mL	0.001 litre
1 microlitre	1 µL	0.000001 litre

Example 4.9 Convert 3643 millilitres into litres

To convert from millilitres to litres, divide by 1000.

3643 ÷ 1000 = 3.643 litres

Example 4.8 Convert 6.7 litres into millilitres

To convert from litres to millilitres, multiply by 1000:

6.7 × 1000 = 6700 millilitres

Example 4.10 Convert 5.5 microlitres into litres

Using the table illustrated in Key Skill 4.3, attempt the calculation in stages. First convert from microlitres to millilitres:

5.5 ÷ 1000 = 0.0055 millilitres

Then convert from millilitres to litres:

0.0055 × 1000 = 0.0000055 litres (5.5 × 10^{-6})

when written by hand may be mistaken for the letter 'm'. Furthermore, it is also best practice when referring to volumes in multiples of litres to write the word 'litre' or 'litres' in full. This will assist in reducing any confusion with the unit 'one' ('1').

Converting between the main volume units is as important as mastering the conversions between weight units. As with weight conversions, volume conversions are easy as they are all based around 1000 times multiplications or divisions of the base unit.

Key Skill 4.3 Conversion between base volume units

To convert between the base volume units, multiply or divide the figure by 1000. For conversions between more than one base unit (e.g. microlitres to litres), convert via any intermediate units (e.g. millilitres).

Conversion from litres to microlitres	Conversion from microlitres to litres
1 litre	1 microlitre
1 millilitre × 1000	1 millilitre ÷ 1000
1 microlitre × 1000	1 litre ÷ 1000

4.1.4 Measures

Any vessel that is used to measure accurately an ingredient must comply with the current Weights and Measures Regulations and should be stamped accordingly.

There are two main types of vessel used within pharmacy for measuring liquids:

- Conical measures
- Syringes.

In addition to these, pipettes are also used in the preparation of some pharmaceutical products. For more information on pipettes see Chapter 5, Section 5.3.4.

Conical measures

In general, conical measures rather than cylindrical measures are used in pharmacy practice. They have a number of advantages over cylindrical measures. For example:

- They are easier to fill without spilling liquid on the sides above the required level.
- It is easier to drain out the preparation.
- It is easier to rinse out the residue left after draining viscous liquids into the preparation.
- They are easier to clean after use.

 See Picture 16

On the other hand, it must be borne in mind

that compared to cylindrical measures, with conical measures:

- It is harder to read the meniscus accurately.
- It is more difficult to estimate volumes between graduations (although in practice, owing to the error, this would be considered poor professional practice and is never done).

It is not good practice to use a conical measure to measure a volume that is smaller than half of the total volume of the measure. Because of the shape of the measure, it is more accurate, for example, to measure 10 mL in a 10 mL conical measure than it would be to measure 10 mL in a 100 mL conical measure.

Stamped conical measures can be used to measure any marked amount but it is sensible to select the smallest measure for the desired volume. For volumes less than 1 mL, a syringe is used (see below) although a 5 mL syringe can be used to measure graduated volumes up to 5 mL.

The markings on a beaker are only approximations and cannot ever be used to measure any volume accurately.

Remember, when measuring liquids, that the bottom of the meniscus should be in line with the desired graduation mark (Figure 4.1). When reading the volume of the liquid, ensure that your eye is in line with the meniscus. This will avoid any parallax errors. If your eye line is not level with the meniscus (for example you are looking down onto the meniscus) errors in

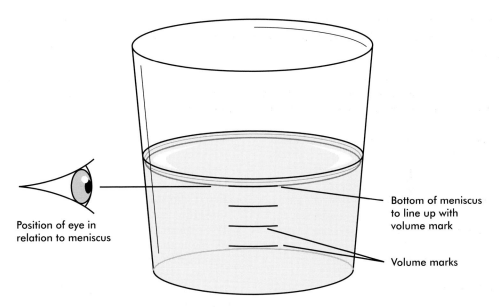

Figure 4.1   Diagram to show which edge of the meniscus is to line up with the volume mark (note – the meniscus has been exaggerated in this diagram)

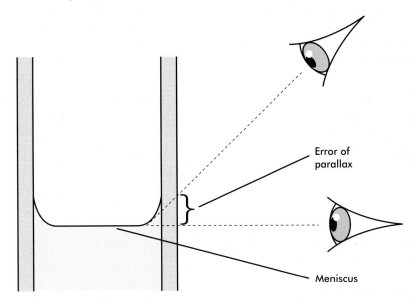

Figure 4.2   Diagram to show how an error of parallax can occur

reading the correct volume will occur (see Figure 4.2).

In addition to ensuring that your eye is in line with the meniscus, it is important that the measure remains on a flat surface. In many cases, this will involve moving your head down to the correct level. Do not lift the measure to the level of your head as it will not be possible to read the volume accurately with the liquid moving about in the measure. Even if the liquid appears stationary, it is unlikely that the measure will be level.

Example 4.11 Measuring a colourless liquid: 25 mL potable water

1. Select an appropriately sized conical measure.
2. Check that the measure is clean and dry.
3. Obtain a beaker of potable water to use as stock.
4. Measure 25 mL potable water in the conical measure. Check the volume and sign your initials in the 'Dispensed by' box on the product worksheet.
5. Ask for a second check from another member of staff. Once the check has been performed, the member of staff initials the 'Checked by' box on the product worksheet.

Extract from product worksheet:

Ingredient	Batch number	Quantity	Dispensed by	Checked by
Potable water	N/A	25 mL		

When measuring certain dark or coloured liquids it may be difficult to see the bottom of the meniscus clearly. In these cases, placing a piece of white or coloured card or paper behind the measure may help.

Finally, it is important to avoid spilling any liquid down the side of the measure as this could result in the incorrect amount of liquid being added to the preparation. It is also poor pharmaceutical practice.

When measuring a viscous liquid (e.g. Syrup BP), it is important once measured that the measure is drained properly to ensure all of the measured liquid is transferred. This will involve holding the measure above the vessel that the ingredient is to be transferred to for several seconds.

Syringes

Traditionally, small volumes have been measured in pharmacy using a graduated pipette (see Section 5.3.4). However, more recently, 1 mL syringes have been used to measure graduated volumes less than 1 mL, and 5 mL syringes to measure graduated volumes up to 5 mL. It must

be remembered that although their use is commonplace, syringes are less accurate than pipettes.

For all syringes, the following technique should be employed:

1. Select an appropriate syringe.
2. Move the plunger up and down a couple of times to check that it moves smoothly without sticking.
3. Draw up liquid in excess of the required volume.
4. Invert the syringe so the nozzle is pointing upwards.
5. Draw the plunger back a little further to allow all the liquid in the nozzle to enter the main chamber.
6. Tap the syringe to allow all the trapped air to come together at the top of the syringe.
7. Expel the air.
8. Re-invert the syringe over the stock liquid and push the plunger until the desired volume is reached. The desired volume is reached when the measuring edge of the plunger is in line with the desired volume mark in the syringe barrel (see Figure 4.3).
9. Add the measured liquid to the preparation. Do NOT expel the liquid left in the nozzle. The syringe is calibrated to allow for this excess.

4.2 Medication strength

There are a number of different ways that the strength of active ingredients in a medicinal product can be expressed. It is important that all practitioners are able to perform calculations using the different methods outlined in this section as all are in common use today in pharmacy.

4.2.1 Millimoles

The strength of active ingredient within a pharmaceutical preparation can be expressed as the number of millimoles per unit volume or mass of product. The mole is the unit of amount

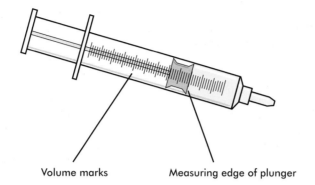

Volume marks   Measuring edge of plunger

Figure 4.3   Diagram to show which edge of the plunger is to line up with the volume mark when using a syringe

of substance and there are 1000 millimoles in a mole. To calculate the number of millimoles of an ingredient in a medicinal product, you will first need to know the molecular weight of the ingredient.

The number of moles of ingredient is the mass of ingredient divided by the molecular mass (see Key Skill 4.4).

To calculate the number of moles of active ingredient, you need to know its molecular mass. Molecular masses for different ingredients are listed in the British Pharmacopoeia, Martindale – The Extra Pharmacopoeia and the British Pharmaceutical Codex, within the relevant ingredient monographs.

Sometimes a compounder will be asked to prepare a pharmaceutical preparation with a specified amount of active ingredient, expressed in millimoles, per unit of preparation. Preparation calculations for this type of product use the same basic principles, the only difference being that you know the number of millimoles required and so have to calculate the mass of active ingredient to be included in the preparation (see Example 4.12).

4.2.2 Milliequivalents and equivalent weights

When solutions are formulated, sometimes the compounder is only interested in one half of an ion pair (for example, the number of H^+ ions present in a solution of HCl). One of the best ways to express this is by stating the number of equivalents (Eq).

Example 4.12   How much Sodium Chloride BP is required to prepare 100 mL of Sodium Chloride BP solution containing 1.5 mmol sodium chloride per mL

First, you will need to know the molecular weight of sodium chloride. Reference texts quote the molecular weight as 58.44. Therefore a 1 molar solution would contain 58.44 g of sodium chloride in 1 litre.

- In a final solution of 1.5 millimoles (mmol) per mL, each millilitre will contain 1.5 mmol.
- If 1 mole of solution contains 58.44 g, 1 mmol contains 0.05844 g (58.44 ÷ 1000).
- Therefore 1.5 mmol contains 0.05844 × 1.5 = 0.08766 g.
- If the final solution contains 1.5 mmol per mL, there will be 0.08766 g per mL of solution.
- We need to dispense 100 mL of solution to the patient and so the product will need a total of 0.08766 × 100 = 8.766 g of Sodium Chloride BP.

Key Skill 4.4   Calculating the number of moles of an ingredient or product

---

$$\text{Number of moles} = \frac{\text{Mass in grams}}{\text{Molecular mass}}$$

The term 'equivalents' refers to the number of univalent counter ions required to react with each molecule of the substance. In the example given above, HCl has one equivalent of H^+ ions per mole as one mole of a univalent ion (e.g. OH^-) reacts with one mole of H^+. Sulphuric acid (H_2SO_4) contains two equivalents of H^+ ions per mole because two moles of a univalent ion (e.g. OH^-) are required to react with one mole of sulphuric acid.

Because of the small quantities of electrolytes often used in pharmaceutical solutions, the more common term milliequivalents is used (there are 1000 mEq per Eq and so it follows that the number of Eq/mol is equal to the number of mEq/mmol). This is a common method for expressing the amount of electrolyte that is needed to be administered to a patient to correct an electrolyte imbalance.

Following on from the above, the equivalent weight of an element or compound is the weight that combines chemically with one equivalent of another element or compound. The equivalent weight (for molecules) is given by:

$$\text{Equivalent weight (g/Eq)} = \frac{\text{Atomic or molecular weight (g/mol)}}{\text{Equivalents per atomic or molecular weight}}$$

4.2.3 Isotonicity

It is important for some pharmaceutical solutions that the osmotic pressure of the solution should be approximately the same as the osmotic pressure of the body tissue to which the solution is applied, for example solutions intended for application to the eye. If the osmotic pressure is different (i.e. the solutions are either hypo- or hypertonic with respect to body tissues), swelling or contraction of the body tissue may occur.

If no net movement of solvent molecules occurs for two solutions separated by a perfect semi-permeable membrane, the solutions are said to be iso-osmotic. Within the body, tissues do not behave as true semi-permeable membranes (i.e. some solute molecules are able to pass across the membrane as well as solvent molecules). If the two iso-osmotic solutions are able to remain in equilibrium across a biological membrane, they are described as being isotonic with respect to the membrane in question.

One of the most common pharmaceutical solutions that the compounder will encounter is a sodium chloride solution that is isotonic with human blood. A solution containing 0.9 g of sodium chloride per 100 mL of solution is isotonic. This is more commonly referred to as a 0.9% w/v solution (also known as normal saline).

Although the adjustment of solutions to make them isotonic is beyond the scope of this book, it is worth indicating that if isotonicity is required, any adjustment to the tonicity must take place after the addition of all the other ingredients to the solution owing to their own individual effect on the osmotic pressure of the solution.

4.2.4 Percentage strength

Expressing the strength of a pharmaceutical product by 'percentage' can have a number of different meanings. These meanings are indicated by the addition of suffixes, such as w/w or w/v, following the percentage symbol. It is important to be able to distinguish between the different types of percentage, as all are in common use in modern pharmacy.

The following terms are commonly used:

- % w/w or percentage weight in weight (or % m/m – percentage mass in mass) – This expresses the amount in grams of solute in 100 g of product.
- % w/v or percentage weight in volume – This expresses the amount in grams of solute in 100 mL of product.
- % v/v or percentage volume in volume – This expresses the number of millilitres of solute in 100 mL of product.
- % v/w or percentage volume in weight – This expresses the number of millilitres of solute in 100 g of product.

The strength of solutions of solids in liquids is usually expressed as % w/v and of liquids in liquids as % v/v. When the type of percentage is not specified, by convention the above rule will apply (i.e. % solid in liquid is interpreted as % w/v).

4.2.5 Parts and solubility

Parts

Another common method for expressing the strength of a pharmaceutical product is through the use of the term 'parts', for example 'parts' of solute in 'parts' of product. This is interpreted as parts by weight (grams) of a solid in parts by volume (millilitres) of the final solution; or in parts by volume (millilitres) of a liquid in parts by volume (millilitres) of the final solution. In addition to expressing the concentration of a medicinal product, this terminology is also a common method for expressing the solubility of ingredients.

Solubility

Solubilities are quoted in reference works in terms of the number of parts of solvent by volume required to dissolve one part (by weight for solids or volume for liquids) of the medicament in question. The solubility value for a substance at 20 °C is generally quoted unless otherwise stated.

Reference texts often quote solubilities in a range of solvents. For example, iodine is soluble 1 in 3500 of water, 1 in 125 of glycerol, 1 in 8 of alcohol and 1 in 5 of ether. In this case 1 g iodine would dissolve in 3500 mL water, whereas the same weight of iodine would dissolve in only 5 mL of ether.

It is also common to see the solubilities of medicaments described by a scale of terms derived by convention that range from 'very soluble' to 'practically insoluble' (Table 4.4).

Table 4.4   Numerical value of different solubility descriptions

Solubility description	Numerical value
Very soluble	1 in less than 1
Freely soluble	1 in 1 to 1 in 10
Soluble	1 in 10 to 1 in 30
Sparingly soluble	1 in 30 to 1 in 100
Slightly soluble	1 in 100 to 1 in 1000
Very slightly soluble	1 in 1000 to 1 in 10000
Practically insoluble	1 in greater than 10000

It should be borne in mind that when a solute is added to a solvent the liquid volume does not necessarily increase summatively. For example, if a solid was soluble 1 in 11 this would mean that 1 g of solute would dissolve in 11 mL of solvent. The resulting solution will be greater in volume than 11 mL but not necessarily as much as 12 mL. It would appear that during the solution process the solute must be fitting into 'spaces' within the solvent.

The process of dissolution in simple terms can be broken down into three stages:

1. Removal of a molecule from the solute.
2. Preparation of a 'space' in the solvent ready for the transfer of the dislodged solute molecule.
3. Positioning the solute molecule in the solvent space.

 Example 4.13 What volume of potable water is required to dissolve 4 g of sodium bicarbonate?

To calculate the required amount of solvent to dissolve 4 g of sodium bicarbonate, you need to know the solubility of the solute. The solubility of sodium bicarbonate in water can be found by reference to any official text. In the British Pharmacopoeia it is quoted as 1 in 11. This means that 1 g of sodium bicarbonate is soluble in 11 mL of water.

Multiplying the amount of sodium bicarbonate required in the preparation by the solubility gives the quantity of solvent required:

$4 \times 11 = 44$ mL of water

 Example 4.14 What volume of potable water is required to dissolve 3 g of a solid which is soluble in 2.5 parts of water?

1 g dissolves in 2.5 mL of water. Therefore, 3 g dissolves in $3 \times 2.5 = 7.5$ mL of water.

Dissolution of more than one solute

Questions arise when there are two or more soluble solids to be incorporated into a single solution. Should each solid be dissolved individually in the solvent and then the two solutions combined, or alternatively should the least soluble solid be dissolved first followed by the most soluble solid, or vice versa?

It should be remembered that the rapidity of solution does not depend entirely on the degree of solubility of the solid. Some substances are very soluble but are slowly soluble; others dissolve more rapidly but to a smaller extent. The problem is also compounded by consideration of the use of each of the soluble solids. For example, if one compound is an antioxidant and the other a compound susceptible to oxidation, the addition of the antioxidant as the first solid introduced to the vehicle would seem the commonsense answer to prevent oxidation of the second; this would be regardless of the ease of solubility.

Historically this problem has been dealt with in differing ways. In the late 1800s and early 1900s the two powders would be transferred to a mortar and thoroughly mixed together (using the 'doubling-up' technique – see Key Skill 7.1). A small amount of vehicle would be added to the mortar and mixed with the powders using a pestle; the saturated solution thus formed would be decanted off and the process repeated until all of the soluble solids had been incorporated into small amounts of saturated solution.

By the 1950s this advice had been changed. The idea was now to add the soluble powders to the vehicle at the same time. The quantity of vehicle used did not reflect the solubility of any of the soluble powders to be incorporated. The assumption made was that three-quarters of the vehicle would be a suitable volume for dissolution. This decision was based on two factors:

- The volume occupied by other ingredients in the preparation would rarely exceed the remaining one quarter, but if it should, the quantity of vehicle used for dissolution must be reduced.
- Solution is hastened by using as much of the solvent as is convenient.

Although each of these methods has its merits, the choice of the most appropriate method is based on the solubility of the solids. First dissolve the least soluble solid in slightly more than the minimum amount of liquid required for dissolution and then add in any other soluble solids in increasing order of solubility. Normally this will be achieved just using the amount of vehicle required for the least soluble solid. In simplistic terms, the 'spaces' occupied by the molecules of the least soluble compound will be different from the 'spaces' occupied by the molecules of the more soluble compounds. This would be a logical conclusion, as the degree of solubility generally decreases with an increase of molecular weight; therefore the least soluble molecules will be larger than the more soluble molecules and will therefore occupy bigger 'spaces' than those needed by the more soluble compounds.

In some cases the dissolution of certain medicaments can only be achieved within a particular pH range. The final pH of a solution must be considered in conjunction with the intended use of the product.

There is some latitude when compounding solutions intended for oral use, as the gastro-intestinal tract can accommodate solutions with a wide range of pH values. For example, aqueous solutions of potassium citrate have a pH between 7.5 and 9. It should be noted, though, that markedly hypertonic solutions for oral use should be diluted with water before administration. Potassium Citrate Mixture BP contains 3 g potassium citrate and 500 mg citric acid in each 10 mL dose, which must be mixed with approximately 200 mL potable water immediately before administration.

Where solutions are compounded for external use on mucous membranes or broken skin, appropriate buffering agents should be included to adjust the final pH to neutral in order to avoid irritation. Similarly, such solutions should be rendered isotonic, usually by the addition of an appropriate amount of sodium chloride.

4.2.6 Dilutions

It is not uncommon for a compounder to have to dilute a concentrated stock product to make either an ingredient for incorporation into a pharmaceutical product or a product itself.

Additionally, some products are dispensed to patients for further dilution at home, for example dressing soaks. In both cases it is necessary to specify the required amount of concentrated product that needs to be mixed with a specified amount of diluent.

There are two main ways to express dilutions (where '*x*' is the volume in millilitres):

- 1 in *x* (e.g. 1 in 10)
- 1:*x* (or 1 to x) (e.g. 1:10 or 1 to 10).

It is important to understand the difference between these because they appear initially to be the same. However, any misinterpretation can lead to large errors of final concentration. For example, a dilution expressed as 1 in 10 means that there is one part of solvent in 10 parts of final solution (e.g. 1 mL of concentrate and 9 mL vehicle with a final volume of 10 mL). However, a dilution expressed as 1:10 means that there is one part of solvent to 10 parts of solvent (or 1 in 11) (e.g. 1 mL of concentrate and 10 mL vehicle with a final volume of 11 mL). Although useful in some cases, for example communicating to patients how much of a concentrate is to be diluted with a specified amount of diluent, this is a rigid approach to dilution that will always result in a final solution of a specified strength. Problems arise when it is necessary to produce differing strengths of solution from a concentrate. If a variability of strength is required, each diluted preparation will have to be either individually

Key Skill 4.5 Dilutions

There are two main methods for expressing dilutions. It is important that the two are not mixed up as there is a key difference between them.

- 1 in x – 1 part of solute *in* x parts of final solution
- 1:x (or 1 to x) – 1 part of solute *to* x parts of solvent

Example 4.15 Prepare 500 mL of a 0.1% w/v solution using a 20% w/v concentrated stock solution

First, you need to calculate the total amount of active ingredient required in the final solution:

0.1% w/v solution = 0.1 g in 100 mL

Therefore, there is 0.5 g in 500 mL. Next, you need to calculate the quantity of the concentrated solution that contains the same amount of active ingredient.

20% w/v solution = 20 g in 100 mL

So there are 2 g in 10 mL, 1 g in 5 mL and 0.5 g in 2.5 mL. Therefore 2.5 mL of a 20% w/v solution would be required to make 500 mL of a 0.1% w/v solution.

Example 4.16 How much solute is required to produce 5 litres of a 0.9% w/v solution?

0.9% = 0.9 g in 100 mL

Therefore, there are 9 g in 1000 mL and you would need 45 g in 5000 mL.

Example 4.17 How much solute is required to produce 20 mL of a 5% solution?

5% = 5 g in 100 mL

Therefore you would need 1 g in 20 mL.

Example 4.18 What quantity of a 40% w/v solution would be required to produce 1 litre of a 1 in 1000 solution?

1 in 1000 = 1 g in 1000 mL

What volume of a 40% w/v solution contains 1 g?

40% w/v = 40 g in 100 mL

There are 4 g in 10 mL, therefore 1 g in 2.5 mL. Therefore, 2.5 mL of a 40% solution would be required to produce 1 litre of a 1 in 1000.

prepared or a concentrate given and supplied with comprehensive and often complex dilution instructions, making it more suitable for use in a hospital setting. It is therefore essential that all practitioners are able to calculate both the quantity of a concentrated solution and the quantity of diluent that needs to be mixed to produce a specified quantity of the correct strength of a final product.

5

Extemporaneous dispensing

5.1 Guide to general good practice requirements

It is of paramount importance that, during the compounding process, the compounder adheres to strict procedures to ensure the safety of the patient for whom the extemporaneous formulation is intended. The measures indicated below, although fairly simple, are designed to ensure that the compounding process is undertaken in a logical and safe manner for both the intended recipient of the medication and the compounder.

Because of the diversity of the types and number of preparations that can be formulated extemporaneously, compounder experience and expertise are significant factors in the production of safe and effective extemporaneous formulations.

5.1.1 Standards for extemporaneous dispensing

As indicated above, patients who visit a pharmacy with a prescription for a product needing to be extemporaneously prepared are entitled to expect the standards within a pharmacy to be comparable to those of a licensed manufacturing unit. The products produced in the pharmacy must be suitable for use, accurately prepared, and prepared in such a way as to ensure the products meet the required standard for quality assurance. So although this is small-scale production, the same careful attention to detail is required as would be found in a manufacturing unit.

The following measures must be taken into consideration when preparing a product extemporaneously.

Personal hygiene

Personal hygiene is extremely important. Hygiene standards in a pharmaceutical environment should be as high as, if not higher than, those found in food kitchens. This is because medications are being prepared for patients who may already be ill.

Personal protective equipment

A clean white coat should be worn to protect the compounder from the product and, conversely, the product from contamination from the compounder. During the compounding process, safety glasses should always be worn and, depending on the nature of the ingredients to be incorporated into the preparation, additional safety equipment (e.g. facemasks, gloves) may also be required. It is the responsibility of the individual compounder to assess the risk posed by any pharmaceutical ingredient and to ensure that the correct safety equipment is in use. Similarly, long hair should be tied back and hands washed, ensuring any open cuts are covered.

Clean work area and equipment

The cleanliness of the work area and equipment used during the compounding procedure is of paramount importance. The risk of contaminating the final product with either dirt or microorganisms from the surroundings, or from ingredients from a previous preparation can be considerable if attention is not paid to the cleanliness of the work area and equipment. Before starting to compound a product, the work

area and equipment should be cleaned with a suitable solution (e.g. industrial methylated spirits (IMS)), which must be allowed to dry fully.

Appropriate work area

In addition to the cleanliness of the work area, consideration needs to be given to the work area itself to ensure that it is suitable for its intended purpose. Both lighting and ventilation need to be adequate. Some pharmaceutical ingredients are highly volatile and if the ventilation within the work area is inadequate this could cause problems for the compounding staff. For additional premises standards, see Section 5.1.2.

Label preparation

The label for any pharmaceutical product must be prepared before starting the compounding procedure. This will enable the product to be labelled as soon as it has been manufactured and packaged, eliminating the possibility that an unlabelled product will be left on the bench. It also reduces the possibility of the product being mislabelled and given to the wrong patient. For further details on the preparation of a suitable label, see Section 5.6.2.

Weighing and measuring procedure

During weighing and measuring, unless strict guidelines are followed, it can be very easy to mix up different pharmaceutical ingredients as many ingredients resemble each other. It is preferable to incorporate a weighed or measured ingredient into a product as soon as possible to prevent any accidental switching. If this is not possible, when weighing or measuring more than one ingredient, place each on a piece of labelled paper as soon as it has been weighed or measured. This will avoid any accidental cross-over of ingredients.

5.1.2 Premises standards

In addition to the points highlighted in Section 5.1.1, the premises where an extemporaneous product is being prepared needs to be of an appropriate standard.

- Premises decoration should be of a good basic standard.
- The floor should be covered but in such a manner as to be easily cleaned, surfaces should be smooth, impervious to dirt and moisture, and should be clean and uncluttered.
- Sinks should be clean and have a supply of hot and cold water.
- There should be a functioning, clean refrigerator.
- There should be a supply of mains (potable) water.

5.1.3 Equipment requirements

A dispensary should have sufficient equipment available in order to be able to operate effectively. As a guide, the following items should be available:

- Heating ring (means of boiling water)
- Hot water bath (see Section 5.3.7)
- Class II dispensing balance or electronic equivalent (see Section 4.1.2)
- Range of glass and earthenware mortars and pestles (see Section 5.3.1)
- Range of glass beakers
- Range of accurate graduated conical measures (stamped by the weights and measures inspector) (see Section 4.1.4)
- Range of graduated syringes and/or pipettes (see Sections 4.1.4 and 5.3.4)
- Large and small glass or ceramic tiles (see Section 5.3.2)
- Range of spatulas and glass stirring rods (see Section 5.3.3)
- Thermometers
- Suppository moulds (see Section 5.3.5)
- Tablet and capsule counting equipment (see Section 5.3.6)
- Range of suitable containers for prepared products (see Section 5.7)
- Range of suitable information sources
- Electronic labelling system.

5.1.4 Avoidance of contamination

To avoid contamination of any extemporaneously prepared product, compounders should adhere to the following guidelines:

- Ensure all equipment is clean and dry prior to use.
- Keep the dispensing area clear of unnecessary items.
- Do not leave lids off stock bottles: always replace immediately after use.
- Do not return material to stock containers once removed.
- Do not leave weighed and measured items unlabelled on the work surface.
- Do not allow raw materials or the final product to come in contact with the hands (if necessary wear gloves).

The procedure to be followed on receipt of a prescription for extemporaneous preparation is described in Box 5.1.

5.2 Suitable record keeping

Suitable record keeping is a vital part of good extemporaneous preparation. Poor record keeping can lead to dispensing errors which could result in the patient receiving a product other than that intended by the prescriber. Therefore the completion of the record will be another safety check for the patient and is an essential part of any standard operating procedure for extemporaneous dispensing. A suggested layout for a dispensing record sheet is given in Figure 5.1 (p. 68).

In addition to recording the compounding process for extemporaneously dispensed items, other records (e.g. fridge temperatures) should be routinely recorded. Refrigerators used in pharmacies must be capable of storing medicines between 2 °C and 8 °C and must be equipped with a maximum/minimum thermometer. This should be checked each day the premises are open and the maximum/minimum temperatures recorded to ensure that the equipment is operating correctly and that patient safety is not compromised.

The notes section is added to allow for any special instructions with regard to method of preparation.

Service Specification 21 from the Royal Pharmaceutical Society's Code of Ethics and

---

Box 5.1   Dispensing procedure on receipt of a prescription for extemporaneous preparation

Upon receipt of a prescription, the basic procedure to be followed is always the same:

1. Check the prescription is legally valid and contains the following information:

   a. Name and address of the patient.
   b. Age or date of birth of the patient if under 12 years.
   c. Signed by the prescriber.
   d. Suitably dated by the prescriber.

2. Check your interpretation of the prescriber's instructions.

   a. Is the formula official or unofficial?
   b. Are all ingredients within a safe dosage limit?
   c. Are all ingredients compatible?

3. Prepare a label for the product.
4. Copy out the formula onto the extemporaneous work record sheet (which must be kept in the pharmacy for a minimum of 2 years) (see Section 5.2, Figure 5.1).
5. Recheck any calculations made.
6. Test the dispensing balance before use (particularly important if the scales have not been used for some time).
7. Select the equipment to be used for the preparation of the product.
8. Select the container to be used for the completed product.

9. Select the first item to be measured or weighed and make a note of the batch number used. Note when selecting an ingredient from stock, check the label, check it again when measuring/weighing the ingredient, and a third check should be made when returning it to the stock shelf.

   a. When measuring a liquid keep the label into the palm of the hand. This will prevent any liquid running down the outside of the bottle and staining the label.
   b. When weighing on a traditional Class II dispensing beam balance, remember:

      i.   Place a white piece of paper under the scale pan before weighing.
      ii. Keep the drawer of the balance closed. Powder that is spilt into the drawer sticks to the weights and renders them inaccurate.
      iii. Use a spatula when weighing (remember to clean the spatula between each different powder that is weighed).
      iv. Ensure the scale pan is cleaned between each weighing procedure.
      v.   Remove the weights from the scale pan immediately after use.

10. When the preparation is ready to be dispensed, transfer it to the final container and label.

Standards states that extemporaneous record sheets should be kept for a minimum of two years, although ideally five years would be advisable.

5.3 Equipment

A wide variety of equipment is used in extemporaneous dispensing, depending on the product type to be prepared (see Section 5.1.3).

5.3.1 Mortars and pestles

Mortars and pestles are used to:

- Reduce the particle size of powders
- Grind crystals into powder form
- Mix powders
- Mix powders and liquids
- Make emulsions.

It should be noted that the mortar is the bowl and the pestle is the pounding/shearing/grinding implement, so compounders mix in a mortar with a pestle.

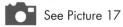 See Picture 17

In pharmacy two main types of mortar and pestle are used:

- **Glass** – These are not usually used for the production of large quantity products as they are usually fairly small. The surfaces of a glass mortar and its pestle are very smooth, making them less suitable for size reduction of powders, although they are efficient when grinding crystals into powder form. Glass mortars are particularly useful when dissolving small amounts of medicament or when incorporating substances such as potassium permanganate or dyes that are absorbed by and stain porcelain mortars.
- **Porcelain** – Generally much larger than their glass counterparts, these lend themselves to larger-scale production. They are ideal for the size reduction of powders, for mixing powders with other powders, for mixing powders with liquids, and for the preparation of emulsions.

When using a mortar and pestle to reduce substances to fine particles, the powder is placed in the mortar and the pestle is used to rub down in a lateral shearing manner on the powder. The pestle is given a circular motion accompanied by downward pressure (not too much pressure as the powder can become compacted on the bottom of the mortar). The most effective way to use the pestle is to start in the centre of the mortar and make a circular motion on the powder, gradually increasing the diameter of the circle with each revolution until the sides of the mortar are touched, then reverse the process, making the circles smaller with each revolution until the centre is reached again. Repeat the process until the powder size is suitably reduced. The pestle therefore follows a spiral track around the mortar.

Mortars and pestles need to be matched. Some mortars are flat bottomed and need a flat-headed pestle to produce efficient mixing. Similarly a round-bottomed mortar will need a round-headed pestle to produce efficient mixing. Ideally the pestle should have as much bearing on the interior surface of the mortar as size will permit, as the speed at which mixing or grinding will occur depends on the amount of contact of the surfaces. The use of a round-headed pestle in a flat-bottomed mortar or a flat-headed pestle in a round-bottomed mortar is very inefficient and frustrating as the required result will either not be achieved or will take a comparatively long time to achieve.

5.3.2 Tiles

Ointment tile or slab is the term used to describe the piece of equipment used to prepare ointments by means of trituration (see Section 9.2.1) or levigation (see Section 9.2.2). Tiles are usually made of glazed porcelain or glass and should be large enough for the quantity of ointment to be prepared. As a guide, a 300 mm square is a suitable size for around 500 g of ointment.

 See Picture 18

5.3.3 Stirring rods

Stirring rods are used to agitate liquids to speed up the process of dissolution of solids. These are normally between 20 and 30 mm in length and made of glass. Care must be taken not to stir too vigorously as this may cause the stirring rod to break.

5.3.4 Pipettes

When measuring small volumes a syringe is used, which is designed to deliver a set amount of the liquid. Syringes have a high degree of accuracy and are readily available in most pharmacies (see Section 4.1.4). However, syringes are less accurate than pipettes and so traditionally small volumes have been measured using pipettes. Graduated pipettes were used to measure volumes from 5 mL to 0.1 mL and, as with measures, they must be stamped by a weights and measures inspector.

 See Picture 19

Two types of pipette are employed, either 'drainage' or 'blow out'. Their use is described in Box 5.2.

Extemporaneous Dispensing Record				Number:	
Date:		Pharmacist in charge:		Compounder:	
Patient name:			Prescriber's name:		
Patient address:			Prescriber's address:		
Item ordered and dosage:					
Master formula and source:					
Dose check and reference:					

Figure 5.1   Example of a dispensing record sheet

	Compounder's signature:	
	Pharmacist's signature:	

Calculation:

	Compounder's signature:	
	Pharmacist's signature:	

Product formula

Item:		Quantity:	

Ingredient:	Batch number:	Quantity:	Dispensed by:	Checked by:

Notes:

Label:

Figure 5.1   Continued

Box 5.2   How to use a pipette

---

1. Select a pipette that is suitable for the required volume to be measured and graduated suitably, i.e. the one that has a maximum volume nearest to the volume to be measured.
2. Check whether the pipette is a 'drainage' type or 'blow out' variety.
3. Check that the pipette is clean and dry.
4. Attach a bulb or teat over the mouth of the pipette (never use mouth suction).
5. Pour some of the solution to be measured into a small clean, dry beaker (never pipette from a stock bottle).
6. Insert the tip of the pipette into the liquid and suck up a sufficient amount of the liquid so that it is well over the required volume.
7. Adjust the meniscus as required to measure the appropriate volume.
8. Remove any excess droplets of fluid on the outside of the pipette by wiping with a non-shed disposable towel.
9. Transfer the volume required to the final admix of the product.

5.3.5 Suppository moulds

Traditionally, suppository moulds come in a range of sizes: 1 g, 2 g, 4 g and 8 g. These weights are nominal and imply calibration with Theobroma Oil BP. For accurate calibration a mould would need to be filled with base alone, the individual suppositories formed weighed, and the mean weight taken as the true capacity (see Section 11.2.1). Suppositories and pessaries are made using the same moulds; when no weight is specified a 1 g mould is used for suppositories and the larger 4 g and 8 g moulds are used for pessaries.

 See Picture 20

The traditional moulds for small-scale production are made of metal with two or three sections held together with a screw fixing. As the moulds open longitudinally, they can be lubricated easily before use, if necessary, and removal of the suppositories should be relatively easy. It should be noted that each part of the mould is designed to match and will be marked accordingly to show this.

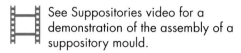 See Suppositories video for a demonstration of the assembly of a suppository mould.

Metal moulds allow the suppositories to set quickly because of their efficient heat transfer. This is an advantage when making suppositories that contain an insoluble medicament, because it does not allow time for the suspended solids to settle by sedimentation.

After removal from the mould the suppositories used to be dispensed in partitioned boxes of paperboard, metal or plastic and lined with waxed paper. Nowadays, in small-scale production the use of aluminium foil is recommended for wrapping.

Alternatively, disposable plastic moulds are available. These are relatively cheap and can even be used to dispense the finished suppositories without removal and the requirement to rewrap.

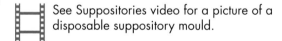 See Suppositories video for a picture of a disposable suppository mould.

5.3.6 Tablet and capsule counting equipment

Tablets and capsules can either be counted manually or using some kind of device, such as a tablet triangle or a capsule counter, a perforated counting tray, or by electronic counting with an electronic balance or photo-electric counter. All of these methods have their advantages and disadvantages, but the main factor is that during the counting process, the medicines are not touched by hand.

Manual counting

The last edition of the (British) Pharmaceutical Codex (12th edition) outlines the manual methods of counting tablets or capsules. This method involves pouring out some tablets or capsules onto a piece of white demy paper which is overlapping another sheet of white demy. The number of tablets or capsules required is counted in tens using a spatula and transferred to the second piece of paper. Once the required number to be dispensed is achieved, the paper is transferred into a trough or funnel and the tablets or capsules transferred to a suitable container. Problems with this method are that demy paper is becoming increasingly difficult to obtain and therefore also quite expensive, and the degree of concentration that must be maintained to ensure accuracy.

Counting triangle/capsule counter

The counting triangle is a fast and accurate way of counting tablets based on Pascal's triangle. Likewise, the capsule counter was designed to allow easy counting of capsules in rows of 10. In each case the tablets or capsules are placed on the counter and any excess removed using a spatula. These simple pieces of equipment speed up the counting process and are easy to clean. Sugar-coated tablets and soft gelatin capsules are more difficult to count using these methods.

 See Picture 21

Perforated counting tray

This is a box of clear Perspex which has trays of perforations of varying sizes. The tray can be used to count tablets or capsules but has the disadvantage of requiring the trays to be changed for different sizes and types of product. An experienced operator can count quite quickly using this type of counter but the novice can find it quite frustrating. The other disadvantage of this type of counter is that cleaning is more complicated and time consuming.

Electronic counters

Electronic balances

A weight reference sample of between 5 and 20 tablets/capsules is weighed and from this a microprocessor computes the total number as further tablets/capsules are added to the balance pan or scoop. The main disadvantage is the reliance on the individual dosage forms being of a consistent individual weight. This is more problematic when dealing with very small tablets or sugar-coated tablets. Between counting the balance needs to be recalibrated for each type and size of dosage form counted. This causes very little problem in practice and does not really detract from the speed of counting. Some problems are encountered if the balance is not well sited as it is very sensitive to vibration and air movement.

Photoelectric counters

The item to be counted is poured through a hopper at the top of the machine, and as the dosage form passes down it interrupts the passage of a light to a photoelectric cell. The main limitation with this type of tablet counter is its inability to discriminate between whole tablets and fragments of tablets, and also its inaccuracy when counting transparent capsules such halibut liver oil capsules. A major drawback with these systems is the necessity to dismantle the system in order to clean it effectively.

The Council for the Royal Pharmaceutical Society of Great Britain issued the following advice regarding the use of tablet counters: 'Severe allergic reactions can be initiated in previously sensitised persons by very small amounts of certain drugs and of excipients and other materials used in the manufacture of tablets and capsules. In order to minimise that risk, counting devices should be carefully cleaned after each dispensing operation involving any uncoated tablet, or any coated tablet or capsule from a bulk container holding damaged contents. As cross-contamination with penicillins is particularly serious, special care should be taken when dispensing products containing those drugs' ((British) Pharmaceutical Codex, 12th edition, 1994, pages 413–414).

5.3.7 Water baths

A heat supply is needed for the production of suppositories and pessaries. It is also required if an ointment or cream is to be prepared from first principles. Normally the item to be melted is placed in an evaporating basin over a water bath containing hot water and allowed to melt. As most products only need to be melted gently, there is no necessity for the water in the bath to be boiling rapidly.

The heat source for the water bath was traditionally a Bunsen burner, but latterly this has been replaced by an electric hotplate. It is important when using a water bath to ensure that enough water is placed in the bath and that it is replaced when necessary, to prevent the bath boiling dry.

 See Picture 22

5.4 Product formulae

Product formulae used in pharmaceutical practice can be divided into two distinctly different categories: official formulae and unofficial formulae.

5.4.1 Official formulae

Traditionally in the UK, official formulae are those that can be found in the British Pharmacopoeia (BP) (see Section 5.5.1), the British Pharmaceutical Codex (BPC), the European Pharmacopoeia (EP) or the British Veterinary Codex (BVetC). A product is deemed 'official' if the full formula can be found in one of these official texts. This is usually indicated by the presence of the designation after the product name (e.g. the 'BP' in the name 'Kaolin Mixture BP').

As the formula for any official product can be found by examining the relevant official text, it is not necessary to include a list of ingredients and their respective quantities on the label for any official product that is compounded extemporaneously (see Section 5.6.2). However, if the formula is not taken from the current edition of the official text in question, it is usual to include the year of the reference in the product title (e.g. Paediatric Chalk Mixture BP 1988).

5.4.2 Unofficial formulae

If the formula of the product that is to be made extemporaneously cannot be found in any official text, this is termed an unofficial formula. In these cases, it is necessary to include a list of the ingredients and their respective quantities on the product label (see Section 5.6.2). Even if the quantity of one of the ingredients differs only slightly from that of an official formula, the product will be deemed unofficial.

The term 'magistral formula' is also used in extemporaneous dispensing. A magistral formula is any medicinal product prepared in a pharmacy in accordance with a prescription for an individual patient.

It should be stressed that when compounders are presented with unofficial formulae, steps must be taken to ensure that the formulation is stable and that there are no compatibility issues (see Chapter 13).

5.5 Ingredients

5.5.1 The British Pharmacopoeia

The British Pharmacopoeia is published on the recommendation of the Medicines Commission in accordance with Section 99(6) of the Medicines Act 1968. It is the authoritative collection of standards for medicines in the UK, providing details of the quality of substances, preparations and articles used in medicine and pharmacy. It incorporates the British Pharmacopoeia (Veterinary) and contains monographs from the European Pharmacopoeia.

All European entries in the British Pharmacopoeia are identified by the use of the European Chaplet of stars alongside the name (Figure 5.2). The entire European Pharmacopoeia text is then bounded by two horizontal lines bearing the symbol 'Ph Eur'. In addition, statements that are relevant to UK usage have been added (e.g. action and use statement and a list of British Pharmacopoeia preparations). Should there be any discrepancy between the entries in the European Pharmacopoeia and the British Pharmacopoeia (or any other official text), the entry in the European Pharmacopoeia would take precedence.

The inclusion of a triangle within the Chaplet of stars denotes monographs that have been adopted by the European Pharmacopoeia

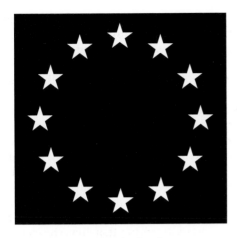

Figure 5.2 The European Chaplet of stars

Commission following their preparation according to a procedure of harmonisation agreed between the bodies responsible for the European Pharmacopoeia and those of Japan and the United States of America (Figure 5.3).

The British Pharmacopoeia:

- Provides standards concerning the quality of a product or ingredient demonstrable at any time during its accepted shelf life.
- Does not give minimum production standards but takes into account that products or ingredients may deteriorate over time.
- Gives minimum standards for efficacy and

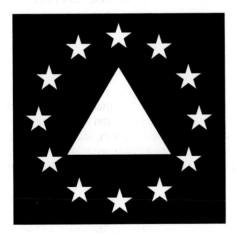

Figure 5.3 The European Chaplet of stars with a triangle denoting monographs that have been adopted by the European Pharmacopoeia Commission from Japan or the United States of America

acceptability for inclusion in a medicinal product.

Anything that is subject to a monograph must comply with the complete monograph for the whole of its period of use.

5.5.2 Solvents and vehicles

A number of liquids can act as pharmaceutical solvents. The most common solvent used in pharmacy is water.

Water

In the pharmaceutical context, there are a number of terms used to describe water, each reflecting the source, quality and purity of the water described. Care must be taken to select an appropriate water type when preparing aqueous vehicles when compounding.

Some drugs are insoluble or only poorly soluble in water. In such cases it is necessary to employ an organic compound, either alone or as a co-solvent with water as the vehicle.

Potable water

Water that is taken directly from the mains drinking water supply is termed 'potable water'. It should be palatable and suitable for drinking. In most cases, potable water is suitable for compounding preparations intended for either internal or external use. Potable water is not suitable for preparations used for systemic injection. Care should be taken to identify that the source of water used originates in a suitable mains supply rather than a storage system, as the latter may contain a potentially dangerous range and number of pathogens. It should be noted that in some geographical areas water from the mains supply may be inappropriate for use in compounding certain products owing to excessive hardness, extremes of pH or the presence of solid contaminants.

On the use of potable water, the British Pharmacopoeia states:

The term Water used without qualification in formulae for formulated preparations means either potable water freshly drawn direct from the public supply and suitable for drinking or freshly boiled and cooled Purified Water. The latter should be used if the public supply is from a local storage tank or if the potable water is unsuitable for a particular preparation.

Purified Water BP

Purified water is prepared from potable water by de-ionisation or distillation. Purified water supports the rapid growth of microbiological organisms on standing for even short periods and therefore should be freshly boiled and cooled when used for compounding pharmaceuticals.

The British Pharmacopoeia definition of Purified Water BP is as follows:

> Purified water is water for the preparation of medicines, other than those that are required to be sterile and apyrogenic, unless otherwise justified and authorised.

Water for preparations

Either freshly drawn potable water or freshly boiled and cooled purified water would qualify as water for preparations.

Water for Injections BP

This water is distilled, pyrogen free and sterilised. Although this water type is used chiefly when compounding aqueous preparations for parenteral use, commercially produced Water for Injections BP constitutes a convenient, albeit expensive, source of water of known high quality, which may be used in situations where other water sources are questionable.

The British Pharmacopoeia definition for Water for Injections BP is as follows:

> Water for injections is water for the preparation of medicines for parenteral administration when water is used as vehicle (water for injections in bulk) and for dissolving or diluting substances or preparations for parenteral administration (sterilised water for injections).

Alcohol

After water, this is probably the next most important solvent used pharmaceutically. Although ethanol (ethyl alcohol) is rarely used as a lone solvent for preparations for internal use, it

is used in the manufacture of some of the galenicals used in pharmacy (e.g. tinctures, see Chapter 2). In extemporaneous dispensing it is normally used for the production of lotions for external application to unbroken skin. It is particularly useful if rapid evaporation is required (e.g. for insecticidal lotions applied to hair for the treatment of lice). In most cases in the formulation of products for external use Industrial Methylated Spirits (IMS) is used. IMS is ethanol that has been 'denatured' by the addition of wood naphtha, rendering it unfit for internal use because of the toxicity of the methanol (methyl alcohol). As IMS is 'denatured' it is free from excise duty and is therefore cheaper than Ethanol BP.

There are problems with the use of ethanol in medicines intended for internal use. The main recipients of liquid medicines tend to be young children, for whom the use of alcohol in such preparations must be questioned. For patients of certain faiths (e.g. Muslims), a medicine containing alcohol may also be unacceptable. Therefore the use of alcohol is generally limited.

When used in products for external use, problems have been encountered because of the volatile nature of the solvent. Asthma attacks have been precipitated in susceptible individuals when using alcohol-based lotions. This was highlighted by the use of alcoholic insecticidal preparations for the treatment of head lice. The problem was considered so serious that a number of aqueous formulations were designed for use by asthmatics.

Glycerol

Glycerol is another solvent used in pharmaceutical preparations although its use is not as wide-ranging as that of water or alcohol. It is often used in preparations to treat the throat or the mouth because its viscosity prevents rapid dilution with saliva, and hence local action of the drug is prolonged. Its viscosity also makes it suitable for use as a solvent for ear drops.

Propylene glycol

This is widely used as a substitute for glycerol. It is used as a vehicle for ear drops and as a co-solvent in aqueous vehicles. It produces less viscous solutions than glycerol.

Oils

Oils such as arachis oil have been used as solvents for fat-soluble ingredients. Fractionated coconut oil has also been used as a vehicle for fat-soluble ingredients. Arachis oil is also known as peanut oil, and latterly the use of this oil as a vehicle has declined because of the increase in cases of allergy to nuts and the subsequent increase in risk of anaphylaxis in susceptible individuals.

5.5.3 Ointment bases

Ointment bases are usually fatty, waxy or synthetic in nature. They are intended to soften but not melt when applied to the skin. There are two distinct purposes for an ointment base.

- As a vehicle from which drugs may be absorbed by the skin.
- As a protective or emollient for the skin.

The base employed will depend on the intended use of the ointment but all should have the following properties:

- Stable
- Easily removable from the skin
- Equally efficient on wet or dry skin
- Miscible with skin secretions
- Miscible with water-soluble and fat-soluble medicaments
- Capable of allowing transference of medicaments rapidly to the skin
- Approximately neutral with regard to pH.

The base should not:

- Cause sensitisation to the skin
- Irritate the skin
- Dehydrate the skin
- Retard wound healing
- Interfere with the normal functioning of the skin by preventing radiation of heat from the skin or preventing the excretion of various secretions. (i.e. not 'clog up' the pores)
- Inactivate or interfere in any way with any incorporated medicament.

Ointment bases can be divided into five main groups:

1. Hydrocarbon bases
2. Fats and fixed oil bases
3. Absorption bases
4. Emulsifying bases
5. Water-soluble bases.

Hydrocarbon bases

Paraffin bases are usually used when the medicament is not intended to be absorbed systemically. Various mixtures of hard, soft or liquid paraffins may be combined to produce a base of suitable consistency. These bases are very stable as they are a mixture of hydrocarbons, chiefly saturated, which have virtually no tendency to react with either the medicament or the atmospheric conditions of storage.

The paraffins inhibit water loss from the skin by forming a greasy layer, and this in turn improves hydration of the skin in dry scaly conditions. Ointments are preferred for the treatment of such conditions and also for overnight use. Mixtures of 50% White Soft Paraffin BP and 50% Liquid Paraffin BP are regularly used for the treatment of very dry skin.

Common hydrocarbon bases include:

1. **Yellow/White Soft Paraffin BP** – Both Yellow and White Soft Paraffin BP are widely used ointment bases. They are both semi-solid mixtures of hydrocarbons obtained from petroleum. White Soft Paraffin BP has been highly refined and is decolourised (bleached Yellow Soft Paraffin BP). Both have similar properties with a melting point range of 38–56 °C (the melting point range is because the melting point may vary slightly from batch to batch). Traditionally Yellow Soft Paraffin BP has been used when an ointment includes dark-coloured ingredients (e.g. Coal Tar BP or Ichthammol BP). White Soft Paraffin BP was reserved for products with colourless, white or pale ingredients. It is accepted nowadays that although White Soft Paraffin BP may produce products that are more 'pleasing to the eye', the unbleached form, Yellow Soft Paraffin BP, is less likely to cause sensitivity reactions in susceptible patients.

2. **Hard Paraffin BP** – This is used as a stiffening agent in ointment bases. It is a mixture of solid hydrocarbons obtained from petroleum or shale oil. It has a solidifying point of 50–57 °C. Because of its relatively high melting point it is also added to other paraffins to increase the melting point of a product and therefore increase its suitability for use in warm climates.

3. **Liquid Paraffin BP** – As the name suggests, this is a mixture of the liquid hydrocarbons obtained from petroleum. Its main use in ointment bases is to reduce their viscosity.

4. **Paraffin Ointment BP** – This is an 'official' hydrocarbon ointment base consisting of:

Hard Paraffin BP	30 g
White Soft Paraffin BP	900 g
White Beeswax BP	20 g
Cetostearyl Alcohol BP	50 g

The Cetostearyl Alcohol BP is added to the hydrocarbon base to increase its emollient properties and the White Beeswax BP is added to help stiffen the ointment. These ingredients help to produce a homogeneous mixture of the Hard Paraffin BP and the White Soft Paraffin BP.

Fats and fixed oil bases

Ointment bases can include oils of vegetable origin such as arachis oil, olive oil, almond oil, soya or maize oil. Such oils can decompose on exposure to air, light and high temperatures and turn rancid. For example, in the 1932 British Pharmacopoeia, Olive Oil BP was an accepted ingredient in Ung. Aquosum BP (Hydrous Ointment BP). Because of the problems of rancidity and because it facilitates bacterial growth, the formulation was updated in the Sixth Addendum to the 1932 British Pharmacopoeia and Olive Oil BP was replaced by Liquid Paraffin BP.

Absorption bases

These bases are capable of absorbing water and aqueous solutions to form water in oil (w/o) emulsions. They consist of one or more of the paraffins combined with a sterol type of emulsifying agent such as:

1. Beeswax.
2. Wool fat (lanolin) – which can absorb about 50% of its weight of water. (N.B. patients can become sensitised to lanolin.)
3. Wool alcohols. This is the emulsifying component of wool fat obtained by fractionation.

Examples of this type of ointment base include Wool Alcohols Ointment BP and Simple Ointment BP.

Emulsifying bases

These are anhydrous bases that contain sufficient emulsifying agent (oil in water) to make them miscible with water and therefore 'washable'. They are easy to remove from the skin and therefore also make suitable bases for application to the scalp. There are three types of emulsifying base – anionic, cationic and non-ionic – and the ionic nature of the base is determined by its charge (i.e. it has a negative, positive or no charge, respectively) (Table 5.1).

All of these bases are miscible with water; the choice of base is determined by the chemical nature of the active ingredient to be incorporated (i.e. it is the overall charge on an ingredient to be incorporated that dictates which type of emulsifying base is appropriate to use).

Water-soluble bases

Polyethylene glycols are stable, hydrophilic substances that are non-irritant to the skin. The name applied to them in the BP is 'macrogols' and the solid grades (1000 and above) are used as ointment bases. There are a number of different molecular weight macrogols and by combining various ones a product with the consistency of an ointment can be produced. The advantages of macrogols include:

- They are water miscible and therefore allow medications to mix with skin secretions and exudates.
- They are non-occlusive.
- They are non-staining to clothes or bed linen.
- They are easily washed off.
- They do not hydrolyse or deteriorate.
- They do not support mould growth.
- They are non-irritant to the skin.

Examples include Macrogol Ointment BP.

Table 5.1   Examples of different emulsifying bases

Ionic nature of emulgent	Emulgent example	Base produced
Anionic	Emulsifying Wax BP	Emulsifying Ointment BP
Cationic	Cetrimide Emulsifying Wax BP	Cetrimide Emulsifying Ointment BP
Non-ionic	Cetomacrogol Emulsifying Wax BP	Cetomacrogol Emulsifying Ointment BPC

Macrogol bases are used with local anaesthetics such as lidocaine but their use is limited because they are incompatible with many chemicals, including phenols, iodine, potassium iodide and the salts of silver, mercury and bismuth. More significantly they also reduce the antimicrobial properties of quaternary ammonium compounds such as cetrimide.

5.5.4 Suppository and pessary bases

The ideal suppository or pessary base should:

- Either melt after insertion into the body or dissolve in (and mix with) any rectal or vaginal fluid (ideally the melting range should be slightly lower than 37 °C as body temperature may be as low as 36 °C at night)
- Be non-toxic and non-irritant
- Be compatible with any medicament and release it readily
- Be easily moulded and removed from the mould
- Be stable to heating above the melting point
- Be stable on storage and resistant to handling.

Fatty bases

Theobroma Oil BP is a yellowish-white solid that smells like chocolate. It is the solid fat obtained from the crushed and roasted seeds of *Theobroma cacao* and is most commonly obtained as a by-product in the manufacture of cocoa. It has many of the properties of an ideal suppository base but has largely been replaced by synthetic alternatives. The reasons for this are:

- It is particularly susceptible to physical changes with overheating.
- It has a tendency to stick to the mould, which needs lubricating before use.
- Its softening point makes it unsuitable for use in hot climates.
- As a natural product it tends to go rancid on storage owing to oxidation of the unsaturated glycerides.

Synthetic fats

Synthetic fats have all the advantages of Theobroma Oil BP but none of the disadvantages. They are prepared by hydrogenating suitable vegetable oils and examples include Hard Fat BP, which is a mixture of triglycerides, diglycerides and monoglycerides.

The drawback is that the low viscosity of the synthetic bases when melted increases the risk of sedimentation of the active ingredient during the preparation of the suppository, but as the difference between melting point and setting point is small (generally 1.5–2 °C) the problem of sedimentation is minimal. Synthetic bases also become very brittle if cooled too quickly. Therefore setting must not be accelerated by refrigeration.

Aqueous bases

The most commonly encountered aqueous base is Glycerin Suppository BP base. The use of this base is limited by the incompatibility of gelatin with medicaments, and as a suppository base it exerts a local purgative action and therefore its usefulness is limited through premature evacuation of the bowel. Macrogol bases are also used as suppository bases for proprietary products.

Other additives are used in the mass manufacture of suppositories, such as emulsifiers, hardening agents or viscosity modifiers and preservatives. When preparing suppositories extemporaneously the synthetic fats are the most commonly used bases, and invariably the suppository consists of the active ingredients and base alone as they are small batch productions and not intended for long-term storage.

5.5.5 Preservatives

Antimicrobial preservatives are added either to kill or slow down the growth of microorganisms. Microorganisms may be present in ingredients used to prepare the product or may be introduced during the compounding process and product use. Preservatives are never added to obscure microbial contamination resulting from unsatisfactory production processes, unsuitable containers or inadequate storage conditions.

Aqueous preparations are the most susceptible to microbial contamination as an aqueous environment is an ideal supporting medium for many microorganisms.

The properties of an ideal antimicrobial preservative are as follows:

- Active at low concentrations with rapid bactericidal and fungicidal action
- Compatible with a wide number of medicaments and systems
- Active and stable over a wide temperature range
- Active and stable over a wide pH range
- Readily soluble at the concentration used
- Compatible with plastics, rubbers and other materials used in packaging
- Free from unpleasant odours
- No unpleasant taste
- Suitable colour (i.e. attractive, not disagreeable)
- Non-toxic at the concentrations necessary for preservative activity
- Non-carcinogenic
- Non-irritant and non-sensitising at the concentration used.

Acids

- Benzoic acid – Used in varying concentrations dependent upon the pharmaceutical form, commonly 0.1% w/v in solutions.
- Sorbic acid – Antimicrobial activity shown in concentrations of 0.05–0.2% in oral and topical pharmaceutical formulations. It is particularly useful as it can be used with gelatin and vegetable gums.
- Sulphurous acid – Used in food preservation as it shows low toxicity in the concentrations used. Pharmaceutical applications include preservation of Blackcurrant Syrup BPC and Liquid Glucose BP.

Alcohols

- Benzyl alcohol – Antimicrobial preservative (2.0% v/v) and a disinfectant (10% v/v).
- Ethyl alcohol (ethanol) – Antimicrobial preservative ($\geq$10% v/v) also used as a disinfectant (60–90% v/v).
- Isopropyl alcohol – Not recommended for oral use owing to toxicity. Shows some antimicrobial activity and is used as a disinfectant as a 70% v/v aqueous solution. It is a more effective antibacterial preservative than alcohol.
- Phenoxyethyl alcohol – Usually used as an antimicrobial preservative in ophthalmic and parenteral formulations (0.25–0.5% v/v) and in some topical formulations (1% v/v).

Hydroxybenzoates

- Butyl hydroxybenzoate – Antimicrobial preservative active over a wide pH, having a broad spectrum of antimicrobial activity but being most effective against yeasts and moulds. Used in varying concentrations dependent upon the pharmaceutical form.
- Ethyl hydroxybenzoate – Active as an antimicrobial preservative between pH 4 and 8.
- Methyl hydroxybenzoate – Active as an antimicrobial preservative between pH 4 and 8.
- Propyl hydroxybenzoate – Used in varying concentrations dependent upon the pharmaceutical form.

Mercurials

- Phenyl mercuric acetate – Used in preference to phenyl mercuric nitrate as it is more soluble. Used in eye drops and parenteral formulations as an antimicrobial preservative (0.001–0.002% w/v) and also used as a spermicide in spermicidal jellies (0.02% w/v).
- Phenyl mercuric nitrate – Used in preference to phenyl mercuric acetate in acidic preparations. Used in eye drops and parenteral formulations as an antimicrobial preservative (0.001–0.002% w/v).
- Thiomersal – Used as an alternative to benzalkonium chloride and other phenyl mercuric preservatives. It has both bacteriostatic and fungistatic activity and is used in a number of preparations in varying concentrations (0.001–0.15%).

Phenols

- Chlorocresol – Used as an antimicrobial preservative in concentrations of up to 0.2% w/v. Only suitable for products not intended for oral route of administration. In higher concentrations it is an effective disinfectant.
- Cresol – Used as an antimicrobial preservative in concentrations 0.15–0.3% v/v. Only suitable for products not intended for oral route of administration.
- Phenol – Mainly used as a preservative in parenteral products (0.5% w/v) although it has also been used in topical preparations.

Quaternary ammonium compounds

- Benzalkonium chloride – Antimicrobial preservative, antiseptic, disinfectant, solubilising agent and wetting agent. Widely used to preserve ophthalmic preparations (0.01–0.02% w/v). In nasal and ophthalmic formulations (0.002–0.02% w/v in combination with thiomersal 0.002–0.005% w/v).
- Cetrimide – Used as an antimicrobial preservative in eye drops (0.005% w/v) and as an antiseptic in aqueous solution (0.1–1.0 %).

Miscellaneous examples

- Bronopol – Antimicrobial preservative (0.01–0.1% w/v).
- Chlorbutol – Used primarily as an antimicrobial preservative in ophthalmic or parenteral preparations. Its antimicrobial activity tends to be bacteriostatic rather than bactericidal and its action is markedly reduced above pH 5.5.
- Chlorhexidine – Antimicrobial agent and antiseptic.
- Chloroform – Chloroform (0.25% v/v) usually included in solutions or mixtures designed for oral use in the form of chloroform water (see Section 2.1.23).
- Glycerol – In addition to its action as an antimicrobial preservative (>20% v/v) glycerol is also an emollient, humectant, solvent and sweetener.
- Propylene glycol – Used as an antimicrobial preservative for solutions and semi-solids (15–30% v/v).
- Sucrose – When sugar is present in high concentrations (≥67%) in, for example, elixirs, fermentation is prevented because of the resultant osmotic pressure.

The commonly used preservatives used in different formations encountered in extemporaneous dispensing are summarised in Table 5.2.

5.5.6 Antioxidants

The decomposition of pharmaceutical products by oxidation can be retarded by the addition of antioxidants (reducing agents). Any antioxidant included in the product must be compatible with the active medicament in the product and also compatible with the formulation itself and not produce unwanted changes in that formulation.

The properties of an ideal antioxidant are similar to those of an ideal antimicrobial and include:

- Active at low concentrations
- Compatible with a wide number of medicaments and systems
- Active and stable over a wide temperature range

Table 5.2 Common preservatives used in extemporaneous dispensing along with examples of extemporaneous preparations containing them

Pharmaceutical formulation	Antimicrobial preservative used	Examples

Solutions for oral administration	Alcohol
	Benzoic acid (0.1% w/v)
	Chloroform (0.25% v/v)
	Included as Chloroform Water BP
	  or Double Strength Chloroform
	  Water BP
		Phenobarbital Elixir BPC
		Kaolin Paediatric Suspension BP
		Ammonia and Ipecacuanha Mixture BP

	Glycerol Methyl hydroxybenzoate Sucrose	Diamorphine Linctus BPC Streptomycin Elixir Paediatric BPC Paediatric Chloral Elixir BP

Solutions for external use	Alcohol
	
	Benzalkonium chloride
	Chlorbutol (0.5% w/v)
	Chloroform (0.25% v/v)
	Included as Chloroform Water BP
	  or Double Strength Chloroform
	  Water BP
	Glycerol
		Chloroxylenol Solution BP 1988
		Soap Liniment BPC
		Phosphates Enema BPC
		Ephedrine Nasal Drops BPC 1973
		Sodium Chloride Mouthwash BP
		
		Sodium Bicarbonate Ear Drops BPC

Suspensions for oral administration	Benzoic acid (0.1% w/v)
	Chloroform (0.25% v/v)
	Included as Chloroform Water BP
	  or Double Strength Chloroform
	  Water BP
		Paediatric Kaolin Mixture BP1980
		Magnesium Trisilicate Mixture BP 1988

Suspensions for external use	Alcohol Liquefied phenol	Compound Sulphur Lotion BPC 1973 Calamine Lotion BP

Emulsions for oral administration	Benzoic acid (0.1% w/v)
	Chloroform (0.25% v/v)
	Included as Chloroform Water BP
	  or Double Strength Chloroform
	  Water BP
		Liquid Paraffin Emulsion BP 1968
		
		Liquid Paraffin Emulsion BP 1968

Creams and external emulsions	Cetrimide Chlorocresol Hydroxybenzoates Phenoxy ethyl alcohol	Cetrimide cream BP 1988 Cetomacrogol Cream (Formula A) BP Dimethicone Cream BPC Buffered Cream BPC Cetomacrogol Cream (Formula B) BP Aqueous Cream BP Oily Cream BP

- Active and stable at a range of pH
- Readily soluble at the concentration used
- Compatible with plastics, rubbers and other materials used in packaging
- Free from unpleasant odours
- No unpleasant taste
- Suitable colour (i.e. attractive not disagreeable)
- Non-toxic at the concentrations necessary for antioxidant activity
- Non-carcinogenic
- Non-irritant and not sensitising at the concentration used.

Antioxidants can be grouped according to their mechanism of action.

Antioxygens

These are thought to block chain reactions by reacting with free radicals. They provide the necessary electrons and easily available hydrogen ions to stop the chain reaction in auto-oxidation. Examples include:

- Alpha-tocopherol acetate – Although this acts as an antioxidant, its inclusion in most pharmaceutical formulae is as a source of vitamin E.
- Butylated hydroxyanisole (BHA) – In addition to its antioxidant properties this also has some antimicrobial activity similar to that of the parabens (hydroxybenzoates). It is used to prevent or delay oxidative rancidity of fats and oils, and is particularly used to prevent loss of activity of oil-soluble vitamins. Often used in conjunction with butylated hydroxytoluene and the alkyl gallates and chelating agents such as citric acid.
- Butylated hydroxytoluene (BHT) – Used to prevent or delay oxidative rancidity of fats and oils, and particularly to prevent loss of activity of oil-soluble vitamins.
- Alkyl gallates (dodecyl, propyl and octyl gallate) – Primarily used to prevent rancidity in fats and oils. Used in concentrations up to 0.1% w/v. Also possess some antimicrobial activity against both Gram-negative and Gram-positive bacteria and also fungi. They have been reported to give an 'off' flavour to corn and cottonseed oils when used as an antioxidant. Alkyl gallates can be used for internal and external products but their inclusion is not recommended in preparations for oral administration to children and babies.

Reducing agents

Reducing agents are more readily oxidised than the medicament and therefore can be used if oxidising agents are present. They protect a drug until they themselves are used up or until all the oxygen in the container is used up. Reducing agents are therefore also useful in blocking chain reactions that occur in the auto-oxidation of drugs. Examples include:

- Ascorbic acid – Used as an antioxidant in concentrations of 0.01–0.5%.
- Sodium metabisulphite – Used in oral, parenteral and topical formulations. Mainly used in preparations that are acidic in nature. Sodium metabisulphite also has some preservative properties and is often used to preserve oral preparations such as syrups. As an antioxidant it is used in concentrations of 0.01–0.1%.
- Sodium sulphite – Used in preference to sodium metabisulphite in alkaline preparations.

Chelating agents

These enhance the effects of antioxidants but have little use as sole agents as they work by chelating with heavy metal ions which often catalyse autoxidations.

- Citric acid – Also used as an acidifying agent, buffering agent and flavour enhancer. As an antioxidant synergist it is used in concentrations of 0.005–0.01%.
- Disodium edetate (disodium dihydrogen ethylenediaminetetra-acetate dihydrate – EDTA) – Used in concentrations of 0.002–0.1%.
- Sodium citrate – Also used as an alkalising agent and buffering agent.
- Tartaric acid – Also used as an acidifier and flavour enhancer. It is widely used in conjunction with bicarbonates as the acidic component of effervescent granules and tablets. As an antioxidant synergist it is used in concentrations of 0.01–0.02%.

Choice of antioxidant

There is no perfect antioxidant as all have their limitations. The choice is determined by a number of factors.

Formulation

The type of formulation may well influence the effectiveness of an antioxidant. For example, in two-phase systems such as emulsions and creams, the oily (lipid) phase may be susceptible to oxidation and therefore an antioxidant added to the formula should be preferentially soluble in the oily phase. The addition of an antioxidant is also important as some of the emulsifying agents themselves can be subject to oxidation by atmospheric oxygen. Atmospheric oxidation is controlled by the use of antioxidants such as butylated hydroxyanisole (BHA), butylated hydroxytoluene (BHT) or ethyl, propyl or dodecyl gallate. These are also often used as antioxidants in ointments, pastes, gels, suppositories and pessaries. In a suspension, consideration must be given to the likelihood of adsorption of the antioxidant onto particles of the drug or interaction with the suspending agent.

Packaging

The antioxidant chosen must not react with the packaging as its effectiveness can be reduced if it is adsorbed by the container or the closure, which is especially true of plastic and rubber closures.

Time of addition of the antioxidant

It is important to add the antioxidant as early as possible in the preparation of a product to help slow down auto-oxidation. It is also important to ensure that the antioxidant is incorporated evenly throughout the product.

Concentration of the antioxidant

The concentration of antioxidant used is normally determined by previous experience with that antioxidant. Generally the more antioxidant added, the greater the antioxidant effect (however, in higher concentrations the antioxidant effect may be less because of the reaction of the antioxidant with peroxides to form free radicals).

5.5.7 Buffers

Buffers are often added to solutions to prevent pronounced variations of pH during use and storage. Buffers dissolve in the solvent and then resist changes in pH should an acid or an alkali be added to the formulation. The pH and buffering capacity required will determine the choice of buffer.

Most pharmaceutical buffers are based on carbonates, phosphates, citrates, lactates, gluconates and tartrates. Borates have been used for external products but not in those intended for abraded skin or membranes.

The pH of most bodily fluid is 7.4 and therefore this is the pH for which most products will be buffered.

Borate buffers

A borate buffer (boric acid/borax) pH range 6.8–9.1, is used to buffer Chloramphenicol Eye Drops BP 1993 (pH 7.5) and Hypromellose Eye Drops BPC 1973 (pH 8.4) (Table 5.3).

Borate buffers are not included in topical preparations used on abraded skin or membranes

Table 5.3   Quantity of boric acid, borax and sodium chloride that is required for a given pH value

pH (25 °C)	Boric acid (g/L)	Borax (g/L)	Sodium chloride to make iso-osmotic (g/L)
6.8	12.03	0.57	2.7
7.2	11.66	1.15	2.7
7.4	11.16	1.91	2.7
7.7	10.54	2.87	2.6
7.8	9.92	3.82	2.6
8.0	9.30	4.78	2.5
8.1	8.68	5.73	2.4
8.2	8.06	6.69	2.3
8.4	6.82	8.60	2.1
8.6	5.58	10.51	1.9
8.7	4.96	11.46	1.8
8.8	3.72	13.37	1.4
9.0	2.48	15.28	1.1
9.1	1.24	17.20	0.7

because of their potential toxicity when systemically absorbed.

Phosphate buffers

A phosphate buffer (sodium acid phosphate/sodium phosphate) pH range 4.5–8.5 is used to buffer Neomycin Eye Drops BPC 1973 (pH 6.5) and Prednisolone Sodium Phosphate Eye Drops BPC 1973 (pH 6.6) (Table 5.4).

5.5.8 Thickening and suspending agents

The amount of suspending agent used in any given formulation depends on the volume of vehicle being thickened. It does not vary with the amount of powder in the preparation. A suspending agent is intended to increase the viscosity of the vehicle and therefore slow down sedimentation rates. This outcome could also be achieved by decreasing the particle size of the powder in suspension.

Natural polysaccharides

Acacia BP
This is a natural gummy exudate from the stems and branches of some species of acacia tree. A viscous mucilage of acacia in water is prepared by using acacia gum 4 parts by weight and water 6 parts by volume. Acacia is normally used in combination with tragacanth and starch in Compound Tragacanth Powder BP (Acacia BP 20%, Tragacanth BP 15%, Starch BP 20% and Sucrose BP 45%). Compound Tragacanth Powder BP is a suitable suspending agent for products for internal use but because of the high sucrose content it is unsuitable for external products as it renders them too sticky.

Tragacanth BP
This is the dried gummy exudate from some species of the *Astralagus* shrub. Like acacia, when it is combined with water it forms a viscous liquid or gel depending on the concentration used. Tragacanth can be used as a sole suspending agent, and as it is less sticky it may be used for external as well as internal products. Tragacanth is used to suspend heavy insoluble powders.

The appropriate quantities of Tragacanth BP and Compound Tragacanth Powder BP to use to form suspensions are listed in Key Skill 5.1.

The main problem with natural products is that their natural variability can cause differences between batches, and also because they are natural products there is a greater chance of microbial contamination.

Semi-synthetic polysaccharides

Methylcellulose BP
Methylcellulose is a methyl ether of cellulose. The name 'methylcellulose' is followed by a

Table 5.4 Quantity of sodium acid phosphate, sodium phosphate and sodium chloride that is required for a given pH value

pH	Sodium acid phosphate (g/L)	Sodium phosphate (g/L)	Sodium chloride to make iso-osmotic (g/L)
5.9	9.4	2.4	5.2
6.2	8.3	4.8	5.1
6.5	7.3	7.2	5.0
6.6	6.2	9.5	4.9
6.8	5.2	11.9	4.8
7.0	4.2	14.3	4.6
7.2	3.1	16.7	4.5
7.4	2.1	19.1	4.4
7.7	1.0	21.5	4.3
8.0	0.5	22.7	4.2

 Key Skill 5.1 Appropriate quantities of tragacanth to use to form suspensions

Often, the quantity of suspending agent is not given on a prescription and so the compounder needs to know how much suspending agent to use.

- 0.2 g Tragacanth BP powder for 100 mL suspension.
- 2 g Compound Tragacanth Powder BP for 100 mL suspension.

number, which indicates the approximate viscosity of a 2% solution. Methylcellulose 2500 and methylcellulose 4500 are used as thickening agents. Methylcellulose is suitable for products intended for both internal and external use.

To form a suspension 0.5–2% methylcellulose is needed, depending on the polymer used.

Clays

A number of naturally occurring clays are used as thickening agents. Because these clays hydrate easily and often absorb many times their weight in water, they produce gels of varying thickness depending on the concentration of clay used. Although these clays do not support microbial growth neither do they inhibit it, therefore a preservative must also be added. The clays themselves are prone to contamination with microbial spores (for example, Bentonite BP may be contaminated with *Clostridium tetani*) as they are natural products. It is therefore essential that any clays used for pharmaceutical manufacture be sterilised prior to use as a suspending agent.

Bentonite BP
This is a very pale buff-coloured powder. The colour may make it unsuitable for use in some products. It is used in suspensions for external use such as calamine lotion. To form a suspension for external use 2–3% of Bentonite BP is required.

Synthetic thickeners

Synthetic thickeners have been developed as standardised products that can easily be reproduced. This overcomes the problem of variability of naturally occurring suspending agents.

Carbomer
The main advantage with carbomer is that it is used in very low concentrations, normally 0.1–0.4%. It is mainly used in products intended for external use although some grades of this product can be used internally.

5.5.9 Wetting agents

Wetting agents may also be added to aid suspension of powders. Some powders tend to float on the surface of the preparation. This is because air becomes trapped in the solid particles and prevents them from being dispersed through the vehicle. A film of unwettable solid forms at the liquid/air interface. If a wetting agent is added this is adsorbed at the solid/liquid interface, making the particles have more affinity for the surrounding vehicle. Wetting agents used for internal mixtures include polysorbates and sorbitan esters, although acacia and tragacanth can also be used. Wetting agents suitable for products for external use include quillaia tincture, as in Sulphur Compound Lotion BPC 1973, or sodium lauryl sulphate.

5.5.10 Emulsifying agents and emulsifying waxes

Emulsifying agents for internal use should ideally be non-toxic and non-irritant. Many of the substances described as thickeners in the formulation of suspensions also act as emulgents. Both water-in-oil and oil-in-water emulsions will need an emulsifying agent.

Emulsifying agents

Acacia BP
This is the most widely used emulsifying agent for extemporaneously prepared oral emulsions. Acacia stabilises emulsions by forming a film around each oil globule, slowing down any coalescence of the globules. Because of the low viscosity of any emulsions formed using acacia, creaming may occur (see Section 8.4). To help prevent this, tragacanth, a thickening agent, is often also added as an emulsion stabiliser.

Methylcellulose BP
Some grades of methylcellulose can be used as emulsifying agents and emulsion stabilisers. For example, 2% of Methylcellulose 20 is used in Liquid Paraffin Oral Emulsion BP.

Wool Alcohols BP
This is made by treating Wool Fat BP with alkali and separating the fraction containing cholesterol and other alcohols. It is a good emulsifying agent for water-in-oil emulsions and is chosen in

preference to Wool Fat BP, as emulsions made with Wool Alcohols BP do not have an objectionable odour in hot weather, as is often the case with Wool Fat BP.

Wool Fat BP

This is obtained from sheep wool. It is made up of the fatty acid esters of cholesterol and other sterols and alcohols. One problem with this as an emulgent is that, although it is similar to human sebum, it can cause sensitisation in some people. It is used mainly as an emulsion stabiliser.

Emulsifying waxes

These are the main emulsifiers used in external products. These are termed anionic, cationic and non-ionic emulsifying waxes. Each consists of two ingredients, cetostearyl alcohol and a surface active agent (surfactant).

Anionic surfactants

Anionic surfactants are often used to produce oily lotions, for example Oily Calamine Lotion BPC 1973. Examples include:

- Alkali metal and ammonium soaps, e.g. sodium stearate
- Alkyl sulphates, e.g. sodium lauryl sulphate
- Amine soaps, e.g. triethanolamine oleate
- Soaps of divalent and trivalent metals e.g. calcium oleate.

Cationic surfactants

Usually these are used in the preparation of oil-in-water emulsions for external use, for example cetrimide and benzylkonium chloride. Cationic surfactants also have antimicrobial activity.

Non-ionic surfactants

These are synthetic materials. Some are oil-soluble stabilising water-in-oil (w/o) emulsions, others are water soluble and stabilise oil-in-water (o/w) emulsions. Examples include:

- Fatty alcohol polyglycol ethers
- Glycol and glycerol esters
- Polysorbates
- Sorbitan esters.

Three types of emulsifying wax encountered in extemporaneous dispensing are described in Table 5.5.

5.5.11 Colourings and flavourings

Colourings

Colourings are used in pharmaceutical preparations to increase the acceptability of a product to a patient and to also ensure a consistent appearance of a product that may have ingredients that can vary slightly in appearance from batch to batch. The introduction of a colour can also mask an unattractive colour of an inconsequential

Table 5.5 Composition of three types of emulsifying wax

Product	Oil-soluble component	Water-soluble component	Ratio CSA/SAA	Notes
Cetomacrogol Emulsifying Wax BP (non-ionic)	Cetostearyl Alcohol BP	Cetomacrogol BP	8:2	Cetomacrogol 1000 is a condensate of cetyl and stearyl alcohol with ethylene oxide and is non-ionised
Cetrimide Emulsifying Wax BP (cationic)	Cetostearyl Alcohol BP	Cetrimide BP	9:1	On dissociation the 'cetyl trimethyl ammonium' group of cetrimide is the cation
Emulsifying Wax BP (anionic)	Cetostearyl Alcohol BP	Sodium Lauryl Sulphate BP	9:1	On dissociation the 'lauryl sulphate' group of sodium lauryl sulphate is the anion.

CSA, cetostearyl alcohol; SAA, surface active agent.

Table 5.6 Flavourings associated with each of the different colourings used in pharmaceutical preparations intended for internal use

Colour	Flavour
Red	Cherry, strawberry, raspberry
Yellow	Citrus fruits, banana
Green	Mint flavours

degradation product that, despite its not affecting the efficacy of the product, may hamper patient compliance. Generally the colorant of choice is determined by the flavour of the product if it is for internal use (Table 5.6).

Colorants can also be added to products for external use to indicate that they should not be taken internally, for example the addition of colouring to mineralised methylated spirit. In hospitals different antiseptics may be coloured according to their use, e.g. disinfection of skin, instruments, syringes, etc.

Colourings used in pharmaceutical preparations are either natural agents or synthetic dyes. Natural agents include:

- Caramel (burnt sugar) – Prepared by heating a suitable water-soluble carbohydrate with or without a suitable accelerator until a black viscous mass is formed. It is then adjusted to the required standard by the addition of water and strained. Caramel is capable of producing a wide range of colours, from a pale straw colour to dark brown.
- Carmine – A preparation of cochineal (see below) containing about 50% carminic acid. Carmine is used for colouring ointments, tooth powders, mouthwashes, dusting powders, medicines and other preparations. If in solid form prolonged trituration with a powder is necessary to obtain a good colour and an even distribution. To obtain the maximum colour carmine should be dissolved in a small quantity of strong ammonia solution before triturating with the powder. The colouring matter is precipitated in acidic solution.
- Chlorophyll – The green colouring matter in plants. Its principal use is as a colouring agent for soaps, oils and fats.

- Cochineal – Made from the dried bodies of the female insect *Dactylopius coccus* (or the crushed eggs in the case of cochineal extract).
- Saffron – The dried stigmas and tops of the styles of *Crocus sativus*. Saffron exerts no therapeutic effects and is used as a colouring and flavouring in some pharmaceutical products.
- Turmeric – The dried rhizome of *Curcuma domestica*.

The choice of colorant can be affected by the country of use, as different countries have different legislation with regard to colorant use. This problem is exacerbated by the various synonyms used for the same dye. For example, amaranth, a common ingredient for extemporaneous dispensing, is also known as:

- Bordeaux S
- CI Acid Red 27
- CI Food Red 9
- Colour Index Number 16185 (by Society of Dyers and Colourists and the American Association of Textile Chemists and Colorists)
- E123 (Council of European Communities)
- FD and C Red Number 2 (by USA Food, Drug and Cosmetics Act).

Generally within the UK, the E number specification is most commonly used. .

Examples of colours permitted for use in the UK are listed in Table 5.7.

The use of colorants for oral medication is falling out of favour because of the association of additives with rare allergic reactions and cases of hypersensitivity and hyperactivity. Tartrazine, for example, has been associated with hypersensitivity reactions and intolerance, particularly in those sensitive to aspirin. Its use in medicinal preparations is therefore diminishing and any official formula calling for the addition of tartrazine may be prepared without it if sensitivity may be an issue with the intended patient.

Flavourings

Liquid preparations for oral use are usually flavoured and occasionally coloured to improve their acceptability to the patient. Masking an unpleasant flavour may prevent the feeling of nausea or the incidence of vomiting. Flavourings

Table 5.7   Examples of permitted colours for inclusion in pharmaceutical products in the UK

E numbers	Colour range	Examples
100–110	Yellows	E101 Riboflavin
		E102 Tartrazine
		E110 Sunset Yellow
120–128	Reds	E120 Cochineal carminic acid
		E123 Amaranth
		E127 Erythrosine
131–133	Blues	E131 Patent Blue V
140–142	Greens	E140 Chlorophylls
		E142 Acid Brilliant Green
150–155	Black and browns	E150 Caramel
		E153 Carbo medicinalis vegetabilis (charcoal)
170–175	Metallic	E172 Iron Oxides

are often derived from natural products and are available in a number of formulations for use in the extemporaneous preparation of products. These include the aromatic waters, concentrated extracts, syrups or spirits. Often the addition of syrup will be sufficient to mask unpleasant tastes.

Syrup (a solution of sucrose in water) may be used as a co-solvent or as a solvent in its own right in a number of oral medicines, e.g. elixirs and linctuses. It acts as a sweetening agent to mask unpleasant-tasting ingredients. Unfortunately it has the disadvantage of promoting dental decay. It is also unsuitable for diabetic patients who need to monitor their carbohydrate intake.

Examples of flavoured syrups that are often used to mask unpleasant tastes along with examples of preparation that contain them are listed in Table 5.8.

Flavouring is particularly important in paediatric formulations, as the correct choice of flavouring can ensure patient compliance. In addition to providing sweetness and flavour, the texture of the product can also be enhanced, giving a more pleasant sensation in the mouth.

In addition to the flavoured syrups described above, various other ingredients are used to flavour pharmaceutical preparations. These are also listed in Table 5.8.

Choice of flavouring

The choice of flavouring is affected by a number of factors:

- The intended recipient – Children generally prefer fruit or sweet flavours, whereas adults tend to prefer slightly acidic flavouring and older people often find mint or wine-flavoured products preferable.

- The use of the product – Products intended for the relief of indigestion, for example, are often flavoured with peppermint. This is because traditionally mint has been used for its carminative effect. Nowadays, although the action of the product may be dependent on a totally different active ingredient, peppermint flavouring is added because the smell and taste of mint is strongly associated with antacid action.

- The type of unpleasant taste to be masked:

  a. A **bitter** taste can be masked by anise, chocolate, mint, passion fruit, wild cherry. The effect of a bitter aftertaste has also been reduced by addition of flavour enhancers such as monosodium glutamate.

  b. **Saltiness** can be counteracted by apricot, butterscotch, liquorice, peach or vanilla. Butterscotch and caramel combined have been found to be particularly successful in masking the taste of salty drugs.

Table 5.8   Flavourings and examples of preparations in which they are used

	Example of use
Flavoured syrups	
Blackcurrant Syrup BP	Ipecacuanha and Squill Linctus Paediatric BPC
	Paediatric Chloral Elixir BPC
Ginger Syrup BP	Rhubarb Mixture Paediatric BP
	Sodium Bicarbonate Mixture Paediatric BP
Lemon Syrup BP	Codeine Linctus BP
Orange Syrup BP	Ferrous Sulphate Mixture Paediatric BP
Raspberry Syrup BP	Kaolin Mixture Paediatric BP
Tolu Syrup BP	Squill Opiate Linctus BP
	Methadone Linctus BP
Aromatic waters	
Concentrated Anise Water BP	Ammonia and Ipecacuanha Mixture BP
	Belladonna and Ephedrine Mixture Paediatric BP
Concentrated Cinnamon Water BP	Chalk Mixture Paediatric BP
Concentrated Dill Water BP	Sodium Bicarbonate Mixture Paediatric BP
Concentrated Peppermint Water BP	Kaolin Mixture BP
(latterly replaced by Concentrated	Magnesium Carbonate Mixture BP
Peppermint Emulsion BP)	Magnesium Trisilicate Mixture BP
Double Strength Chloroform Water BP	Although its primary use in extemporaneous dispensing is as a preservative, it is also considered to provide a pleasant flavouring
Spirits	
Compound Orange Spirit BP	Belladonna Mixture Paediatric BP
	Ferric Ammonium Citrate Mixture Paediatric BP
	Ipecacuanha and Squill Linctus Paediatric BP
Lemon Spirit BP	Diabetic Codeine Linctus BP
	Potassium Citrate Mixture BP
	Sodium Citrate Mixture BP
Concentrated extracts	
Liquid Liquorice Extract BP	Ammonia and Ipecacuanha Mixture BP
	Ammonium Chloride Mixture BP
	Ipecacuanha and Morphine Mixture BP

c. A **sour** taste can be masked by citrus fruits, liquorice or raspberry.

d. **Sweetness** can be toned down using vanilla, fruits or berries.

Other additives used to affect flavour include:

• Citric Acid BP – This obscures some bitter tastes and has the added advantage of improving the ability of citrus flavours to mask acid tastes.

• Menthol BP and Peppermint Oil BP – These have a slightly anaesthetic action locally and therefore numb the taste buds.

• Sodium Chloride BP and Sodium Citrate BP – These help to reduce bitterness.

The traditional flavourings previously highlighted are obtained from natural products. Numerous other flavourings have been produced synthetically and as these tend to be a cheaper alternative to the natural products it is the synthetic flavours that tend to be employed commercially.

Further information on both colourings and flavourings can be found in the following pharmaceutical texts:

1. The British Pharmacopoeia (current edition).
2. *Martindale – The Extra Pharmacopoeia* (current edition).
3. Wade A, Weller P J (ed.) 1994, *Handbook of Pharmaceutical Excipients*. The Pharmaceutical Press, London.

Quantities of flavourings to use

Table 5.9 lists suggested doses of some suitable flavourings for extemporaneously prepared products. Note the inclusion of Concentrated Peppermint Emulsion BP, which has superseded Concentrated Peppermint Water BP as the flavouring of choice.

In the absence of a dosage guide for individual flavourings, another way to decide on the amount of flavouring to include in a product is to compare the quantities used of the flavouring of choice in official products. For example, many indigestion mixtures have a peppermint flavouring, and in the absence of any other data concerning the quantity of Concentrated Peppermint Emulsion BP to use to safely flavour a magistral formula, one could compare the

amounts used in formulae such as Magnesium Trisilicate Mixture BP and Kaolin Mixture BP, where the formulae would suggest using 25 mL of Concentrated Peppermint Emulsion BP in 1000 mL of mixture. Therefore if you use Concentrated Peppermint Emulsion BP in the same proportions in a magistral formula as the proportions in an official formula the dose you use is likely to be safe.

5.6 Storage and labelling requirements

5.6.1 Storage

All products dispensed extemporaneously require some form of additional storage instructions to be detailed on the label. This information can be the addition of just a product expiry date through to a number of important additional auxiliary labels.

The summary list given in Table 5.10 can be used as a guide in the absence of any guidance from the official pharmaceutical texts, but it should be used as a guide only – any information on additional labelling or expiry dates in the official texts will take precedence. The suggested expiry dates in Table 5.10 are based on historical practice. Nowadays, it is common to assign a maximum of a 2-week discard to any extemporaneously prepared product, and consideration should always be given to assigning a shorter discard date.

5.6.2 General principles of labelling

Every pharmaceutical preparation requires a label to be produced before the product can be dispensed or sold to the patient. The accuracy of the label is of paramount importance as it conveys essential information to the patient on the use of the preparation.

Although the pharmacist or other healthcare practitioner may counsel the patient when the medication is handed over, it is unlikely that the patient will be able to remember all the information that they are given verbally. The label

Table 5.9 Guide to suggested doses of different flavourings commonly used in pharmaceutical products

Flavouring	Suggested dose
Blackcurrant Syrup BP	5–10 mL
Concentrated Anise Water BP	0.3–1 mL
Concentrated Caraway Water BP	0.3–1 mL
Concentrated Cinnamon Water BP	0.3–1 mL
Concentrated Dill Water BP	0.3–1 mL
Concentrated Peppermint Emulsion BP	0.25–1 mL
Concentrated Peppermint Water BP	0.25–1 mL
Double Strength Chloroform Water BP	5–15 mL
Ginger Syrup BP	2.5–5 mL
Lemon Syrup BP	2.5–5 mL
Liquid Liquorice Extract BP	2–5 mL
Orange Syrup BP	2.5–5 mL
Raspberry Syrup BP	1 mL
Tolu Syrup BP	2–10 mL

Table 5.10   Guide to auxiliary labels and discard dates for extemporaneous preparations

Preparation	Container	Important auxiliary labels	Suggested discard date
Applications	Amber fluted bottle with CRC	For external use only	4 weeks
Capsules	Amber tablet bottle with CRC	See BNF for advisory labels recommended for active ingredient	3 months
Creams and gels	Amber glass jar or collapsible metal tube	For external use only	4 weeks
Dusting powders	Plastic jar, preferably with a perforated, reclosable lid	For external use only Not to be applied to open wounds or raw weeping surfaces Store in a dry place	3 months
Ear drops	Hexagonal amber fluted glass bottle with a rubber teat and dropper closure	For external use only	4 weeks
Elixirs	Plain amber medicine bottle with CRC		4 weeks
Emulsions	Plain amber medicine bottle with CRC	Shake the bottle	4 weeks
Enemas	Amber fluted bottle with CRC	For rectal use only[a] Warm to body temperature before use	4 weeks
Gargles and mouthwashes	Amber fluted bottle with CRC	Not to be taken[a] Do not swallow in large amounts	4 weeks
Inhalations	Amber fluted bottle with CRC	Not to be taken[a] Shake the bottle	4 weeks
Linctuses	Plain amber medicine bottle with CRC		4 weeks
Liniments and lotions	Amber fluted bottle with CRC	For external use only Shake the bottle Avoid broken skin	4 weeks
Mixtures and suspensions	Plain amber medicine bottle with CRC	Shake the bottle	4 weeks
Nasal drops	Hexagonal amber fluted glass bottle with a rubber teat and dropper closure	Not to be taken[a]	4 weeks
Ointments	Amber glass jar	For external use only	3 months
Pastes	Amber glass jar	For external use only	3 months
Pessaries	Wrapped in foil and packed in an amber glass jar	For vaginal use only[a]	3 months
Powders (individual)	Wrapped in powder papers and packed in a cardboard carton	Store in a dry place Dissolve or mix with water before taking See BNF for advisory labels recommended for active ingredient	3 months
Suppositories	Wrapped in foil and packed in an amber glass jar	For rectal use only[a] See BNF for advisory labels recommended for active ingredient	3 months

BNF, British National Formulary; CRC, child-resistant closure.
[a]See Section 5.6.2 (General principles of labelling).

therefore acts as a permanent reminder of the key points that the patient needs to know.

The functions of a label are to indicate clearly:

- The contents of the container
- How and when the medicinal product should be taken or used
- How the product should be stored and for how long
- Any warnings or cautions that the patient needs to be made aware of.

Appearance

Positioning

It is important to position the label with care, making sure that the patient can open the container without destroying the label (e.g. when labelling cartons) and placing the label straight, not crooked.

- Medicine bottles – The label should be on the front of a medicine bottle about a third of the way down the container. The front of an internal bottle is the curved side and the front of a fluted bottle is the plain side.
- Cartons – The label should be placed on the large side of the carton. If there is not enough room on a single side of the carton for the entire label, it should be placed around the carton, ensuring that all the information is visible.
- Ointment jars – The label should be placed on the side of the jar, ensuring that the contents of the label are visible when the top is placed on the jar.

Cleanliness

Ensure the container is clean before packing the product, then clean the outside before affixing the label. Never pour any liquids into a pre-labelled container as this risks spoiling the label with drips of the medicament.

Security

Make sure that the label is secure before dispensing the product to the patient. The main reason for labels not sticking to product containers is dirt or grease on the outside of the container.

Information

The information on the label should be:

- Legible – Always check label print size and quality to ensure that it can be read clearly. If there is too much information to place on one label, consider placing the additional information on a secondary label, rather than reducing the size of the print or trying to cram too much information onto one label.
- Concise – Although it is important that sufficient information is placed on the label, it must be remembered that it is important not to confuse the patient by placing too much information on the label. If the label contains too much information, rather than assisting the patient, they may feel overwhelmed and this may result in the patient reading none of the information.
- Adequate – Ensure that sufficient information is given, for example the term 'when required' leaves the questions How much? How often? When required for what?
- Intelligible – The wording of the information on the label must be in plain English, be easily understandable and use unambiguous terms. Patients may feel embarrassed to ask for further clarification on the meaning of complicated words used on the label.
- Accurate – Ensure that the title is accurate, the instructions are accurate and the patient's name is complete and accurate.

Dispensed type labels

In the UK detailed requirements for labelling of medicinal products are contained in the Medicines Act 1968 and in amendments to that Act made by Statutory Instrument. The legislation distinguishes between labelling of a medicinal product for sale and the labelling for a dispensed product, when lesser requirements apply.

1. All labels for dispensed medicines must have the name of the patient, preferably the full name, not just initials, and if possible the title of the patient (Mr, Mrs, Miss, Master, Ms, etc.) as this helps to distinguish between family members. The date and the name and address of the pharmacy are also legally required. This will normally automatically appear on most

computer labelling systems, with the date being reset automatically. The words 'Keep out of the reach of children' are also legally required, but most labels used for dispensing purposes are already pre-printed with these words.

2. All labels must state the name of the product dispensed, the strength where appropriate, and the quantity dispensed.

3. a. **Products for internal use** – The title of an extemporaneous preparation if it is an official product (i.e. one with an accepted formula that can be found in an official text – see Section 5.4.1). The title should be as quoted in the official text (for example, Ammonia and Ipecacuanha Mixture BP).

   If it is an unofficial product (that is, a product made from an individual formula, for example a doctor's own formula – see Section 5.4.2) it may be labelled 'The Mixture' or 'The Solution' etc. Unofficial products must state the full quantitative particulars on the label (i.e. the formula must be stated on the label). For preparations intended for internal use this is expressed as the amount of ingredient per unit dose.

   For example, a Sodium Chloride BP solution 4% with a dose of 10 mL bd could be labelled as:

   > The Solution
   > Each 10 mL dose contains:
   > Sodium Chloride BP 400 mg
   > Freshly boiled and cooled purified water to 10 mL

   b. **Products for external use** – Labels for preparations not intended for oral use require slightly different labelling. If the product being made is official the official title should be used (e.g. Sodium Bicarbonate Ear Drops BP or Sodium Chloride Mouthwash BP – see Section 5.4.1).

   If the product is an unofficial one (see Section 5.4.2) the label title may reflect the type of external product, for example 'The Nose Drops', 'The Ear Drops', 'The Mouthwash', 'The Lotion', 'The Enema', etc.

   As with preparations intended for oral use, unofficial products for external use need to be labelled with the full quantitative particulars.

In the case of products for external use, the quantitative particulars are expressed as the complete formula. Therefore, 100 mL Sodium Chloride BP Lotion 4% would be labelled:

> The Lotion
> Containing:
> Sodium Chloride BP 4 g
> Freshly boiled and cooled purified water to 100 mL

Similarly, 200 mL of Sodium Chloride BP Lotion 4% would be labelled:

> The Lotion
> Containing:
> Sodium Chloride BP 8 g
> Freshly boiled and cooled purified water to 200 mL

4. Labels must also include an expiry date. See Table 5.10 for guidance. The Medicines Act 1968 (as amended) requires medicinal products to specify a month and year after which the product should not be used. However, in practice this can cause confusion and an alternative format is to show expiry as a single discard date: for example 'Discard after 31.01.07'.

5. Warning labels may also be required. These may be pharmaceutical or pharmacological warnings (see labelling appendix in the British National Formulary). Generally, if there is a choice between two warning labels with equivalent meanings, the positive one should be chosen (e.g. 'For rectal use only' is preferable to 'Do not swallow' for suppositories).

   Table 5.10 gives guidance on the use of additional auxiliary labels. In the UK, the term 'For external use only' is used on any preparation intended for external use. The Medicines Act 1968 defines products for external use as embrocations, liniments, lotions, liquid antiseptics, other liquids or gels for external use. However, traditionally, for the following dosage forms, alternative labels have been employed instead of 'For external use only' to more closely reflect the intended purpose of the product. These alternative labels (indicated in Table 5.10 by '[a]') are:

- Enemas – 'For rectal use only'.
- Gargles and mouthwashes – 'Not to be taken'.
- Inhalations – 'Not to be taken'.
- Nasal drops – 'Not to be taken'.
- Pessaries – 'For vaginal use only'.
- Suppositories – 'For rectal use only'.

Pharmacists should use their professional judgement when deciding which auxiliary labels should be applied to different pharmaceutical dosage forms. As it is accepted practice in the UK to use the terms outlined above, these will be the terms used in each of the product chapters.

6. All directions on labels should use active rather than passive verbs, for example 'Take two' (not 'Two to be taken'), 'Use one' (not 'One to be used'), 'Insert one' (not 'One to be inserted') etc.

7. Where possible adjacent numbers should be separated by the formulation name. For example, 'Take two three times a day' could easily be misinterpreted by the patient, therefore ideally the wording on this label would include the formulation, e.g. 'Take two tablets three times a day'. The frequency and quantity of individual doses is always expressed as a word rather than a numeral (i.e. 'two' not '2').

8. Liquid preparations for internal use usually have their dose expressed as a certain number of 5 mL doses. This is because a 5 mL spoon is the normal unit provided to the patient to measure their dose from the dispensed bottle. Therefore, if a prescription called for the dosage instruction 10 mL tds this would be expressed as 'Take two 5 mL spoonfuls three times a day'.

     Paediatric prescriptions may ask for a 2.5 mL dose. In this case the label would read 'Give a 2.5 ml dose using the oral syringe provided'. Note here the use of the word 'Give' as the preparation is for a child and would be given to the patient by the parent or guardian.

9. Remember the label on a medicine is included

so that the item can be identified and the patient instructed as to the directions for use. Simple language should be used.

a. Never use the word 'Take' on a preparation that is not intended for the oral route of administration.
b. Use 'Give' as a dosage instruction on products for children, as a responsible adult should administer them.
c. Only use numerals when quoting the number of millilitres to be given or taken. All other dosage instructions should use words in preference to numerals.
d. Always be prepared to give the patient a verbal explanation of the label.

5.7 Pharmaceutical packaging

All dispensed medicinal products will need to be dispensed to the patient in a suitable product container. The function of a container for a medicinal product is to maintain the quality, safety and stability of its contents.

The ideal container should be:

- Robust enough to protect the contents against crushing during handling and transport.
- Convenient to use in order to promote good patient compliance (i.e. encourage the patient to take their medication at the correct times).
- Easy to open and close, if required, especially if the medication is for an elderly or arthritic patient.
- Constructed of materials that do not react with the medicine, so the materials of construction should be inert.
- Sufficiently transparent to allow for inspection of the contents in the case of liquid preparations.

Although different pharmaceutical preparations will be packaged in different containers depending on the product type, pharmaceutical packaging can largely be grouped into a few main types.

5.7.1 Tablet bottles

Tablet bottles come in a variety of shapes and sizes and are usually made of either glass or plastic. They are usually coloured amber to reduce the likelihood of the contents reacting with light. They are used for solid, single-dose preparations that are intended for oral use (i.e. tablets and capsules).

 See Picture 23

In normal circumstances, all tablet bottles should be fitted with child-resistant closures. Although they are not child-proof, these closures reduce the possibility of access to medication by children. There are a number of different types of child-resistant closures on the market. Consideration should be given to the patient when using child-resistant closures, as some patient groups (e.g. the elderly and arthritic patients) may not be able to open the container to access their medication. This can lead to non- or reduced compliance.

5.7.2 Medical bottles

Plain amber medicine bottles

Plain amber medicine bottles can be used to package all internal liquid preparations. Traditional amber medicine bottles used in the UK have two different sides, one curved and one flat. The label or labels are usually placed on the curved side of the bottle as the natural action by the patient will be to pick the bottle up with the curved side of the bottle facing the inside of the palm. By placing the label on the curved side, this will mean the label is on the upper side of the bottle when in use. This will prevent the label becoming damaged by any dribbles of liquid running down the side of the bottle during pouring of a dose.

Plain amber medicine bottles come in a variety of sizes. The capacity of each bottle is traditionally marked on the bottom of the container in millilitres. In the UK, plain amber medicine bottles come in the following sizes: 50 mL, 100 mL, 150 mL, 200 mL, 300 mL and 500 mL.

 See Picture 24

As with tablet bottles (see Section 5.7.1), child-resistant closures should be used whenever possible.

Fluted amber medicine bottles

Fluted (or ribbed) amber medicine bottles are similar to the plain amber medicine bottles but instead of having a flat plain side, this side is curved and contains a number of ridges or grooves running from the top of the bottle down to the bottom. The ridges or grooves are intended to be both a visual and tactile warning to the patient or carer that the contents of the bottle are not to be administered via the oral route. For this reason, these types of container are often referred to as 'external medicine bottles'. There is a legal requirement (Medicines Act 1968) in the UK that fluted bottles be used with specific types of pharmaceutical preparation: embrocations, liniments, lotions, liquid antiseptics, other liquids or gels for external use.

As with plain amber medicine bottles, the label is placed on the smooth curved side of the bottle and the capacity of each bottle is traditionally marked on the bottom of the container in millilitres. In the UK, fluted amber medicine bottles typically come in the following sizes: 50 mL, 100 mL and 200 mL, although other sizes may be available.

 See Picture 25

As with tablet bottles (see Section 5.7.1), child-resistant closures should be used whenever possible.

Calibrated containers for liquid preparations

Liquid preparations are normally made up to volume in a conical measure (see Chapter 4). There are occasions where a tared or calibrated bottle may be used. A tared bottle is normally only employed when, because of the viscosity of the final product, the transference loss from the measure to the container would be unacceptable. For example, Kaolin Mixture BP (see Chapter 16) is a very dense suspension and transference may cause problems; similarly, a thick emulsion will also prove difficult and time consuming to transfer in its entirety because of the viscosity of the finished product.

To tare a container:

1. Measure a volume of water equal to that of the product being prepared. This must be measured accurately using a conical measure.
2. Pour the water into the container and mark the meniscus using a small adhesive label.
3. Remove the water from the bottle and drain the bottle.
4. Transfer the prepared mixture into the calibrated bottle. Rinse the measure or mortar used in the preparation of the product with more vehicle and add this to the bottle.
5. Add any liquid ingredients and make the mixture up to volume using the vehicle.
6. Remove the meniscus marker before dispensing the preparation to the patient.

Please note that unless the bottle is thoroughly dried after taring, this method can only be used where water is one of the ingredients of the mixture, as putting medicines into a wet bottle is considered to be bad practice.

5.7.3 Cartons

Cardboard cartons come in a variety of sizes, depending on the manufacturer. They tend to be rectangular in shape and the label is placed on the larger side of the box. They are used to package blister strips of tablets or capsules, powder papers and other pharmaceutical products that may be of a shape that is not suitable for labelling. Although it is good dispensing practice to label the primary container of a medicinal product, in some cases this is not possible. Placing the primary container into a labelled carton is the next best method for labelling the product in question (for example the labelling of very small eye dropper bottles). Additional care must be exercised in the storage of pharmaceutical products in cardboard cartons as they do not come with child-resistant closures.

 See Picture 26

5.7.4 Ointment jars

Ointment jars come in a variety of different sizes and can either be made of colourless glass or amber glass. Amber ointment jars are used for preparations that are sensitive to light. They are used to package ointments, creams, and individually-wrapped suppositories. As with cartons, additional care must be exercised in the storage of ointment jars as they do not come with child-resistant closures.

 See Picture 27

6

Solutions

6.1 Introduction and overview

Solutions are one of the oldest dosage forms used in the treatment of patients and afford rapid and high absorption of soluble medicinal products. Therefore, the compounding of solutions retains an important place in therapeutics today. Owing to the simplicity and hence the speed of preparation of an ad hoc formulation, they are of particular use for individuals who have difficulty in swallowing solid dosage forms (for example paediatric, geriatric, intensive care and psychiatric patients), where compliance needs to be checked on administration (for example in prisons or psychiatric pharmacy) and in cases where precise, individualised dosages are required.

Essentially a solution is a homogeneous liquid preparation that contains one or more dissolved medicaments. Since, by definition, active ingredients are dissolved within the vehicle, uniform

doses by volume may be obtained without any need to shake the formulation. This is an advantage over some other formulation types (e.g. suspensions, see Chapter 7).

In general, water is chosen as the vehicle in which medicaments are dissolved, as it is non-toxic, non-irritant, tasteless, relatively cheap, and many drugs are water soluble. Problems may be encountered where active drugs are not particularly water soluble or suffer from hydrolysis in aqueous solution. In these cases it is often possible to formulate a vehicle containing water mixed with a variety of other solvents.

In the British Pharmacopoeia (BP), Oral Solutions are defined as 'Oral Liquids containing one or more active ingredients dissolved in a suitable vehicle'.

Solutions provide a number of distinct advantages and disadvantages compared with other dosage forms. The advantages of solutions as pharmaceutical products are that:

- The drug is immediately available for absorption. When solid dosage forms are taken orally, the drug needs to dissolve before absorption into the body can take place. By providing the drug in a solution, the dissolution phase of the absorption process can be bypassed, providing quicker absorption.
- Flexible dosing is possible. The active ingredient within the solution will be present in a certain concentration per unit volume. If alterations to the quantity of active ingredient to be administered are required, a simple alteration to the quantity of solution to be taken is all that is required.
- They may be designed for any route of absorption. Although when discussing solutions the oral route of administration is often considered, solutions can be administered via a number of other routes. Parenteral preparations (injections), enemas for rectal use, topical (for use on the skin) preparations and ophthalmic preparations can all be solutions.
- There is no need to shake the container. Unlike some liquid preparations (e.g. suspensions), as the active ingredient is dissolved within the vehicle there is no need to shake the container to ensure a uniform dose is measured.
- They facilitate swallowing in difficult cases. Some patients may find it hard to swallow traditional solid dosage forms (e.g. infants or the elderly). In these situations, it may be easier for the patient to take a liquid dosage form.

The disadvantages of solutions as pharmaceutical products are that:

- Drug stability is often reduced in solution by solvolysis, hydrolysis or oxidation. The stability of the active ingredient needs to be taken into consideration when formulating a solution. For this reason, it is common for solutions to attract a shorter expiry date than equivalent solid dosage forms.
- It is difficult to mask unpleasant tastes. Although liquid dosage forms may be ideal for small children who are unable to swallow solid dosage forms, many drugs taste unpleasant when formulated into a solution. It is possible to attempt to mask any unpleasant tastes by the addition of a flavouring, but this will not always be successful.
- They are bulky, difficult to transport and prone to breakages. A major disadvantage of all liquid dosage forms is that they are always much larger and more bulky than their comparable solid formulation. This makes them heavier and more difficult to transport. Coupled with this is the fact that, traditionally, pharmaceutical liquids are packed in glass bottles. These are obviously prone to breakage which can be hazardous and cause the loss of the preparation.
- Technical accuracy is needed to measure the dose on administration. Although the dose can be titrated without the need to produce additional preparations (see point 2 from the advantages above), patient accuracy in measuring a dose is required. It is accepted that patients' abilities to measure an accurate dose can vary considerably and this needs to be taken into consideration when preparing a liquid preparation. This is especially important when the volume of liquid to be administered is very small, where small changes in the volume administered may result in large increases or decreases in dose.
- Some drugs are poorly soluble. The solubility of a drug needs to be taken into consideration when preparing a solution to ensure that the final volume produced is not excessive. In some cases it may be necessary to alter the vehicle or drug form (for example the free alkaloid or its salt) in order to be able to formulate a convenient preparation.
- A measuring device is needed for administration. Although not a major disadvantage, it must be borne in mind that a measuring device will need to be supplied to the patient in order for them to be able to measure an accurate dose (this will have cost implications), and in addition the patient will need counselling on the use of the measuring device.

The advantages and disadvantages of solutions as dosage forms are summarised in Box 6.1.

Box 6.1   Advantages and disadvantages of solutions as dosage forms

Advantages	Disadvantages
Drug available immediately for absorption	Drug stability often reduced in solution
Flexible dosing	Difficult to mask unpleasant tastes
May be designed for any route of administration	Bulky, difficult to transport and prone to container breakages
	Technical accuracy needed to measure dose on administration
No need to shake container	Measuring device needed for administration
Facilitates swallowing in difficult cases	Some drugs poorly soluble

6.2 General principles of solution preparation

Historically, a range of solutions have been developed in order to fulfil a wide variety of pharmaceutical functions. It is therefore common to find solutions classified according to their intended use (e.g. oral internal, topical, ophthalmic, nasal or parenteral), by the nature of their formulation (e.g. simple or complex), or to be categorised by a traditional name that relates to the solvent system used and/or their intended function (e.g. spirits, tinctures, aromatic waters, syrups and elixirs).

Although the precise characteristics of different types of solution may vary, the essential principles governing their preparation remain similar. The two key characteristics that need to be considered when compounding solutions are solubility and stability.

6.2.1 Solubility

The following points relating to the solubility of the drug element(s) of the formulation need to be taken into consideration:

- Will the drug(s) dissolve in the solvent or a component of the solvent system?
- What quantity of drug will dissolve?
- How long will dissolution take?
- Will the drug(s) remain in solution and for how long?
- What is the pH of solvent required for dissolution?

Answers to many of the above questions will require the compounder to perform a solubility calculation, as described in Chapter 4.

When preparing a solution, the solid(s) will need to go through a dissolution phase. During compounding, it is worth remembering that dissolution rates generally increase with:

- Smaller particle sizes
- Effective stirring
- Lower viscosities
- Increased temperature.

6.2.2 Stability

In addition to the solubility of the drug element(s) of the formulation, other considerations regarding the physical stability of the preparation will need to be taken into consideration (e.g. temperature variation, photosensitivity, etc.), as will the chemical stability and time period, and the microbiological stability and need for a preservative.

6.2.3 General method

The following general method should be used in the preparation of a solution:

1. Write out the formula either from the prescription (unofficial) or from an official text (official).
2. Calculate the quantities required for each ingredient in the formula to produce the required final volume. Remember, it is not

usual to calculate for an overage of product in the case of solutions as it is relatively easy to transfer the entire final contents of the conical measure. Also, as far as is practically possible, the product will be assembled in the final measure, thus reducing any transference losses.

3. Complete all sections of the product worksheet (see Section 5.2).
4. Prepare a suitable label (see Section 5.6.2).
5. Weigh all solids.
6. Identify the soluble solids and calculate the quantity of vehicle required to fully dissolve the solids. If more than one solid is to be dissolved, they are dissolved one by one, in order of solubility (i.e. the least soluble first, see Section 4.2.5). In almost all cases, dissolution will take place in a glass (or occasionally plastic) beaker, not a conical measure. Remember that the solubility of the soluble solids will be dependent on the vehicle used.
7. Transfer the appropriate amount of vehicle to a glass beaker.
8. If necessary, transfer the solid to a glass mortar and use the glass pestle to reduce particle size to aid dissolution.
9. Transfer the solid to the beaker and stir to aid dissolution. If a mortar and pestle have been used to reduce particle size, ensure that the mortar is rinsed with a little vehicle to ensure completer transfer of the powders.
10. When all the solid(s) have dissolved, transfer the solution to the conical measure that will be used to hold the final solution.
11. Rinse out the beaker in which the solution was made with a portion of the vehicle and transfer the rinsings to the conical measure.
12. Add any remaining liquid ingredients to the conical measure and stir.
13. Make up to final volume with remaining vehicle.
14. Transfer to a suitable container, label and dispense to the patient.

 See Solutions video for a demonstration of the preparation of a solution.

Key points from the method

*   Dissolution will normally take place in a glass beaker, not a conical measure, for a number of reasons. First, owing to the shape of the conical measure, any solid added will tend to 'cake' at the bottom of the measure and hamper any attempt to stir the solid around with the stirring rod, which aids dissolution. Second, the action of the stirring rod may scratch the inside of the glass, permanently altering the internal volume of the measure.
*   During the dissolution phase, solutions should be stirred gently and uniformly to avoid air entrapment, which may result in foaming of the solution. If available, automatic stirring devices may be useful in assisting the production of a uniform product and can be timesaving. If stirring devices are used to assist dissolution (e.g. rod, magnetic stirrers), remember to remove them before adjusting to final volumes.
*   It is best to stir continuously when combining ingredients into a solution (either liquid or solid ingredients). By stirring continually during incorporation, high concentration planes within the fluid body, which might increase the likelihood of incompatibilities, will be avoided.

Further considerations during the preparation of a solution:

*   To aid dissolution, high-viscosity liquid components should be added to those of lower viscosity.
*   Completely dissolve salts in a small amount of water prior to the addition of other solvent elements.
*   In complex solutions, organic components should be dissolved in alcoholic solvents and water-soluble components dissolved in aqueous solvents.
*   Aqueous solutions should be added to alcoholic solutions with stirring to maintain the alcohol concentration as high as possible – the reverse may result in separation of any dissolved components.

6.3 Oral solutions

This section describes the different types of pharmaceutical solution that are used orally. Although all are prepared using the same general techniques highlighted above, there are important differences between the different solution types.

6.3.1 Elixirs

An elixir is a liquid oral preparation that usually contains either potent or unpleasant-tasting drugs. The formulation is clear and generally contains a high proportion of sugar or other sweetening agent, included to mask offensive or nauseating tastes. Paediatric elixirs are usually formulated with a fruit syrup as a base flavouring agent.

Generally, non-aqueous solvents (alcohol, glycerin or propylene glycol) form a significant proportion of the vehicle used in elixirs, or alternatively solubilising agents are included.

6.3.2 Linctuses

A linctus is a liquid oral preparation that is chiefly used for a demulcent, expectorant or sedative purpose, principally in the treatment of cough. As such, a linctus is intended to be sipped slowly and allowed to trickle down the throat in an undiluted form. Consequently, linctuses are formulated as viscous solutions which contain sugars.

6.3.3 Syrups

A syrup is a concentrated, viscous solution containing one or more sugar components, chiefly sucrose, and is described in more detail in Section 2.1.20.

6.3.4 Mixtures

Simple liquid preparations intended for oral use containing dissolved medicaments may be described as oral solutions or mixtures, although the term 'mixture' may also be applied to a suspension.

6.3.5 Draughts

A draught is an older term used to describe a liquid preparation formulated as a single dose, in a volume which is larger than generally utilised in traditional mixture formulations. Each draught was usually supplied in a 50 mL unit dose container.

6.3.6 Spirits

Spirits are solutions containing one or more active medicaments dissolved in either absolute or dilute ethanol.

6.3.7 Paediatric drops

These are an oral liquid formulation of potent drugs usually in solution, intended for administration to paediatric patients, though they may be useful in other patients with swallowing difficulties. The formulation is designed to have very small dose volumes which must be administered with a calibrated dropper.

6.4 Gargles and mouthwashes

Gargles and mouthwashes are aqueous solutions that are intended for treatment of the throat (gargles) and mouth (mouthwashes) and are generally formulated in a concentrated form.

These preparations must be diluted before use and care should be taken to ensure that appropriate instructions are included in labelling and that the container used will be easily distinguishable from those containing preparations intended to be swallowed.

6.5 Enemas and douches

These liquid preparations are often formulated as solutions (though may be presented as an emulsion or suspension) and are intended for instillation into the rectum (enema) or other orifice, such as the vagina or nasal cavity (douche). The volumes of these preparations may vary from 5 mL to much larger volumes. When the larger volumes are used it is important that the liquid is warmed to body temperature before administration.

6.6 External solutions

As with internal solutions, owing to the versatility of the solution, a number of different preparation types have been developed for external use.

6.6.1 Lotions

Lotions are solutions, but may also be suspensions or emulsions, that are intended to be applied to the skin without friction on a carrier fabric such as lint and covered with a waterproof dressing. In some cases lotions are applied to the scalp, where the vehicle for the medication is alcohol based, allowing for rapid drying of the hair and thus making the product more acceptable to the patient (e.g. Salicylic Acid Lotion 2%

BPC). In these cases, problems of flammability are addressed by suitable labelling.

6.6.2 Liniments

A liniment is a liquid preparation intended to be rubbed with friction and massaged onto the skin to obtain analgesic, rubefacient or generally stimulating effects. Liniments should not be used on broken skin. They are usually solutions of oils, alcohols or soaps, but may be formulated as emulsions.

6.6.3 Applications

Applications are solutions, though they may also be suspensions or emulsions, intended to be applied without friction to the skin and to be used without any dressing or covering material.

6.6.4 Collodions

These are principally solutions of pyroxylin in a vehicle of ether and alcohol that are intended to be painted onto the skin and left to dry. When dry, the collodion leaves a flexible film of cellulose on the skin which may be used to seal minor injuries or retain a dissolved drug in contact with the skin for an extended period.

Collodions are highly volatile and highly inflammable and care should be taken to label any preparation appropriately.

6.7 Worked examples

Example 6.1 Preparation of 150 mL of Alkaline Gentian Mixture BP

Product formula (British Pharmacopoeia 1988, page 736):

	1000 mL	100 mL	50 mL	150 mL
Concentrated Compound Gentian Infusion BP	100 mL	10 mL	5 mL	15 mL
Sodium Bicarbonate BP	50 g	5 g	2.5 g	7.5 g
Double Strength Chloroform Water BP	500 mL	50 mL	25 mL	75 mL
Potable water	to 1000 mL	to 100 mL	to 50 mL	to 150 mL

Interim formula for Double Strength Chloroform Water BP (see Section 2.1.23):

Concentrated Chloroform Water BPC 1959	5 mL
Potable water	to 100 mL

Method:

1. Using the master formula from the British Pharmacopoeia for 1000 mL of final product, calculate the quantity of ingredients required to produce the final volume needed (150 mL).

   Point of clarity – Step 1
   Rather than attempt this conversion in one stage, it may be simpler to take the calculation through a number of stages. In the example given here, the quantities in the master formula are first divided by 10 to give a product with a final volume of 100 mL. These quantities are then halved to give a product with a final volume of 50 mL. The quantities in the 100 mL product and 50 mL product are then added together to give the quantities of ingredients in a product with a final volume of 150 mL. By using this method, the compounder is less likely to make a calculation error.

2. Calculate the composition of a convenient quantity of Double Strength Chloroform Water BP, sufficient to satisfy the formula requirements but also enabling simple, accurate measurement of the concentrated component. To compound Double Strength Chloroform Water BP:

   a. In this case, 75 mL of Double Strength Chloroform Water BP is required and so it would be sensible to prepare 100 mL. To prepare 100 mL Double Strength Chloroform Water BP, measure 5 mL of Concentrated Chloroform water BPC 1959 accurately using a 5 mL conical measure.

   b. Add approximately 90 mL of potable water to a 100 mL conical measure (i.e. sufficient water to enable dissolution of the concentrated chloroform component without reaching the final volume of the product).

   c. Add the measured Concentrated Chloroform Water BPC 1959 to the water in the conical measure.

   d. Stir gently and then accurately make up to volume with potable water.

   e. Visually check that no undissolved chloroform remains at the bottom of the measure.

   See Solutions video for a demonstration of the preparation of Double Strength Chloroform Water BP.

Noting that sodium bicarbonate is soluble 1 in 11 with water, a minimum of 11 mL of water would be required to dissolve 1 g of sodium bicarbonate. The final volume of Gentian Alkaline Mixture BP required (150 mL) will

Example 6.1 Continued

contain 7.5 g of Sodium Bicarbonate BP. As 1 g of sodium bicarbonate is soluble in 11 mL, 7.5 g is soluble in 82.5 mL (7.5 × 11 = 82.5 mL). Therefore a minimum of 82.5 mL of vehicle would be required to dissolve the 7.5 g of Sodium Bicarbonate BP in this example. For ease of compounding choose a convenient volume of vehicle, say 90 mL, in which to initially dissolve the solute. When choosing the amount of vehicle to use for dissolution, it is important to consider the total amount of each liquid ingredient in the preparation to ensure that only the correct amounts are added or the final product does not go over volume.

3. Weigh 7.5 g Sodium Bicarbonate BP on a Class II or electronic balance.
4. Accurately measure 75 mL Double Strength Chloroform Water BP using a 100 mL measure. To this add approximately 15 mL potable water in order to produce 90 mL of vehicle which should be poured into a beaker (in order to produce sufficient volume to dissolve the 7.5 g Sodium Bicarbonate BP).

    Point of clarity – Step 4
    As discussed above, in this example 90 mL of vehicle is required to dissolve the Sodium Bicarbonate BP. It is important to consider the total amount of each liquid ingredient in the product to ensure that only the correct amounts are added. In this example, it would be incorrect to dissolve the Sodium Bicarbonate BP in 90 mL of Double Strength Chloroform Water BP as the final volume of the preparation only contains 75 mL. In this case, all the Double Strength Chloroform Water BP is used (75 mL) along with enough potable water to reach the desired volume (approximately 15 mL).

5. The Sodium Bicarbonate BP (7.5 g) should be added to the vehicle, thus following the principle of adding solutes to solvents.
6. Stir to aid dissolution.
7. Transfer the solution to a 250 mL conical measure.
8. Rinse the beaker with potable water, adding the rinsings to the Sodium Bicarbonate BP solution.
9. Accurately measure 15 mL of Concentrated Compound Gentian Infusion BP in an appropriately sized conical measure and add to the Sodium Bicarbonate BP solution in the 250 mL measure. Rinse out the small conical measure with potable water and add the rinsings to the mixture.
10. Make up to volume (150 mL) accurately with potable water and stir.
11. Transfer the solution to a 150 mL amber flat medical bottle with a child-resistant closure and label.

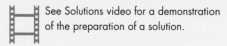

See Solutions video for a demonstration of the preparation of a solution.

Example 6.2 Preparation of 50 mL Ammonium Chloride Mixture BP

Product formula (British Pharmacopoeia 1988, page 720):

	1000 mL	500 mL	50 mL
Ammonium Chloride BP	100 g	50 g	5 g
Aromatic Ammonia Solution BP	50 mL	25 mL	2.5 mL
Liquorice Liquid Extract BP	100 mL	50 mL	5 mL
Potable water	to 1000 mL	to 500 mL	to 50 mL

Method:

1. Calculate the quantity of ingredients required to produce the final volume needed. As with Example 6.1, this calculation is best attempted in stages.
2. Weigh 5 g Ammonium Chloride BP accurately on a Class II or electronic balance. As ammonium chloride is soluble 1 part in 2.7 parts of water, the 5 g required for this product would only dissolve in a minimum initial volume of 13.5 mL aqueous vehicle. Therefore we should choose a convenient volume of vehicle to dissolve the solute, say 15 mL.
3. Measure approximately 15 mL potable water and transfer to a beaker.
4. Add the Ammonium Chloride BP to the water in the beaker and stir until dissolved.
5. Transfer to a 50 mL conical measure with rinsings.
6. Measure 5 mL Liquorice Liquid Extract BP accurately in a 5 mL conical measure and add, with rinsings, to the 50 mL measure containing ammonium chloride solution.
7. Measure 2.5 mL Aromatic Ammonia Solution BP accurately in a syringe and transfer to the 50 mL measure containing the composite solution.
8. Make up to the final volume of 50 mL with potable water and stir.
9. Pack into a 50 mL amber flat medicine bottle and label.

 See Solutions video for a demonstration of the preparation of a solution.

Example 6.3 Preparation of 150 mL of Sodium Chloride Compound Mouthwash BP

Product formula (British Pharmacopoeia 1988, page 703):

	1000 mL	100 mL	50 mL	150 mL
Sodium Bicarbonate BP	10 g	1 g	500 mg	1.5 g
Sodium Chloride BP	15 g	1.5 g	750 mg	2.25 g
Concentrated Peppermint Emulsion BP	25 mL	2.5 mL	1.25 mL	3.75 mL
Double Strength Chloroform Water BP	500 mL	50 mL	25 mL	75 mL
Potable water	to 1000 mL	to 100 mL	to 50 mL	to 150 mL

Interim formula for Double Strength Chloroform Water BP (see Section 2.1.23):

Concentrated Chloroform Water BPC 1959   5 mL
Potable water   to 100 mL

Method:

1. Using the master formula from the British Pharmacopoeia for 1000 mL of final product, calculate the quantity of ingredients required to produce the final volume needed (150 mL).
2. Calculate the composition of a convenient quantity of Double Strength Chloroform Water BP, sufficient to satisfy the formula requirements but also enabling simple, accurate measurement of the concentrated component. Method of compounding for Double Strength Chloroform Water BP:

    a. In this case, 75 mL of Double Strength Chloroform Water BP is required and so it would be sensible to prepare 100 mL. To prepare 100 mL Double Strength Chloroform Water BP, measure 5 mL of Concentrated Chloroform water BPC 1959 accurately using a 5 mL conical measure.
    b. Add approximately 90 mL of potable water to a 100 mL conical measure (i.e. sufficient water to enable dissolution of the concentrated chloroform component without reaching the final volume of the product).
    c. Add the measured Concentrated Chloroform Water BPC 1959 to the water in the conical measure.
    d. Stir gently and then accurately make up to volume with potable water.
    e. Visually check that no undissolved chloroform remains at the bottom of the measure.

    See Solutions video for a demonstration of the preparation
    of Double Strength Chloroform Water BP.

Noting that sodium bicarbonate is soluble 1 in 11 with water, a minimum of 11 mL of water would be required to dissolve 1 g of sodium bicarbonate. The final volume of Sodium Chloride Compound Mouthwash BP required (150 mL) will contain 1.5 g of Sodium Bicarbonate BP. As 1 g of sodium bicarbonate is soluble in 11 mL, 1.5 g is soluble in 16.5 mL (1.5 × 11 = 16.5 mL). The sodium chloride is soluble 1 in 2.8 with water. Therefore a minimum of 2.8 mL of water would be required to dissolve 1 g of sodium chloride. The final volume of Sodium Chloride Compound Mouthwash BP required (150 mL) will contain 2.25 g of Sodium Chloride BP. As 1 g of sodium chloride is soluble in 2.8 mL, 2.25 g is soluble in 6.3 mL (2.25 × 2.8 = 6.3 mL). Therefore a minimum of 16.5 mL of vehicle would be required to dissolve the 1.5 g of sodium bicarbonate and a minimum of 6.3 mL of vehicle would be required to dissolve the 2.25 g of sodium chloride in this example. For ease of compounding choose a convenient volume of vehicle, say 30 mL, in which to initially dissolve the solute. When choosing

Example 6.3 Continued

the amount of vehicle to use for dissolution, it is important to consider the total amount of each liquid ingredient in the preparation to ensure that only the correct amounts are added or the final product does not go over volume.

3. Weigh 2.25 g Sodium Chloride BP on a Class II or electronic balance.
4. Weigh 1.5 g Sodium Bicarbonate BP on a Class II or electronic balance.
5. Measure 75 mL of Double Strength Chloroform Water BP in a 100 mL conical measure.
6. Transfer approximately 30 mL of Double Strength Chloroform Water BP to a beaker, add the Sodium Bicarbonate BP and stir to aid dissolution.
7. When the Sodium Bicarbonate BP has dissolved, add the Sodium Chloride BP and stir to aid dissolution.
8. Transfer the solution from the beaker to a 250 mL conical measure.
9. Rinse out the beaker with some Double Strength Chloroform Water BP and add the rinsings to the conical measure.
10. Measure 3.75 mL of Concentrated Peppermint Emulsion BP using a 5 mL and a 1 mL syringe.
11. Add the Concentrated Peppermint Emulsion BP to the conical measure.
12. Make up to volume with the remaining Double Strength Chloroform Water BP and potable water.
13. Transfer to a 200 mL amber fluted bottle and label.

 See Solutions video for a demonstration of the preparation of a solution.

Example 6.4 Preparation of a magistral formulation (150 mL of Potassium Permanganate Solution 0.2% w/v) from a doctor's prescription

Given that 0.2% w/v is equal to 0.2 g in 100 mL, there are 200 mg of Potassium Permanganate BP in every 100 mL of solution.

Product formula:

	100 mL	50 mL	150 mL
Potassium Permanganate BP	200 mg	100 mg	300 mg
Freshly boiled and cooled purified water	to 100 mL	to 50 mL	to 150 mL

Method:

Point of clarity – product formula

Rather than attempt the above conversion in one stage, it may be simpler to take the calculation through a number of stages. In the example given above, the quantities in the master formula are first divided by 2 to give a product with a final volume of 50 mL. The quantities in the 100 mL product and 50 mL product are then added together to give the quantities of ingredients in a product with a final volume of 150 mL. By using this method, the compounder is less likely to make a calculation error.

Note that Potassium Permanganate is soluble in cold water and freely soluble in boiling water. Freshly boiled and cooled purified water is used as the vehicle as no other preservative is included and the preparation is intended for application to an open wound.

1. Weigh 300 mg Potassium Permanganate BP on a Class II or electronic balance.
2. Transfer to a glass mortar as the Potassium Permanganate BP is crystalline and for ease of dissolution needs to be ground into a powder.

   Point of clarity – Step 2

   Potassium Permanganate BP is an oxidising substance therefore there is risk of explosion. To prevent this add approximately 20 mL of freshly boiled and cooled purified water to a glass mortar (Potassium Permanganate BP stains and so a porcelain mortar would not be suitable) and grind under water.

3. Transfer the solution to a 250 mL conical measure.
4. Rinse the mortar with freshly boiled and cooled purified water and add the rinsings to the conical measure.
5. Make up to volume with freshly boiled and cooled purified water.
6. Transfer the solution to a 150 mL amber fluted medical bottle with a child-resistant closure and label.

See Solutions video for a demonstration of the preparation of a solution.

6.8 Summary of essential principles relating to solutions

This section recaps the main principles relating to solutions that have been covered in other sections of the book. To assist compounders in understanding the extemporaneous preparation of solutions, this section contains the following:

- Further notes on the packaging of extemporaneously prepared solutions.
- Specific points relevant to the expiry of extemporaneously prepared solutions.
- Additional key points related to the labelling of pharmaceutical solutions.

6.8.1 Packaging

The packaging of extemporaneous preparations has been covered in Section 5.7. A brief overview of the main considerations for the packaging of solutions will be given here.

When selecting packaging for extemporaneously prepared solutions, consideration should be given to the route or method of administration. Liquid preparations that are intended for the oral route should be packed in plain (smooth) amber bottles. External preparations and preparations that are not intended to be taken internally (e.g. mouthwashes) should be packaged in fluted amber bottles (i.e. amber bottles with vertical ridges or grooves). This will enable simple identification, by both sight and touch, of preparations that are not to be taken via the oral route.

Pharmaceutical bottles come in a variety of different sizes and it is important to choose a suitably sized container to match the volume of preparation to be dispensed. Obviously it is important not to use a container that is too large for the volume of preparation to be dispensed for both cost and appearance issues (see Table 6.1).

6.8.2 Discard dates

Extemporaneously compounded solutions are often relatively unstable for physical, chemical (hydrolysis) and microbiological reasons. The exact impact of such processes on a compounded solution will depend largely upon the storage conditions, the formulation and its intended purpose. Commercially available manufactured

Table 6.1 Summary of packaging for pharmaceutical solutions

		Typical sizes	Pharmaceutical product examples include
Oral liquids	Amber flat medical bottle	50 mL, 100 mL, 150 mL, 200 mL, 300 mL, 500 mL	Draughts Elixirs Linctuses Mixtures Spirits Syrups
	Amber round medical bottle with dropper top	10 mL	Paediatric drops
External liquids	Amber fluted medical bottle	50 mL, 100 mL, 200 mL	Applications Collodions Enemas and douches Gargles and mouthwashes Liniments Lotions
	Amber fluted medical bottle with dropper top	10 mL	Ear drops Nose drops

products generally have long shelf lives because of strictly controlled manufacturing environments supported by rigorous quality assurance testing. Because of the lack of complete control of conditions and inability to perform retrospective stability tests on extemporaneously compounded solutions, much shorter shelf lives must be attributed.

For official preparations, the BP employs two definitions that are useful when extemporaneously compounding solutions:

- **'Freshly Prepared'** refers to a preparation that has been compounded less than 24 hours prior to issue for use.
- **'Recently Prepared'** should be applied to compounded items that are likely to deteriorate if stored for a period greater than 4 weeks when maintained at 15–25 °C.

In practical terms it is suggested that an expiry date of 2 weeks is applied to oral solutions that need to be Freshly Prepared or that contain an infusion or other vegetable matter. A 4-week expiry should be applied to oral solutions that require to be Recently Prepared.

Remember that because patients frequently misunderstand the term 'expiry' it is suggested that a preferred method of indicating shelf life on the label of extemporaneously compounded products is to apply the term 'Discard after' followed by a definite date and/or time.

When dealing with unofficial preparations, the compounder must take a number of considerations into account. As a general rule, an expiry of 7–14 days would be given to any of the following preparations:

- A solution that does not contain a preservative.
- A solution where there are no stability data available.
- A new solution or ad hoc preparation.

Further guidance on expiry dates for pharmaceutical preparations can be found in Section 5.6.1.

6.8.3 Labelling

The labelling of extemporaneous preparations has been covered previously in Section 5.6.2. An overview of the main considerations for the labelling of solutions will be given here.

In addition to the standard requirements for the labelling of extemporaneous preparations, the following points need to be taken into consideration:

- **'Not to be taken'** and **'Do not swallow in large amounts'** – This warning must be added to gargles and mouthwashes.
- **'Not to be taken'** – This warning should be added to inhalations and nasal drops.
- **'For rectal use only'** and **'Warm to body temperature before administration'** – These warnings should be added to large-volume enemas.
- **'For external use only'** – This warning must be added to the label of any other preparation that is not intended for administration via the oral route.

Further guidance on auxiliary labelling can be found in Section 5.6.1, Table 5.10.

7

Suspensions

7.1 Introduction and overview

Suspensions are an important pharmaceutical dosage form that are still widely in use. Owing to their versatility they are often used in situations where an 'emergency' formulation is required (see Section 7.2.5).

Common pharmaceutical products that are suspensions include:

- Ear drops
- Enemas
- Inhalations
- Lotions
- Mixtures for oral use.

A pharmaceutical suspension is defined as a preparation where at least one of the active ingredients is suspended throughout the vehicle. In contrast to solutions (see Chapter 6), in a suspension at least one of the ingredients is not dissolved in the vehicle and so the preparation will require shaking before a dose is administered.

The British Pharmacopoeia (BP) defines oral suspensions as: 'Oral Liquids containing one or more active ingredients suspended in a suitable vehicle. Suspended solids may slowly separate on standing but are easily redispersed.'

Suspensions provide a number of distinct advantages and disadvantages compared to other dosage forms. The advantages of suspensions as pharmaceutical products are that:

- Insoluble derivatives of certain drugs may be more palatable than their soluble equivalent.
- Insoluble derivatives of drugs may be more stable in the aqueous vehicle than the equivalent soluble salt.
- Suspended insoluble powders are easy to swallow.

- Bulky insoluble powders such as Kaolin BP and Chalk BP can be administered in suspension and can act as adsorbents of toxins in the gastrointestinal tract.
- Suspended drugs will be more rapidly absorbed from the gastrointestinal tract than the equivalent solid dosage form (although absorption will be slower than from the equivalent solution).
- Lotions that are suspensions leave a thin layer of medicament on the skin. The liquid part of the suspension evaporates, giving a cooling effect to the skin and leaving the thin layer of powder behind (for example Calamine Lotion BP).
- Sustained-release preparations can be prepared in suspension (but because of the difficulty of formulation they are rarely encountered).

The disadvantages of suspensions as pharmaceutical products are that:

- They must be well shaken prior to measuring a dose.
- The accuracy of the dose is likely to be less than with the equivalent solution.
- Conditions of storage may adversely affect the disperse system and in the case of indiffusible solids clumping may occur, leading to potential dosing inaccuracy.
- Like all liquid dosage forms, they are always much larger and more bulky than their comparable solid formulations. This makes them heavy and difficult to transport. Coupled with this is the fact that traditionally, pharmaceutical liquids are packed in glass bottles. These are obviously prone to breakage which can be hazardous and cause the loss of the preparation.

The advantages and disadvantages of suspensions as dosage forms are summarised in Box 7.1.

7.2 General principles of suspension preparation

Although similar to pharmaceutical solutions in a number of ways, pharmaceutical suspensions differ in that one or more of the solid ingredients are suspended throughout the vehicle rather than dissolved within it. Different pharmaceutical solids have differing abilities to suspend throughout a vehicle. This results in two types of pharmaceutical suspension: diffusible suspensions and indiffusible suspensions.

7.2.1 Diffusible suspensions

These are suspensions containing light powders that are insoluble, or only very slightly soluble, in the vehicle but which on shaking disperse evenly throughout the vehicle for long enough to allow an accurate dose to be poured.

Box 7.1   Advantages and disadvantages of suspensions as dosage forms

Advantages

Insoluble drugs may be more palatable
Insoluble drugs may be more stable
Suspended insoluble powders are easier to swallow
Enables easy administration of bulk insoluble powders
Absorption will be quicker than solid dosage forms
Lotions will leave a cooling layer of medicament on the skin
Theoretically possible to formulate sustained-release preparations

Disadvantages

Preparation requires shaking before use
Accuracy of dose likely to be less than equivalent solution
Storage conditions can affect disperse system
Bulky, difficult to transport and prone to container breakages

Examples of diffusible powders commonly incorporated into pharmaceutical suspensions include:

- Light Kaolin BP – insoluble in water
- Light Magnesium Carbonate BP – very slightly soluble in water
- Magnesium Trisilicate BP – insoluble in water.

7.2.2 Indiffusible suspensions

These are suspensions containing heavy powders that are insoluble in the vehicle and which on shaking do not disperse evenly throughout the vehicle long enough to allow an accurate dose to be poured.

Examples of indiffusible powders commonly incorporated into pharmaceutical suspensions include:

- Aspirin BP
- Calamine BP
- Chalk BP
- Zinc Oxide BP.

In the preparation of indiffusible suspensions, the main difference from diffusible suspensions is that the vehicle must be thickened to slow down the rate at which the powder settles. This is achieved by the addition of a suspending agent.

7.2.3 Formulation of suspensions

The non-soluble ingredients of a suspension are dispersed in the vehicle and, as with pharmaceutical solutions, water is normally the vehicle of choice. The density of the aqueous vehicle can be altered slightly by the addition of sucrose or glycerol and the viscosity can be changed by the addition of thickening agents. The increase in the viscosity means that the rate of sedimentation of the insoluble solid will be slower.

Details of suspending agents have been given in Chapter 5. A summary of the different types of suspending agent used in extemporaneous formulation is shown in Table 7.1.

7.2.4 Other additives

Colourings and flavourings are added to suspensions for the same purposes as they are added to solutions (see Section 5.5.11). It must be remembered that with the large surface area of

Table 7.1   Summary of the different suspending agents used in extemporaneous formulation

Category of suspending agent	Example of suspending agent
Natural polysaccharides (Section 5.5.8)	Acacia Gum BP
	Agar BP
	Carrageenan BP
	Compound Tragacanth Powder BP
	Guar Gum BP
	Powdered Tragacanth BP
	Sodium Alginate BP
	Starch BP
Semi-synthetic polysaccharides (Section 5.5.8)	Hydroxyethylcellulose BP
	Methyllcellulose BP
	Sodium Carboxymethylcellulose BP
Clays (Section 5.5.8)	Aluminium Magnesium Silicate BP
	Bentonite BP
	Magnesium Aluminium Alginate BP
Synthetic agents (Section 5.5.8)	Carbomer BP
	Polyvinyl Alcohol BP
Miscellaneous compounds	Gelatin BP

the dispersed powders some of these additives may be adsorbed onto the powder and therefore the effective concentration in solution may be reduced. For example, a given concentration of dye may produce a paler-coloured product when there is a large amount of finely divided disperse phase in suspension, owing to dye adsorption.

As with solutions, Double Strength Chloroform Water BP is a commonly used preservative for suspensions. Other useful preservatives employed in the manufacture of suspensions include Benzoic Acid BP 0.1%, which is suitable for internal use, and Chlorocresol BP (0.1% w/v), which is suitable for external use.

7.2.5 Suspensions as 'emergency' formulations

In addition to established formulae, compounders may be required to produce a suitable liquid preparation for patients who are unable to swallow tablets or capsules. Occasionally, the medicament required may only be available commercially as a solid dosage form. If a liquid preparation is unavailable, the compounder may be expected to prepare a liquid product from the commercially available solid dosage form. This normally involves crushing of tablets or opening of capsules to provide powdered drug to prepare a suspension.

When preparing a suspension from solid dosage forms, it must always be remembered that tablets and capsules will contain unknown excipients as well as the nominal quantity of drug. The bioavailability of the drug is likely to be unknown, and if possible a pure sample of powdered drug should be obtained in order to produce a suspension without extraneous components. However, in cases where the solid dosage form is the only source of the drug, Tragacanth Powder BP or Compound Tragacanth Powder BP are usually suitable suspending agents.

7.3 Oral diffusible suspensions

7.3.1 General method for the preparation of a suspension containing a diffusible solid

1. Check the solubilities, in the vehicle, of all solids in the mixture.
2. Calculate the quantities of vehicle required to dissolve any soluble solids.
3. Prepare any Double Strength Chloroform Water BP required.
4. Weigh all solids on a Class II or electronic balance.
5. Dissolve all soluble solids in the vehicle in a small glass beaker using the same procedures as outlined in the chapter on solutions (Chapter 6).
6. Mix any insoluble diffusible powders in a porcelain mortar using the 'doubling-up' technique to ensure complete mixing (see Key Skill 7.1).

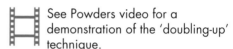 See Powders video for a demonstration of the 'doubling-up' technique.

 Key Skill 7.1 The 'doubling-up' technique

1. Weigh the powder present in the smallest volume (powder A) and place in the mortar.
2. Weigh the powder present in the next largest volume (powder B) and place on labelled weighing paper.
3. Add approximately the same amount of powder B, as powder A in the mortar.
4. Mix well with pestle
5. Continue adding an amount of powder B that is approximately the same as that in the mortar and mix with the pestle, i.e. doubling the amount of powder in the mortar at each addition.
6. If further powders are to be added, add these in increasing order of volume as in steps 3, 4 and 5 above.

7. Add a small quantity of the vehicle (which may or may not be a solution of the soluble ingredients) to the solids in the mortar and mix using a pestle to form a smooth paste.
8. Add further vehicle in small quantities, and continue mixing until the mixture in the mortar is of a pourable consistency.
9. Transfer the contents of the mortar to a conical measure of suitable size.
10. Rinse out the mortar with more vehicle and add any rinsings to the conical measure.
11. Add remaining liquid ingredients to the mixture in the conical measure. (These are added now, as some may be volatile and therefore exposure during mixing needs to be reduced to prevent loss of the ingredient by evaporation.)
12. Make up to final volume with vehicle.
13. Stir gently, transfer to a suitable container, ensuring that all the solid is transferred from the conical measure to the bottle, and label ready to be dispensed to the patient.

> *Point of clarity – Method*
> Alternatively, the contents of the mortar could be transferred directly to a pre-prepared tared container. Rinsings from the mortar and other liquid ingredients could then be added to the bottle before being made up to final volume. This would prevent any possible transference loss caused by powders sedimenting in the conical measure (see Section 5.7.2).

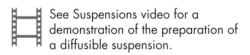
See Suspensions video for a demonstration of the preparation of a diffusible suspension.

7.4 Oral indiffusible suspensions

Oral indiffusible suspensions are prepared using the same basic principles as for oral diffusible suspensions. The main difference is that the preparation will require the addition of a suspending agent. The suspending agent of choice will normally be combined with the indiffusible solid using the 'doubling-up' technique before incorporation into the product.

7.4.1 General method for the preparation of a suspension containing an indiffusible solid

1. Check the solubilities in the vehicle of all solids in the mixture.
2. Calculate the quantities of vehicle required to dissolve any soluble solids.
3. Prepare any Double Strength Chloroform Water BP required.
4. Weigh all solids on a Class II or electronic balance.
5. Dissolve all soluble solids in the vehicle in a small glass beaker.
6. Mix any insoluble indiffusible powders and the suspending agent in a porcelain mortar using the 'doubling-up' technique to ensure complete mixing (see Section 7.3.1, Key Skill 7.1).

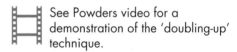
See Powders video for a demonstration of the 'doubling-up' technique.

7. Add a small quantity of the vehicle (which may or may not be a solution of the soluble ingredients) to the solids in the mortar and mix using a pestle to form a smooth paste.
8. Add further vehicle in small quantities, and continue mixing until the mixture in the mortar is a pourable consistency.
9. Transfer the contents of the mortar to a conical measure of suitable size.
10. Rinse out the mortar with more vehicle and add any rinsings to the conical measure.
11. Add remaining liquid ingredients to the mixture in the conical measure. (These are added now, as some may be volatile and therefore exposure during mixing needs to be reduced to prevent loss of the ingredient by evaporation.)
12. Make up to final volume with vehicle.
13. Stir gently, transfer to a suitable container, ensuring that all the solid is transferred from the conical measure to the bottle, and label ready to be dispensed to the patient.

Point of clarity – Method

Alternatively, the contents of the mortar could be transferred directly to a pre-prepared tared container. Rinsings from the mortar and other liquid ingredients could then be added to the bottle before being made up to final volume. This would prevent any possible transference loss caused by powders sedimenting in the conical measure (see Section 5.7.2).

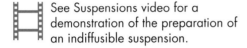

See Suspensions video for a demonstration of the preparation of an indiffusible suspension.

7.5 Suspensions for external use

Suspensions intended for external use can be compounded using the same basic principles as those intended for internal use. There may be differences in the choice of suspending agent used, as outlined in Section 7.2 above.

7.5.1 Inhalations

Inhalations are liquid products that contain volatile ingredients intended to be released and brought into contact with the respiratory lining. Suspensions are a particularly useful way of effecting this transfer as the volatile ingredient can be adsorbed onto a carrier powder (a diffusible solid) and formulated as a suspension which can then provide an accurate dose to be added to hot (about 65 °C) but not boiling water, so that the volatile ingredient is released and inhaled by the patient. Alcoholic solutions are also suitable to use as a 'hot' inhalation. If ingredients are volatile at room temperature they may be inhaled directly from a handkerchief or absorbent pad.

7.5.2 Lotions

Lotions can be suspensions, although they may also be solutions (see Section 6.6.1) or emulsions (see Section 8.5). They are intended to be applied to the skin, without friction, on a carrier fabric such as lint and covered with a waterproof dressing. In some cases, such as Calamine Lotion BP, they may be dabbed onto the skin surface and allowed to dry.

7.5.3 Applications

Applications can be suspensions, although they may also be solutions (see Section 6.6.3) or emulsions (see Section 8.5). They are intended to be applied without friction to the skin and to be used without any dressing or covering material.

7.6 Worked examples

 Example 7.1 Preparation of 150 mL Magnesium Trisilicate Mixture BP

Product formula (British Pharmacopoeia 1988, page 740):

	1000 mL	100 mL	50 mL	150 mL
Magnesium Trisilicate BP	50 g	5 g	2.5 g	7.5 g
Light Magnesium Carbonate BP	50 g	5 g	2.5 g	7.5 g
Sodium Bicarbonate BP	50 g	5 g	2.5 g	7.5 g
Concentrated Peppermint Emulsion BP	25 mL	2.5 mL	1.25 mL	3.75 mL
Double Strength Chloroform Water BP	500 mL	50 mL	25 mL	75 mL
Potable water	to 1000 mL	to 100 mL	to 50 mL	to 150 mL

Interim formula for Double Strength Chloroform Water BP (see Section 2.1.23):

Concentrated Chloroform Water BPC 1959	5 mL
Potable water	to 100 mL

Method:

1. Using the master formula from the British Pharmacopoeia for 1000 mL of final product, calculate the quantity of ingredients required to produce the final volume needed (150 mL).

   Point of clarity – Step 1
   Rather than attempt the above conversion in one stage, it may be simpler to take the calculation through a number of stages. In the example given above, the quantities in the master formula are first divided by 10 to give a product with a final volume of 100 mL. These quantities are then halved to give a product with a final volume of 50 mL. The quantities in the 100 mL product and 50 mL product are then added together to give the quantities of ingredients in a product with a final volume of 150 mL. By using this method, the compounder is less likely to make a calculation error.

2. Calculate the composition of a convenient quantity of Double Strength Chloroform Water BP, sufficient to satisfy the formula requirements but also enabling simple, accurate measurement of the concentrated component. Method of compounding for Double Strength Chloroform Water BP:

   a. In this case, 75 mL of Double Strength Chloroform Water BP is required and so it would be sensible to prepare 100 mL. To prepare 100 mL Double Strength Chloroform Water BP, measure 5 mL of Concentrated Chloroform water BPC 1959 accurately using a 5 mL conical measure.
   b. Add approximately 90 mL of potable water to a 100 mL conical measure (i.e. sufficient water to enable dissolution of the concentrated chloroform component without reaching the final volume of the product).
   c. Add the measured Concentrated Chloroform Water BPC 1959 to the water in the conical measure.
   d. Stir gently and then accurately make up to volume with potable water.
   e. Visually check that no undissolved chloroform remains at the bottom of the measure.

    See Solutions video for a demonstration of the preparation of Double Strength Chloroform Water BP.

Example 7.1 Continued

Noting that sodium bicarbonate is soluble 1 in 11 with water, a minimum of 11 mL of water would be required to dissolve 1 g of sodium bicarbonate. The final volume of Magnesium Trisilicate Mixture BP required (150 mL) will contain 7.5 g of Sodium Bicarbonate BP. As 1 g of sodium bicarbonate is soluble in 11 mL, 7.5 g is soluble in 82.5 mL ($7.5 \times 11 = 82.5$ mL). Therefore a minimum of 82.5 mL of vehicle would be required to dissolve the 7.5 g of sodium bicarbonate in this example. For ease of compounding choose a convenient volume of vehicle, say 90 mL, in which to initially dissolve the solute. When choosing the amount of vehicle to use for dissolution, it is important to consider the total amount of each liquid ingredient in the preparation to ensure that only the correct amounts are added or the final product does not go over volume.

3. Weigh 7.5 g Magnesium Trisilicate BP on a Class II or electronic balance.
4. Weigh 7.5 g Light Magnesium Carbonate BP on a Class II or electronic balance.
5. Weigh 7.5 g Sodium Bicarbonate BP on a Class II or electronic balance.
6. Measure 3.75 mL Concentrated Peppermint Emulsion BP using a 1 mL and 5 mL syringe.
7. Accurately measure 75 mL Double Strength Chloroform Water BP using a 100 mL measure. To this add approximately 15 mL potable water in order to produce 90 mL of vehicle, which should be poured into a beaker (in order to produce sufficient volume to dissolve the 7.5 g Sodium Bicarbonate BP).

   Point of clarity – Step 7
   As discussed above, in this example 90 mL of vehicle is required to dissolve the Sodium Bicarbonate BP. It is important to consider the total amount of each liquid ingredient in the product to ensure that only the correct amounts are added. In this example, it would be incorrect to dissolve the Sodium Bicarbonate BP in 90 mL of Double Strength Chloroform Water BP as the final volume of the preparation only contains 75 mL. In this case, all the Double Strength Chloroform Water BP is used (75 mL) along with enough potable water to reach the desired volume (approximately 15 mL).
   It is also important not to dissolve the Sodium Bicarbonate BP in 90 mL of potable water, as when the 75 mL of Double Strength Chloroform Water BP is added to the preparation, the final volume would be greater than 150 mL.

8. The Sodium Bicarbonate BP (7.5 g) should be added to the vehicle, thus following the principle of adding solutes to solvents.
9. Stir to aid dissolution.
10. Transfer the Magnesium Trisilicate BP to a porcelain mortar.
11. Add the Light Magnesium Carbonate BP to the Magnesium Trisilicate BP in the mortar using the 'doubling-up' technique and stir with a pestle to ensure even mixing.

    Point of clarity – Steps 10 and 11
    The Magnesium Trisilicate BP is added to the mortar first as although the weights of the insoluble solids are identical, the volume occupied by the powders differs markedly. The Magnesium Trisilicate BP occupies the smallest volume and therefore the first powder to be added to the mortar.

12. Add a small amount of the sodium bicarbonate solution to the powder in the mortar and mix with a pestle to make a smooth paste.
13. Slowly, continue adding the sodium bicarbonate solution until the paste is pourable.
14. Transfer the contents of the mortar to a 200 mL conical measure.
15. Rinse out the mortar with more sodium bicarbonate solution and add the rinsings to the conical measure.
16. Add the Concentrated Peppermint Emulsion BP to the mixture in the conical measure.
17. Make up to volume with any remaining solution and potable water.

Example 7.1 Continued

18. Transfer the solution to a 150 mL amber flat medical bottle with a child-resistant closure and label.

See Suspensions video for a demonstration
of the preparation of a suspension.

Example 7.2 Preparation of 100 mL of Chalk Mixture Paediatric BP

Product formula (British Pharmacopoeia 1988, page 724):

	1000 mL	100 mL
Chalk BP	20 g	2 g
Tragacanth BP	2 g	200 mg
Concentrated Cinnamon Water BP	4 mL	0.4 mL
Syrup BP	100 mL	10 mL
Double Strength Chloroform Water BP	500 mL	50 mL
Potable water	to 1000 mL	to 100 mL

Interim formula for Double Strength Chloroform Water BP (see Section 2.1.23):

Concentrated Chloroform Water BPC 1959	2.5 mL
Potable water	to 50 mL

Method:

1. Calculate the composition of a convenient quantity of Double Strength Chloroform Water BP, sufficient to satisfy the formula requirements but also enabling simple, accurate measurement of the concentrated component. Method of compounding for Double Strength Chloroform Water BP:

   a. In this case, 50 mL of Double Strength Chloroform Water BP is required and so it would be sensible to prepare 50 mL. To prepare 50 mL Double Strength Chloroform Water BP, measure 2.5 mL of Concentrated Chloroform water BPC 1959 accurately using a 5 mL and a 1 mL syringe.
   b. Add approximately 45 mL of potable water to a 50 mL conical measure (i.e. sufficient water to enable dissolution of the concentrated chloroform component without reaching the final volume of the product).
   c. Add the measured Concentrated Chloroform Water BPC 1959 to the water in the conical measure.
   d. Stir gently and then accurately make up to volume with potable water.
   e. Visually check that no undissolved chloroform remains at the bottom of the measure.

See Solutions video for a demonstration of the preparation
of Double Strength Chloroform Water BP.

Example 7.2 Continued

2. Weigh 200 mg Tragacanth BP accurately on a Class II or electronic balance.
3. Weigh 2 g Chalk BP accurately on a Class II or electronic balance.
4. Measure 10 mL Syrup BP in a 10 mL conical measure.
5. Measure 0.4 mL Concentrated Cinnamon Water BP using a 1 mL syringe.

   Point of clarity – Step 5
   Although it is a volatile ingredient, it is not bad practice to measure the Concentrated Cinnamon Water BP at this stage of the method as loss by evaporation will be avoided by measuring in a syringe.
   It must always be remembered that when using a syringe to measure ingredients, consideration must be given to the properties of the liquid being measured. This will avoid dissolution of the volume markings from the outside of the syringe, or even parts of the syringe itself, which may occur with some ingredients.

6. Measure 50 mL of Double Strength Chloroform Water BP in a 50 mL conical measure.
7. Transfer the Tragacanth BP to a porcelain mortar.
8. Add the Chalk BP to the mortar using the 'doubling-up' technique to mix the two powders.

   Point of clarity – Steps 7 and 8
   The Tragacanth BP is included in the mixture because Chalk BP is an indiffusible solid and therefore it is necessary to add a suspending agent. They are admixed by the 'doubling-up' technique to ensure even mixing and therefore the successful suspension of the indiffusible chalk.

9. Add the Syrup BP to the mortar and mix to form a smooth paste.
10. Add some of the Double Strength Chloroform Water BP to the paste and mix until pourable.
11. Transfer the contents to a 100 mL conical measure.
12. Rinse out the mortar with more Double Strength Chloroform Water BP or potable water and add the rinsings to the conical measure.
13. Add the Concentrated Cinnamon Water BP to the mixture in the conical measure.

   Point of clarity – Step 13
   The Concentrated Cinnamon Water BP is the last ingredient to be added prior to making up to volume because it is a volatile ingredient.

14. Make up to volume with any remaining Double Strength Chloroform Water BP and potable water.

   Point of clarity – Step 14
   Alternatively a bottle could be tared and the mixture made up to volume in the bottle (see Section 5.7.2).

15. Transfer to an amber flat medical bottle label and dispense.

 See Suspensions video for a demonstration of the preparation of a suspension.

Example 7.3 Preparation of 50 mL of Menthol and Eucalyptus Inhalation BP

Product formula (from the British Pharmacopoeia 1980, page 577):

	1000 mL	100 mL	50 mL
Menthol BP	20 g	2 g	1 g
Eucalyptus Oil BP	100 mL	10 mL	5 mL
Light Magnesium Carbonate BP	70 g	7 g	3.5 g
Potable water	to 1000 mL	to 100 mL	to 50 mL

Method:
1. Weigh 1 g Menthol BP on a Class II or electronic balance.
2. Transfer to a glass mortar.
3. Measure 5 mL Eucalyptus Oil BP in a 5 mL conical measure.
4. Transfer to the mortar and mix with a pestle to dissolve the menthol.

> *Point of clarity – Steps 3 and 4*
> Menthol is freely soluble in fixed and volatile oils. Care should be taken as the oil will dissolve away the graduation markings on the syringe. Alternatively, a conical measure could be used.

5. Weigh 3.5 g Light Magnesium Carbonate BP on a Class II or electronic balance.
6. Add to the mortar and mix well.
7. Add potable water to the mixture in the mortar to form a pourable suspension.
8. Transfer the contents of the mortar to a 50 mL conical measure.
9. Rinse the mortar with potable water and add the rinsings to the conical measure.
10. Make up to volume with potable water.
11. Transfer to a 50 mL amber fluted bottle with a child-resistant closure and label.

> *Point of clarity – Step 11*
> Alternatively a bottle could be tared and the mixture made up to volume in the bottle (see Section 5.7.2).

 See Suspensions video for a demonstration of the preparation of a suspension.

Example 7.4 Preparation of a magistral formulation from a hospital formula

You receive a prescription for Clobazam liquid. Clobazam is only available commercially as 10 mg tablets. The patient is required to take 10 mg at each dose but unfortunately cannot swallow solid dosage preparations. The hospital pharmacy gives you the formula that has been used while the patient was in the hospital:

Tabs qs Clobazam	10 mg
Concentrated Peppermint Water BP	2% v/v
Glycerol BP	6% v/v
Syrup BP	25% v/v
Suspending agent	2% w/v
Freshly boiled and cooled purified water	to 100%

The patient needs to take 10 mg at each dose and the prescriber wants 30 doses. Therefore, if we make the formula as above such that each 5 mL contains 10 mg Cobazam we would need to prepare 150 mL of suspension.
To prepare 150 mL of Clobazam Suspension 10 mg/5 mL:

Product formula:

	5 mL	50 mL	150 mL
Clobazam	10 mg	100 mg	300 mg
	1 tablet	10 tablets	30 tablets
Concentrated Peppermint Water BP	0.1 mL	1 mL	3 mL
Glycerol BP	0.3 mL	3 mL	9 mL
Syrup BP	1.75 mL	17.5 mL	52.5 mL
Compound Tragacanth Powder BP	100 mg	1 g	3 g
Freshly boiled and cooled purified water	to 5 mL	to 50 mL	to 150 mL

Freshly boiled and cooled purified water is used as the vehicle as no preservative is included in the preparation.

Method:
1. Count out 30 Clobazam tablets.
2. Weigh 3 g Compound Tragacanth Powder BP using a Class II or electronic balance.

   Point of clarity – Step 2
   As the quantity of suspending agent required was indicated to be 2%, Compound Tragacanth Powder BP was chosen as the suspending agent as this is a suitable quantity to include to produce a reasonable suspension. Tragacanth BP itself is normally used in concentrations of 0.2%, therefore had Tragacanth BP been used in a 2% strength, the suspension produced would have been unacceptable and more closely related to a solid dosage form than a liquid dosage form.

3. Measure 9 mL of glycerol using a 10 mL conical measure.
4. Measure 52.5 mL Syrup BP using a 50 mL measure and a suitably graduated 5 mL syringe.
5. Transfer the tablets to a glass mortar and grind them to make a smooth powder.
6. Transfer the powder to a porcelain mortar and add the Compound Tragacanth Powder BP using the 'doubling-up' technique. Mix with the pestle.
7. Add the Glycerol BP to the powders in the mortar and mix to make a paste.
8. Add the Syrup BP to the mortar to make a pourable paste.

Example 7.4 Continued

9. Transfer the contents of the mortar to a 200 mL conical measure.
10. Rinse out the mortar with more syrup and freshly boiled and cooled purified water.
11. Add rinsings to the mixture in the conical measure.
12. Measure 3 mL Concentrated Peppermint Water BP using a 5 mL conical measure.
13. Add the Concentrated Peppermint Water BP to the mixture in the conical measure.
14. Make up to volume with freshly boiled and cooled purified water.
15. Stir and transfer to a 150 mL amber flat medical bottle with a child-resistant closure, label and dispense to the patient.

See Suspensions video for a demonstration of the preparation of a suspension.

7.7 Summary of essential principles relating to suspensions

This section recaps the main principles relating to suspensions that have been covered in other sections of the book. To assist compounders in understanding the extemporaneous preparation of suspensions, this section contains the following:

- Further notes on the packaging of extemporaneously prepared suspensions.
- Specific points relevant to the expiry of extemporaneously prepared suspensions.
- Additional key points related to the labelling of pharmaceutical suspensions.

7.7.1 Packaging

The packaging of extemporaneous preparations has been covered previously in Section 5.7. An overview of the main considerations for the packaging of suspensions will be given here.

The packaging for suspensions is based on the same principles as for solutions, as both preparation types are based on liquid administration. When selecting packaging for extemporaneously prepared suspensions, consideration should be given to the route or method of administration.

Liquid preparations that are intended for the oral route should be packed in plain (smooth) amber bottles. External preparations should be packaged in fluted amber bottles (i.e. amber bottles with vertical ridges or grooves). This will enable simple identification, by both sight and touch, of preparations that are not to be taken via the oral route.

Pharmaceutical bottles come in a variety of different sizes and it is important to choose a suitably sized container to match the volume of preparation to be dispensed. Obviously it is important not to use a size of container that is too large for the volume of preparation to be dispensed, for both cost and appearance issues. Consideration should be given to selecting a bottle that will leave sufficient space to allow the product to be shaken adequately before a dose is measured.

Guidelines on the packaging of extemporaneously prepared suspensions are summarised in Table 7.2.

7.7.2 Discard dates

Discard dates for pharmaceutical suspensions typically mirror those for pharmaceutical solutions (see Section 6.8.2). The discard date of official preparations will be advised via the relative official texts.

Table 7.2 Summary of packaging for pharmaceutical suspensions

Oral liquids	Amber flat medical bottle (Typical sizes: 50 mL, 100 mL, 150 mL, 200 mL, 300 mL and 500 mL)
	Pharmaceutical product examples include: Mixtures (suspensions) for oral use
External liquids	Amber fluted medical bottle (Typical sizes: 50 mL, 100 mL, 200 mL)
	Pharmaceutical product examples include: Applications Inhalations Lotions
	Amber fluted medical bottle with dropper top (Typical sizes: 10 mL, 20 mL)
	Pharmaceutical product examples include: Ear drops Nose drops

As with solutions, for official preparations the BP employs two definitions that are useful when extemporaneously compounding suspensions:

- **'Freshly Prepared'** refers to a preparation that has been compounded less than 24 hours prior to issue for use
- **'Recently Prepared'** should be applied to compounded items that are likely to deteriorate if stored for a period greater than 4 weeks when maintained at 15–25 °C.

In practical terms it is suggested that an expiry date of 2 weeks is applied to oral suspensions that need to be Freshly Prepared or that contain an infusion or other vegetable matter. A 4-week expiry should be applied to oral suspensions that need to be Recently Prepared.

Remember that because patients frequently misunderstand the term 'expiry' it is suggested that a preferred method of indicating shelf life on the label of extemporaneously compounded products is to apply the term 'Discard after' followed by a definite date and/or time.

When dealing with unofficial preparations, the compounder must consider the following. As a general rule, an expiry of 7–14 days would be given to any of the following preparations:

- A suspension that does not contain a preservative.
- A suspension where there are no stability data available.
- A new suspension or ad hoc preparation.

Further guidance on expiry dates for pharmaceutical preparations can be found in Section 5.6.1.

7.7.3 Labelling

The labelling of extemporaneous preparations has been covered in Section 5.6.2. An overview of the main considerations for the labelling of suspensions will be given here.

In addition to the standard requirements for the labelling of extemporaneous preparations, the following points need to be taken into consideration:

- **'Shake the bottle'** – All suspensions will require this additional label.
- **'Not to be taken'** – This warning must be added to the label of any inhalations.
- **'For external use only'** – This warning must be added to the label of any other suspension not intended for administration via the oral route.

Further guidance on auxiliary labelling can be found in Section 5.6.1, Table 5.10.

8

Emulsions

8.1 Introduction and overview

The pharmaceutical term 'emulsion' is solely used to describe preparations intended for internal use (i.e. via the oral route of administration). Emulsion formulations for external use are always given a different title that reflects their use (e.g. application, lotion, cream, etc.).

An emulsion is essentially a liquid preparation containing a mixture of oil and water that is rendered homogeneous by the addition of an emulsifying agent. The emulsifying agent ensures that the oil phase is finely dispersed throughout the water as minute globules (Figure 8.1). This type of emulsion is termed an 'oil-in-water'

emulsion. The oily phase (disperse phase) is dispersed through the aqueous phase (continuous phase). Generally all oral dose emulsions tend to be 'oil in water', as the oily phase is usually less pleasant to take and more difficult to flavour. 'Water-in-oil' emulsions can be formed, but these tend to be those with external uses.

According to the British Pharmacopoeia (BP):

Oral Emulsions are Oral Liquids containing one or more active ingredients. They are stabilised oil-in-water dispersions, either or both phases of which may contain dissolved solids. Solids may also be suspended in Oral Emulsions. When issued for use, Oral Emulsions should be supplied in wide-mouthed bottles.

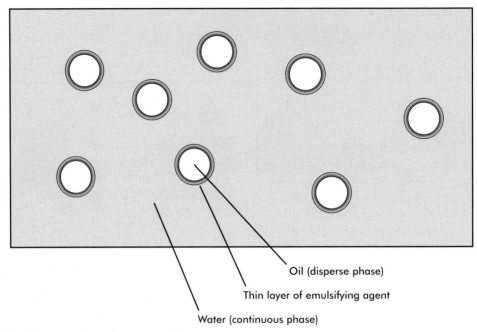

Oil (disperse phase)

Thin layer of emulsifying agent

Water (continuous phase)

Figure 8.1   Illustration of an oil-in-water emulsion

Extemporaneous preparation

In Oral Emulsions prepared according to the formula and directions given for Extemporaneous preparation, the quantity of emulsifying agent specified in individual monographs may be reduced to yield a preparation of suitable consistency provided that by so doing the stability of the preparation is not adversely affected.

There are a number of advantages and disadvantages associated with the use of emulsions as oral dosage forms. The advantages of emulsions as pharmaceutical products are that:

- A dose of an unpalatable drug may be administered in a palatable liquid form (e.g. cod liver oil emulsion).
- An oil-soluble drug can be dissolved in the disperse phase and be successfully administered to a patient in a palatable form.
- The aqueous phase can be easily flavoured.
- The texture/consistency of the product is improved as the 'oily' sensation in the mouth is successfully masked by the emulsification process.
- Emulsification increases the absorption of fats through the intestinal wall. Consider the process of fat digestion, whereby fats are emulsified in the duodenum by bile salts. The efficient absorption of the oil is increased by a process of homogenisation which reduces the size of the oil globules.
- Liquid dosage forms of incompatible ingredients may be formulated by dissolving or suspending each ingredient in one of the phases of an emulsion system.

The disadvantages of emulsions as pharmaceutical products are that:

- They must be shaken well prior to measuring a dose, and even after efficient shaking the accuracy of the dose is likely to be less than with equivalent solutions.
- A measuring device is needed for administration. Although not a major disadvantage, it must be borne in mind that a measuring device will need to be supplied to the patient in order for them to be able to measure an accurate dose (this will have cost implications), and in addition the patient will need counselling on the use of the measuring device.
- Some degree of technical accuracy is needed to measure a dose.

- Conditions of storage may adversely affect the disperse system, leading to creaming or cracking of the emulsion (see Section 8.4).
- Like all liquid dosage forms, they are much more bulky than their comparable solid formulation. This makes emulsions heavier and more difficult to transport than solid dosage forms. Coupled with this is the fact that, traditionally, pharmaceutical liquids are packed in glass bottles. These are obviously prone to breakage which can be hazardous and cause the loss of the preparation.
- They are liable to microbial contamination which can lead to cracking (see Section 8.4).

The advantages and disadvantages of emulsions as dosage forms are summarised in Box 8.1.

8.2 Formulation of emulsions

The theory of emulsification is based on the study of the most naturally occurring emulsion, milk. Milk, if examined closely, will be seen to consist of fatty globules, surrounded by a layer of casein, suspended in water. When a pharmaceutical emulsion is made, the principal considerations are the same. The object is to completely divide the oily phase into minute globules, surround each globule with an envelope of suspending agent (e.g. Acacia BP), and finally suspend the globules in the aqueous phase (Figure 8.1).

As with other liquid preparations for oral use, emulsions will have in the formulation a vehicle, containing added flavouring or colourings as required. There is also the need for a preservative, which is usually chloroform, in the form of Double Strength Chloroform Water BP.

In addition, an emulsion will also need an emulsifying agent (or emulgent).

8.2.1 Continental and dry gum method

Extemporaneously prepared emulsions for oral administration are usually made by the Continental or the dry gum method, where the emulsion is formed by mixing the emulsifying gum (usually Acacia BP) with the oil, which is then mixed with the aqueous phase. The only difference between the Continental and dry gum methods are the proportions of constituents within the primary emulsion (for example, fixed oil emulsions made by the Continental method would use a ratio of 4:3:2 rather than 4:2:1 with the dry gum method – see Section 8.2.2).

Internal emulsions prepared by the dry gum method should contain, in addition to the oil to be emulsified:

- A vehicle (freshly boiled and cooled purified water is normally used because of the increased risk from microbial contamination).
- A preservative (usually added to the product as Double Strength Chloroform Water BP at 50%

Box 8.1   Advantages and disadvantages of emulsions as dosage forms

Advantages	**Disadvantages**
Unpalatable drugs can be administered in palatable form	Preparation needs to be shaken well before use
Unpalatable oil-soluble drugs can be administered in palatable form	Measuring device needed for administration
Aqueous phase easily flavoured	Need a degree of technical accuracy to measure a dose
Oily sensation easily removed	Storage conditions may affect stability
Increased rate of absorption	Bulky, difficult to transport and prone to container breakages
Possible to include two incompatible ingredients, one in each phase of the emulsion	Liable to microbial contamination which can lead to cracking

of the volume of the vehicle). If freshly boiled and cooled purified water is used as the vehicle, it would be appropriate to manufacture the Double Strength Chloroform Water BP using freshly boiled and cooled purified water rather than potable water (see examples in Section 8.6).

- An emulsifying agent (or emulgent). The quantity of emulsifying agent added is determined by the type of oil to be emulsified and the quantity of emulsion to be prepared.
- Additional flavouring if required.
- Additional colouring if required.

Occasionally, finely divided solids have been used to form emulsions. The solid must possess a balance of hydrophilic and hydrophobic properties. Colloidal clays such as bentonite, magnesium hydroxide, aluminium hydroxide, magnesium oxide and silica gel are some of the insoluble substances that have been used as emulsifying agents. If the chosen powder is easily wetted by water then an oil-in-water emulsion is formed, whereas those that are preferentially wetted by the oil phase produce water-in-oil emulsions. The colloidal clays are mainly used as emulsion stabilisers for external lotions or creams, whereas aluminium and magnesium hydroxide have both been used as emulsifying agents for preparations intended for internal use.

All emulsifying agents will exhibit certain physical and chemical characteristics that will determine how effective they are under various conditions of use.

All emulsifying agents will contain a water-attracting or hydrophilic part and an oil-attracting or lipophilic part. If an emulsifying agent was too hydrophilic it would dissolve completely in the aqueous phase and if it was too lipophilic it would totally dissolve in the oily phase. The ideal emulsifying agent must concentrate predominantly at the interface between oil and aqueous phases, where it is positioned such that the hydrophilic portion is in the aqueous phase and the lipophilic portion is in the oily phase. When an emulsifying agent displays these properties it is said to have the proper hydrophil–lipophil balance. If an emulsifying agent is predominantly hydrophilic an oil-in-water emulsion is formed. Conversely, if it is predominantly lipophilic it will favour the production of a water-in-oil emulsion.

The hydrophil–lipophil balance of surface active agents has been categorised into the HLB system of numbering, where high HLB numbers indicate hydrophilic properties and low HLB numbers indicate lipophilic properties (Table 8.1).

The HLB system was developed by WC Griffin in 1949, originally for non-ionic surface active agents, but has been expanded to include cationic and anionic surface active agents. Each emulsifying agent is allocated an HLB number (see Table 8.2 for examples).

When several oils or fats are included in a preparation a blend of emulsifying agents is sometimes employed to produce the best product.

Table 8.1 Different hydrophil–lipophil balance (HLB) ranges and their applications

HLB range	Application
3–6	Water-in-oil emulsifying agents
7–9	Wetting agents
8–18	Oil-in-water emulsifying agents
13–15	Detergents
15–16	Solubilisers

Table 8.2 Hydrophil–lipophil balance (HLB) value of a number of common emulsifying agents

Emulsifying agent	HLB value
Acacia	8.0
Polysorbate 20	16.7
Polysorbate 60	14.9
Polysorbate 80	15.0
Sodium lauryl sulphate	40.0
Sorbitan monolaurate	8.6
Sorbitan monostearate	4.7
Sodium oleate	18.0
Tragacanth	13.2
Triethanolamine oleate	12.0

8.2.2 Calculation of the amount of emulsifying agent to be used in the preparation of an emulsion using the dry gum method

The amount of emulsifying agent used is dependent on the amount and type of oil to be emulsified. Oils can be divided into three categories, fixed oils, mineral oils and aromatic (volatile) oils.

Fixed oils:

Oil	4 parts by volume
Aqueous phase	2 parts by volume
Gum	1 part by weight

Mineral oils:

Oil	3 parts by volume
Aqueous phase	2 parts by volume
Gum	1 part by weight

Aromatic (volatile) oils:

Oil	2 parts by volume
Aqueous phase	2 parts by volume
Gum	1 part by weight

These proportions are important when making the primary emulsion, to prevent the emulsion breaking down on dilution or storage.

The quantities for primary emulsions (in parts) are summarised in Table 8.3.

Accurate weighing and measuring of the components in the primary emulsion are important when making the primary emulsion to prevent the emulsion breaking down on storage or dilution.

8.2.3 Wet gum method

The proportions of oil, water and emulsifying agent for the preparation of the primary emulsion are the same as those used in the dry gum method (see Section 8.2.2). The difference is in the method of preparation.

Using this method the acacia powder would be added to the mortar and then triturated with the water until the gum was dissolved and a mucilage formed. The oil would then be added to the mucilage drop by drop while triturating continuously. When nearly all the oil has been added, the resulting mixture in the mortar may appear a little poor with some of the oil appearing to be absorbed. This can be rectified by the addition of slightly more water. The trituration continues until all the oil has been added, adding extra small amounts of water when necessary. When all the oil has been added, the mixture is triturated until a smooth primary emulsion is obtained.

In the main this method has fallen out of favour as it takes much longer than the dry gum method. It should be noted that there is less chance of failure with this method provided the

Example 8.1 What quantities would be required to produce 100 mL of a 20% emulsion of a fixed oil?

For a 20% emulsion 20 mL of the oil in 100 mL of emulsion would be required.

Therefore 4 parts would be equivalent to 20 mL of oil.

Therefore 2 parts would be equivalent to 10 mL aqueous phase.

Therefore 1 part would be equivalent to 5 g of gum.

The formula for the primary emulsion would therefore be:

Fixed oil	20 mL
Aqueous phase	10 mL
Gum	5 g

Table 8.3 Ratio of oily phase to aqueous phase to gum in a primary emulsion

Type of oil	Examples	Oil	Aqueous	Gum
Fixed	Arachis Oil BP Castor Oil BP Cod Liver Oil BP	4	2	1
Mineral	Liquid Paraffin BP	3	2	1
Volatile	Cinnamon Oil BP Peppermint Oil BP	2	2	1

oil is added very slowly and in small quantities. It also means that the reasons for failure outlined above when using the dry gum method have been eliminated.

8.3 General method of preparation of an emulsion using the dry gum method

It is relatively easy for an emulsion to crack, resulting in a failed product. Remember the following points are critical when preparing emulsions:

- **Clean, dry equipment** – All equipment should be thoroughly cleaned, rinsed with water and dried carefully before use, particularly measures, mortars and pestles.
- **Accurate quantities** – Accurate quantities are essential. Check weighing/measuring technique and minimise transference losses (e.g. allow oil to drain from measure).
- **Have all ingredients ready** – Correct rate of addition is important. Ingredients for the primary emulsion should all be weighed and measured before starting to make the product.

The preparation of an emulsion has two main components:

- Preparation of a concentrate called the 'primary emulsion'.
- Dilution of the concentrate.

8.3.1 Preparation of the primary emulsion

1. Measure the oil accurately in a dry measure. Transfer the oil into a large dry porcelain mortar, allowing all the oil to drain out.
2. Measure the quantity of aqueous vehicle required for the primary emulsion. Place this within easy reach.
3. Weigh the emulsifying agent and place on the oil in the mortar. Mix lightly with the pestle, just sufficient to disperse any lumps. Caution – overmixing generates heat, which may

denature the emulsifying agent and result in a poor product.
4. Add all of the required aqueous vehicle in *one addition*. Then mix vigorously, using the pestle with a shearing action in *one direction*.
5. When the product becomes white and produces a 'clicking' sound the primary emulsion has been formed. The product should be a thick white cream. Increased degree of whiteness indicates a better-quality product. Oil globules/slicks should not be apparent.

8.3.2 Dilution of the primary emulsion

1. Dilute the primary emulsion drop by drop with very small volumes of the remaining aqueous vehicle. Mix carefully with the pestle in one direction.
2. Transfer emulsion to a measure, with rinsings. Add other liquid ingredients if necessary and make up to the final volume.

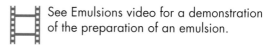 See Emulsions video for a demonstration of the preparation of an emulsion.

8.3.3 Problems encountered when making the primary emulsion

The primary emulsion does not always form correctly and the contents of the mortar may become oily, thin and translucent. This is because of phase inversion. The oil-in-water emulsion has become a water-in-oil emulsion that cannot be diluted further with the aqueous vehicle. The product has failed and must be restarted. Reasons for this include:

- Inaccurate measurement of water or oil.
- Cross-contamination of oil and water.
- Use of a wet mortar.
- Excessive mixing of the oil and gum.
- Poor-quality acacia.
- Insufficient shear between the head of the pestle and the mortar base.
- Too early or too rapid dilution of the primary emulsion.

8.4 Stability of emulsions

Emulsions can break down through cracking, creaming or phase inversion (Table 8.4).

8.4.1 Cracking

This is the term applied when the disperse phase coalesces and forms a separate layer. Re-dispersion cannot be achieved by shaking and the preparation is no longer an emulsion. Cracking can occur if the oil turns rancid during storage. The acid formed denatures the emulsifying agent, causing the two phases to separate.

 See Emulsions video for an example of a cracked emulsion.

8.4.2 Creaming

In creaming, the oil separates out, forming a layer on top of the emulsion, but it usually remains in globules so that it can be re-dispersed on shaking (e.g. the cream on the top of a pint of milk). This is undesirable as the product appearance is poor and if the product is not adequately shaken there is a risk of the patient obtaining an incorrect dose. Creaming is less likely to occur if the viscosity of the continuous phase is increased.

8.4.3 Phase inversion

This is the process when an oil-in-water emulsion changes to a water-in-oil emulsion or vice versa. For stability of an emulsion, the optimum range of concentration of dispersed phase is 30–60% of the total volume. If the disperse phase exceeds this the stability of the emulsion is questionable. As the concentration of the disperse phase approaches a theoretical maximum of 74% of the total volume, phase inversion is more likely to occur.

8.5 Emulsions for external use

Emulsions for external use are designed for application to the skin and may be liquid or semi-liquid in consistency. The formulation of external emulsions differs from that of conventional emulsions in that no primary emulsion is formed. As with internal emulsions, both oil-in-water and water-in-oil emulsions can be produced and applied to the surface of the skin and mucous membranes. The consistency of the formed emulsion determines whether it is a lotion or a much thicker cream product. The advantage of an emulsion as an external application is that it is easily spread over the skin and usually easily removed by washing. For further information, see Chapter 9.

Table 8.4   Summary of the problems encountered in emulsion preparation

Problem	Possible reason for problem	Can the emulsion be saved?
Creaming – Separation of the emulsion into two regions, one containing more of the disperse phase	Lack of stability of the system. Product not homogeneous	The emulsion will reform on shaking
Cracking – The globules of the disperse phase coalesce and there is separation of the disperse phase into a separate layer	Incompatible emulsifying agent. Decomposition of the emulsifying agent. Change of storage temperature	The emulsion will not reform on shaking
Phase inversion – From o/w to w/o or from w/o to o/w	Amount of disperse phase greater than 74%	The emulsion will not reform on shaking

o/w, oil in water; w/o, water in oil.

8.5.1 Vehicles used in the preparation of external emulsions

Vehicles commonly used in the preparation of lotions and liniments are either water miscible or oily.

Water-miscible vehicles

- **Water** – Usually freshly boiled and cooled purified water to reduce the chances of any microbial contamination
- **Alcohol** – Industrial methylated spirit (IMS) is the normal alcoholic constituent of products for external use as it is exempt from excise duty and therefore cheaper than ethanol. Alcohol is sometimes added to increase the cooling effect of the product, owing to the evaporation of the alcohol from the skin's surface.

Oily vehicles

- **Mineral oils** – e.g. Light Liquid Paraffin BP, Liquid Paraffin BP.
- **Vegetable oils** – e.g. Arachis Oil BP, Coconut Oil BP, Olive Oil BP. The problem with these oils is that they tend to go rancid.
- **Synthetic oils** – e.g. Dimethicone (Dimeticone) BP.

8.5.2 Preservatives used in the preparation of external emulsions

The preservatives commonly used in emulsions for external use are the same as those commonly employed in the extemporaneous formulation and production of creams (see Section 5.5.5), namely:

Benzoic Acid BP	0.1%
Chlorocresol BP	0.1%
Cetrimide BP	0.002–0.01%

8.5.3 Emulsifying agents used in the preparation of external emulsions

The range of emulsifying agents used is described in full in Section 5.5.10.

Water-in-oil emulsifiers

- **Beeswax** – Occasionally used and is a traditional water-in-oil emulsifier; it is not a very good emulsifier and nowadays tends to be used as an emulsion stabiliser.
- **Calcium soaps** – Made in situ by mixing a fatty acid and calcium hydroxide solution (Lime Water).
- **Wool alcohol** – Preferable to wool fat as it is purer but still has the problem of creating unpleasant odours in warm weather.
- **Wool fat** – Similar to human sebum and can cause sensitisation problems in some patients. Mainly used as an emulsion stabiliser.
- **Synthetic surface active agents** with low HLB values.

Oil-in-water emulsifiers

- **Emulsifying waxes:**
  - Anionic – Emulsifying wax BP
  - Cationic – Cetrimide Emulsifying Wax BP
  - Non-ionic – Cetomacrogol Emulsifying Wax BP.
- **Soaps:**
  - Soft soap: Sticky green material that produces an oil-in-water emulsion (e.g. Turpentine Liniment BP)
  - Ammonium soaps formed during the preparation of products when the oleic acid and ammonium compounds react to produce ammonium oleate, an oil-in-water emulsifying agent.
- **Synthetic surface active agents** with a high HLB value.

The emulsifying agents used for emulsions for internal use, namely tragacanth and acacia, would not be suitable for an emulsion for external use as they are too sticky.

Other than creams that are thick emulsions, applications, lotions and liniments are often liquid emulsions.

8.6 Worked examples

Example 8.2 The preparation of a magistral formulation of 200 mL of Cod Liver Oil 30% emulsion from a doctor's prescription

Product formula:

	Master (100 mL)	200 mL
Cod Liver Oil BP	30 mL	60 mL
Acacia BP	qs	qs
Double Strength Chloroform Water BP	50 mL	100 mL
Freshly boiled and cooled purified water	to 100 mL	to 200 mL

First it is necessary to calculate the quantity of emulsifying agent (acacia) required to produce 200 mL of the emulsion. As cod liver oil is a fixed oil, the primary emulsion ratio is:

Oil	:	Water	:	Gum
4	:	2	:	1

In this case 60 mL of Cod Liver Oil BP is required, therefore 4 parts = 60 mL. One part will therefore be 60 ÷ 4 = 15. Therefore, the amount of freshly boiled and cooled purified water needed is 2 × 15 mL = 30 mL. The amount of acacia required = 15 g.

Therefore the product formula for 200 mL of Cod Liver Oil 30% emulsion is:

	200 mL
Cod Liver Oil BP	60 mL
Acacia BP	15 g
Double Strength Chloroform Water BP	100 mL
Freshly boiled and cooled purified water	to 200 mL

Interim formula for Double Strength Chloroform Water BP (see Section 2.1.23):

Concentrated Chloroform Water BPC 1959	5 mL
Freshly boiled and cooled purified water	to 100 mL

Method:
1. Calculate the composition of a convenient quantity of Double Strength Chloroform Water BP, sufficient to satisfy the formula requirements but also enabling simple, accurate measurement of the concentrated component. Method of compounding for Double Strength Chloroform Water BP:

    a. In this case, 100 mL of Double Strength Chloroform Water BP is required. To prepare 100 mL Double Strength Chloroform Water BP, measure 5 mL of Concentrated Chloroform water BPC 1959 accurately using a 5 mL conical measure.

    b. Add approximately 90 mL of freshly boiled and cooled purified water to a 100 mL conical measure (i.e. sufficient water to enable dissolution of the concentrated chloroform component without reaching the final volume of the product).

Example 8.2 Continued

Point of clarity – Step b

Although potable water would usually be used in the manufacture of Double Strength Chloroform Water BP, freshly boiled and cooled purified water is used here as emulsions are susceptible to microbial contamination.

c. Add the measured Concentrated Chloroform Water BPC 1959 to the water in the conical measure.
d. Stir gently and then accurately make up to volume with freshly boiled and cooled purified water.
e. Visually check that no undissolved chloroform remains at the bottom of the measure.

 See Solutions video for a demonstration of the preparation of Double Strength Chloroform Water BP.

Point of clarity – Method

Remember the accurate preparation of the primary emulsion is crucial for the full emulsion to be satisfactorily produced.

Primary emulsion:

Cod Liver Oil BP	60 mL
Double Strength Chloroform Water BP	30 mL
Acacia BP	15 g

2. Weigh 15 g of Acacia BP on a Class II or electronic balance.
3. Accurately measure 100 mL Double Strength Chloroform Water BP using a 100 mL measure.
4. Accurately measure 60 mL Cod Liver Oil BP in a conical measure.
5. Transfer the Cod Liver Oil BP to a clean dry porcelain mortar.

Point of clarity – Step 5

Ensure the measure is well drained as the quantities to be used are critical in the formation of the primary emulsion.

6. Measure 30 mL of Double Strength Chloroform Water BP (from the 100 mL measured in Step 3).
7. Transfer the Acacia BP to the mortar and stir gently (approximately three stirs).

Point of clarity – Step 7

This step is to wet the Acacia BP. Gentle stirring is required to ensure that there is no heat production that might denature the gum and prevent the formation of the emulsion.

8. Add the 30 mL of Double Strength Chloroform Water BP to the mortar in one go.
9. Stir vigorously with the pestle in ONE direction only until the primary emulsion is formed.

Point of clarity – Step 9

A characteristic clicking sound will be heard when the primary emulsion is formed. Remember, the whiter the primary emulsion the better it is formed.

10. Add more Double Strength Chloroform Water BP to the primary emulsion until the emulsion is pourable.

Example 8.2 Continued

> *Point of clarity – Step 10*
> The Double Strength Chloroform Water BP needs to be added to the primary emulsion drop by drop until it is pourable to ensure that the primary emulsion does not crack.

11. Transfer to an appropriate conical measure with rinsings.
12. Make up to volume with any remaining Double Strength Chloroform Water BP and freshly boiled and cooled purified water.

> *Point of clarity – Step 12*
> Even though there is a preservative in the preparation, freshly boiled and cooled purified water is used here as emulsions are susceptible to microbial contamination.

13. Stir and transfer to an amber flat medical bottle, label and dispense to the patient.

 See Emulsions video for a demonstration of the preparation of an emulsion.

Example 8.3 Preparation of a magistral formulation of 150 mL of Arachis Oil BP 40% emulsion with a peppermint flavouring from a doctor's prescription

Before deciding the formula for the emulsion, the type and quantity of flavouring must be decided upon. Concentrated Peppermint Emulsion BP (see Section 5.5.11) is a suitable flavouring and the dose is 0.25–1 mL. The dose of the emulsion is 15 mL bd, which means each individual dose is 15 mL, therefore in 150 mL there would be 10 doses. The amount of Concentrated Peppermint Emulsion BP that would be suitable to use would be $10 \times 0.25 = 2.5$ mL.

Product formula:

	Master (100 mL)	50 mL	150 mL
Arachis Oil BP	40 mL	20 mL	60 mL
Acacia BP	qs	qs	qs
Concentrated Peppermint Emulsion BP	qs	qs	2.5 mL
Double Strength Chloroform Water BP	50 mL	25 mL	75 mL
Freshly boiled and cooled purified water	to 100 mL	to 50 mL	to 150 mL

First it is necessary to calculate the quantity of emulsifying agent (Acacia BP) required to produce 150 mL of the emulsion. As Arachis oil is a fixed oil, the primary emulsion ration is:

Oil	:	Water	:	Gum
4	:	2	:	1

In this case 60 mL of Arachis Oil BP is required, therefore 4 parts = 60 mL.

One part will therefore be $60 \div 4 = 15$. Therefore, the amount of freshly boiled and cooled purified water needed is 2×15 mL = 30 mL. The amount of Acacia BP required = 15 g.

Therefore the product formula for 150 mL of Arachis Oil BP 40% emulsion is:

	150 mL
Arachis Oil BP	60 mL
Acacia BP	15 g
Concentrated Peppermint Emulsion BP	2.5 mL
Double Strength Chloroform Water BP	75 mL
Freshly boiled and cooled purified water	to 150 mL

Interim formula for Double Strength Chloroform Water BP (see Section 2.1.23):

Concentrated Chloroform Water BPC 1959	5 mL
Freshly boiled and cooled purified water	to 100 mL

Method:
1. Calculate the composition of a convenient quantity of Double Strength Chloroform Water BP, sufficient to satisfy the formula requirements but also enabling simple, accurate measurement of the concentrated component.

Example 8.3 Continued

Method of compounding for Double Strength Chloroform Water BP:

a. In this case, 75 mL of Double Strength Chloroform Water BP is required and so it would be sensible to prepare 100 mL. To prepare 100 mL Double Strength Chloroform Water BP, measure 5 mL of Concentrated Chloroform water BPC 1959 accurately using a 5 mL conical measure.

b. Add approximately 90 mL of freshly boiled and cooled purified water to a 100 mL conical measure (i.e. sufficient water to enable dissolution of the concentrated chloroform component without reaching the final volume of the product).

> *Point of clarity – Step b*
> Although potable water would usually be used in the manufacture of Double Strength Chloroform Water BP, freshly boiled and cooled purified water is used here as emulsions are susceptible to microbial contamination.

c. Add the measured Concentrated Chloroform Water BPC 1959 to the water in the conical measure.

d. Stir gently and then accurately make up to volume with freshly boiled and cooled purified water.

e. Visually check that no undissolved chloroform remains at the bottom of the measure.

 See Solutions video for a demonstration of the preparation of Double Strength Chloroform Water BP.

Point of clarity – Method
Remember the accurate preparation of the primary emulsion is crucial for the full emulsion to be satisfactorily produced.

Primary emulsion:

Arachis Oil BP	60 mL
Double Strength Chloroform Water BP	30 mL
Acacia BP	15 g

2. Weigh 15 g of Acacia BP on a Class II or electronic balance.
3. Accurately measure 75 mL Double Strength Chloroform Water BP using a 100 mL measure.
4. Accurately measure 60 mL Arachis Oil BP in a conical measure.
5. Transfer the Arachis Oil BP to a clean dry porcelain mortar.

> *Point of clarity – Step 5*
> Ensure the measure is well drained as the quantities to be used are critical in the formation of the primary emulsion.

6. Measure 30 mL of Double Strength Chloroform Water BP (from the 75 mL measured in Step 3).
7. Transfer the Acacia BP to the mortar and stir gently (approximately three stirs).

> *Point of clarity – Step 7*
> This is to wet the Acacia BP. Gentle stirring is required to ensure that there is no heat production that might denature the gum and prevent the formation of the emulsion.

8. Add the 30 mL of Double Strength Chloroform Water BP to the mortar all in one go.
9. Stir vigorously with the pestle in ONE direction only until the primary emulsion is formed.

Example 8.3 Continued

Point of clarity – Step 9
A characteristic clicking sound will be heard when the primary emulsion is formed. Remember, the whiter the primary emulsion the better it is formed.

10. Add more Double Strength Chloroform Water BP to the primary emulsion until the emulsion is pourable.

    Point of clarity – Step 10
    The Double Strength Chloroform Water BP needs to be added drop by drop to the primary emulsion until it is pourable to ensure that the primary emulsion does not crack.

11. Transfer to an appropriate conical measure with rinsings.
12. Measure 2.5 mL of Concentrated Peppermint Emulsion BP using an appropriate syringe.
13. Add the Concentrated Peppermint Emulsion BP to the emulsion in the conical measure.

    Point of clarity – Step 13
    The Concentrated Peppermint Emulsion BP is added just prior to making up to volume as it is a volatile ingredient.

14. Make up to volume with any remaining Double Strength Chloroform Water BP and freshly boiled and cooled purified water.

    Point of clarity – Step 14
    Even though there is a preservative in the preparation, freshly boiled and cooled purified water is used here as emulsions are susceptible to microbial contamination.

15. Stir and transfer to an amber flat medical bottle, label and dispense to the patient.

 See Emulsions video for a demonstration of the preparation of an emulsion.

Example 8.4 The preparation of a magistral formulation of 200 mL of Liquid Paraffin BP 15% emulsion from a doctor's prescription

Product formula:

	Master (100 mL)	200 mL
Liquid Paraffin BP	15 mL	30 mL
Acacia BP	qs	qs
Double Strength Chloroform Water BP	50 mL	100 mL
Freshly boiled and cooled purified water	to 100 mL	to 200 mL

First it is necessary to calculate the quantity of emulsifying agent (Acacia BP) required to produce 200 mL of the emulsion. Liquid Paraffin BP is a mineral oil, therefore the primary emulsion ratio is:

Oil	:	Water	:	Gum
3	:	2	:	1

Since 30 mL of Liquid Paraffin BP is required, 3 parts = 30 mL. One part will therefore be 30 ÷ 3 = 10. Therefore, the amount of freshly boiled and cooled purified water needed is 2 × 10 = 20 mL. The amount of Acacia BP required = 10 g.

Therefore the product formula for 200 mL of Liquid Paraffin BP 30% emulsion is:

	200 mL
Liquid Paraffin BP	30 mL
Acacia BP	10 g
Double Strength Chloroform Water BP	100 mL
Freshly boiled and cooled purified water	to 200 mL

Interim formula for Double Strength Chloroform Water BP (see Section 2.1.23):

Concentrated Chloroform Water BPC 1959	5 mL
Freshly boiled and cooled purified water	to 100 mL

Method:

1. Calculate the composition of a convenient quantity of Double Strength Chloroform Water BP, sufficient to satisfy the formula requirements but also enabling simple, accurate measurement of the concentrated component. Method of compounding for Double Strength Chloroform Water BP:

   a. In this case, 100 mL of Double Strength Chloroform Water BP is required. To prepare 100 mL Double Strength Chloroform Water BP, measure 5 mL of Concentrated Chloroform water BPC 1959 accurately using a 5 mL conical measure.

   b. Add approximately 90 mL of freshly boiled and cooled purified water to a 100 mL conical measure (i.e. sufficient water to enable dissolution of the concentrated chloroform component without reaching the final volume of the product).

   Point of clarity – Step b
   Although potable water would usually be used in the manufacture of Double Strength Chloroform Water BP, freshly boiled and cooled purified water is used here as emulsions are susceptible to microbial contamination.

Example 8.4 Continued

  c. Add the measured Concentrated Chloroform Water BPC 1959 to the water in the conical measure.

  d. Stir gently and then accurately make up to volume with freshly boiled and cooled purified water.

  e. Visually check that no undissolved chloroform remains at the bottom of the measure.

See Solutions video for a demonstration of the preparation of Double Strength Chloroform Water BP.

Point of clarity – Method
Remember, the accurate preparation of the primary emulsion is crucial for the full emulsion to be satisfactorily produced.

Primary emulsion:

Liquid Paraffin BP	30 mL
Double Strength Chloroform Water BP	20 mL
Acacia BP	10 g

2. Weigh 10 g of Acacia BP on a Class II or electronic balance.

3. Accurately measure 100 mL Double Strength Chloroform Water BP using a 100 mL measure.

4. Accurately measure 30 mL Liquid Paraffin BP in a conical measure.

5. Transfer the Liquid Paraffin BP to a clean dry porcelain mortar.

Point of clarity – Step 5
Ensure the measure is well drained as the quantities to be used are critical in the formation of the primary emulsion.

6. Measure 20 mL of Double Strength Chloroform Water BP (from the 100 mL measured in Step 3).

7. Transfer the Acacia BP to the mortar and stir gently (approximately three stirs).

Point of clarity – Step 7
This is to wet the acacia. Gentle stirring is required to ensure that there is no heat production that might denature the gum and prevent the formation of the emulsion.

8. Add the 20 mL of Double Strength Chloroform Water BP to the mortar all in one go.

9. Stir vigorously with the pestle in ONE direction only until the primary emulsion is formed.

Point of clarity – Step 9
A characteristic clicking sound will be heard when the primary emulsion is formed. Remember, the whiter the primary emulsion the better it is formed.

10. Add more Double Strength Chloroform Water BP to the primary emulsion until the emulsion is pourable.

Point of clarity – Step 10
The Double Strength Chloroform Water BP needs to be added drop by drop to the primary emulsion until it is pourable to ensure that the primary emulsion does not crack.

11. Transfer to an appropriate conical measure with rinsings.

Example 8.4 Continued

12. Make up to volume with any remaining Double Strength Chloroform Water BP and freshly boiled and cooled purified water.

> *Point of clarity – Step 12*
> Even though there is a preservative in the preparation, freshly boiled and cooled purified water is used here as emulsions are susceptible to microbial contamination.

13. Stir and transfer to an amber flat medical bottle, label and dispense to the patient.

 See Emulsions video for a demonstration of the preparation of an emulsion.

 Example 8.5 Preparation of 100 mL of Liquid Paraffin Emulsion BP

Product formula (British Pharmacopoeia 1988, page 744):

	1000 mL	100 mL
Liquid Paraffin BP	500 mL	50 mL
Vanillin BP	500 mg	50 mg
Chloroform BP	2.5 mL	0.25 mL
Benzoic Acid Solution BP	20 mL	2 mL
Methylcellulose 20 BP	20 g	2 g
Saccharin Sodium BP	50 mg	5 mg
Freshly boiled and cooled purified water	to 1000 mL	to 100 mL

Method:
1. Heat about 12 mL of freshly boiled and cooled purified water.
2. Weigh 2 g Methylcellulose 20 BP on a Class II or electronic balance.
3. Add the Methylcellulose 20 BP to the heated water.
4. Allow to stand for about 30 minutes to hydrate.
5. Add sufficient freshly boiled and cooled purified water in the form of ice to produce 35 mL and stir.
6. Measure 2 mL of Benzoic Acid Solution BP using a syringe.
7. Measure 0.25 mL of Chloroform BP.
8. Weigh 50 mg Vanillin BP using a sensitive electronic balance (see Section 4.1.2).
9. Mix the Chloroform BP and Benzoic Acid Solution BP together.
10. Dissolve the Vanillin BP in the benzoic acid and chloroform mixture.

> *Point of clarity – Step 10*
> Vanillin BP is only slightly soluble in water but freely soluble in alcohol and soluble in ether. It is therefore more soluble in organic solvents and so is added to the chloroform-containing mixture.

Example 8.5 Continued

11. Add this solution to the previously prepared methylcellulose mucilage and stir for 5 minutes.
12. Prepare a sodium saccharin trituration and add sufficient (5 mL) to provide 5 mg of Sodium Saccharin BP to the mixture.

> *Point of clarity – Step 12*
> The amount of Sodium Saccharin BP cannot be accurately weighed therefore a trituration must be prepared. Water is the diluent chosen as this is also the vehicle for the emulsion.
>
> Trituration for Sodium Saccharin:
>
> | Saccharin Sodium BP | 150 mg |
> |---|---|
> | Freshly boiled and cooled purified water | to 150 mL |
>
> Therefore 5 mL of the trituration will contain 5 mg of Sodium Saccharin BP.

13. Make the volume of the mucilage mixture up to 50 mL with freshly boiled and cooled purified water.
14. Measure 50 mL of Liquid Paraffin BP in a 50 mL conical measure.
15. Mix the 50 mL mucilage and 50 mL of Liquid Paraffin BP together and stir constantly.
16. Pass through a homogeniser to make the emulsion more stable.

> *Point of clarity – Step 16*
> The stability of an emulsion is increased with smaller globule size of the disperse phase. When an emulsion is passed through a homogeniser the emulsion is forced through a fine opening to apply shearing forces to reduce the size of the globules. Although many extemporaneously prepared emulsions do not require the use of a homogeniser, this step may aid in retarding or preventing creaming of the emulsion on long standing.

 See Picture 28

17. Transfer to an amber flat medical bottle with a child-resistant closure, label and dispense.

Example 8.6 Preparation of 200 mL of White Liniment BP

Product formula (British Pharmacopoeia 1988, page 700):

	1000 mL	100 mL	200 mL
Oleic Acid BP	85 mL	8.5 mL	17 mL
Turpentine Oil BP	250 mL	25 mL	50 mL
Dilute Ammonia Solution BP	45 mL	4.5 mL	9 mL
Ammonium Chloride BP	12.5 g	1.25 g	2.5 g
Freshly boiled and cooled purified water	625 mL	62.5 mL	125 mL

Method:
1. Measure 17 mL Oleic Acid BP.
2. Measure 50 mL Turpentine Oil BP.
3. Mix together the Turpentine Oil BP and Oleic Acid BP in a mortar.
4. Measure 9 mL Dilute Ammonia Solution BP and transfer to a beaker.
5. Add an equal volume of warm freshly boiled and cooled purified water to the Dilute Ammonia Solution BP.
6. Add to the oily phase and mix vigorously.
7. Weigh 2.5 g of Ammonium Chloride BP on a Class II or electronic balance.
8. Add the Ammonium Chloride BP to the remaining freshly boiled and cooled purified water in a beaker and stir to dissolve.
9. Add the solution in Step 8 to the emulsion and mix.
10. Measure 200 mL of the emulsion and transfer to an amber fluted medical bottle.

   Point of clarity – Method
   This is an ammonium soap type of emulsion. The interaction between the fatty acid (oleic acid) and ammonia produces ammonium oleate, an oil-in-water emulgent. The ammonium chloride, however, suppresses the ionisation of the soap by the common ion effect and this, combined with the relatively large volume of turpentine oil in the product, causes phase inversion and a water-in-oil emulsion is formed.

8.7 Summary of essential principles relating to emulsions

This section will recap the main principles relating to emulsions that have been covered in other sections of the book. To assist compounders in understanding the extemporaneous preparation of emulsions, this section contains the following:

- Further notes on the packaging of extemporaneously prepared emulsions.
- Specific points relevant to the expiry of extemporaneously prepared emulsions.
- Additional key points related to the labelling of pharmaceutical emulsions.

8.7.1 Packaging

The packaging of extemporaneous preparations has been covered previously in Section 5.7. An overview of the main considerations for the packaging of emulsions will be given here.

With pharmaceutical emulsions intended for internal use, a suitable container would be a flat amber medical bottle. External emulsions (e.g. creams, liniments, lotions, etc.) would be packaged in suitable containers, for example a fluted amber bottle for liniments and lotions and a collapsible tube for a cream (see Section 9.5.1).

Pharmaceutical bottles come in a variety of different sizes and it is important to choose a suitably sized container to match the volume of preparation to be dispensed. Obviously it is important not to use a size of container that is too large for the volume of preparation to be dispensed, for both cost and appearance reasons. Consideration should be given to selecting a bottle that will leave sufficient space to allow the product to be shaken adequately before a dose is measured.

Guidelines on the packaging of extemporaneously prepared emulsions are summarised in Table 8.5.

8.7.2 Discard dates

Discard dates for pharmaceutical emulsions typically mirror those for pharmaceutical solutions (see Section 6.8.2). The discard date of official preparations will be advised via the relative official texts. As with solutions and suspensions, for official preparations the BP employs two definitions that are useful when extemporaneously compounding emulsions:

- **'Freshly Prepared'** refers to a preparation that has been compounded less than 24 hours prior to issue for use.
- **'Recently Prepared'** should be applied to compounded items that are likely to deteriorate if stored for a period greater than four weeks when maintained at 15–25 °C.

Traditionally it was suggested that an expiry date of four weeks be applied to oral emulsions in the absence of any official guidance. Although emulsions usually contain a preservative (Double Strength Chloroform Water BP at 50% v/v), they are liable to microbial contamination. For this reason, consideration should be given to shortening the expiry date to 7–14 days.

Remember that because patients frequently misunderstand the term 'expiry' it is suggested that a preferred method of indicating shelf life on the label of extemporaneously compounded products is to apply the term 'Discard after' followed by a definite date and/or time.

Further guidance on expiry dates for pharmaceutical preparations can be found in Section 5.6.1.

Table 8.5 Summary of packaging for pharmaceutical emulsions

		Typical sizes
Oral emulsions	Amber flat medical bottle (wide-mouthed if available)	50 mL, 100 mL, 150 mL, 200 mL, 300 mL and 500 mL
External emulsions (applications and lotions)	Amber fluted medical bottle (wide-mouthed if available)	50 mL, 100 mL, 200 mL

8.7.3 Labelling

The labelling of pharmaceutical emulsions has been covered in Section 5.6.2. An overview of the main considerations for the labelling of emulsions will be given here.

In addition to the standard requirements for the labelling of extemporaneous preparations, the following points need to be taken into consideration:

- '**Shake the bottle**' – All emulsions will require this additional label.
- '**For external use only**' – This warning must be added to the label of any external emulsion.

Further guidance on auxiliary labelling can be found in Section 5.6.1, Table 5.10.

9

Creams

9.1 Introduction and overview

In pharmacy the term 'cream' is reserved for external preparations. Creams are viscous semi-solid emulsions for external use. Medicaments can be dissolved or suspended in creams.

A cream may be 'water-in-oil' or 'oil-in-water' depending on the emulsifying agent used. A cream is always miscible with its continuous phase.

- **Water-in-oil creams** (oily creams) as bases – These are produced by the emulsifying agents of natural origin (e.g. beeswax, wool alcohols or wool fat). These bases have good emollient properties. They are creamy, white or translucent and rather stiff.
- **Oil-in-water creams** (aqueous creams) as bases – These are produced by the synthetic waxes (e.g. macrogol and cetomacrogol). They are the best bases to use for rapid absorption and penetration of drugs. They are thin, white and smooth in consistency.

The British Pharmacopoeia (BP) definition is as follows:

Creams are formulated to provide preparations that are essentially miscible with the skin secretion. They are intended to be applied to the skin or certain mucous membranes for protective, therapeutic or prophylactic purposes especially where an occlusive effect is not necessary.

9.2 Terminology used in the preparation of creams, ointments, pastes and gels

Two common terms used in the extemporaneous preparation of creams and in the extemporaneous preparation of ointments, pastes and gels (see

Chapter 10) are trituration (= mixing) and levigation (= grinding).

9.2.1 Trituration

This is the term applied to the incorporation, into the base, of finely divided insoluble powders or liquids. The powders are placed on the tile and the base is incorporated using the 'doubling-up' technique. Liquids are usually incorporated by placing a small amount of base on a tile and making a 'well' in the centre. Small quantities of liquid are then added and mixed in. It is important to take care not to form air pockets that contain liquid, which if squeezed when using an inappropriate mixing action, will spray fluid on the compounder and surrounding area.

 See Ointments video for a demonstration of trituration.

Trituration can be successfully achieved using a mortar but this method is usually reserved for large quantities.

9.2.2 Levigation

This is the term applied to the incorporation into the base of insoluble coarse powders. It is often termed 'wet grinding'. It is the process where the powder is rubbed down with either the molten base or a semi-solid base. A considerable shearing force is applied to avoid a gritty product.

9.2.3 Methods for incorporating solids and liquids into cream and ointment bases

Table 9.1 gives a summary of the methods used for incorporating solids and liquids into cream or ointment bases.

9.3 General principles of cream preparation

9.3.1 The preparation of a cream from first principles

- As with other types of emulsion, hygiene is extremely important and all surfaces, spatulas and other equipment must be thoroughly cleaned with industrial methylated spirits (IMS). IMS is better than freshly boiled and cooled purified water as it will quickly evaporate, leaving no residue.
- Always make an excess as it is never possible to transfer the entire cream into the final container.
- Determine which of the ingredients are soluble in/miscible with the aqueous phase and which with the oily phase. Dissolve the water-soluble ingredients in the aqueous phase.
- Melt the fatty bases in an evaporating dish over a water bath at the lowest possible temperature. Start with the base having the highest melting point. These should then be cooled to 60 °C (overheating can denature the emulsifying agent and the stability of the product can be lost).

Table 9.1 Summary of the methods for incorporating solids and liquids into cream and ointment bases

Medicament	Molten base	Solid base
Soluble powder	Fusion – dissolve in base at the lowest temperature possible	Trituration
Insoluble coarse powder	Levigation	Levigation with a small amount of solid base
Insoluble fine powder	Incorporate in small amounts, by trituration, as the base cools and thickens	Trituration
Volatile liquid	Incorporate when the ointment has cooled to below 40 °C by trituration	Trituration
Non-volatile liquid	Incorporate into molten base by trituration	Trituration

- Substances that are soluble/miscible with the oily phase should then be stirred into the melt.
- The temperature of the aqueous phase should then be adjusted to 60 °C.
- The disperse phase should then be added to the continuous phase at the same temperature.
  - Hence, for an oil-in-water (o/w) product add oil to water.
  - For a water-in-oil (w/o) product add water to oil.
- Stir the resulting emulsion without incorporating air, until the product sets. Do not hasten cooling as this produces a poor product.

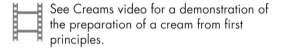 See Creams video for a demonstration of the preparation of a cream from first principles.

9.3.2 Incorporation of ingredients into a cream base

In addition to the preparation of a cream from first principles, it is common to incorporate either liquid or solid ingredients into a cream base.

Incorporation of solids into a cream base

If the cream base has been prepared from first principles (see Section 9.3.1), the solid can be incorporated into the cream as it cools. Alternatively, if using a pre-prepared base, soluble and insoluble solids may be incorporated using the method employed for insoluble solids.

- **Soluble solids** should be added to the molten cream at the lowest possible temperature and the mixture stirred until cold.
- **Insoluble solids** should be incorporated using an ointment tile and spatula. If there is more than one powder to be added these should be triturated together in a mortar using the 'doubling-up' technique prior to transfer to an ointment tile.

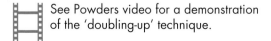 See Powders video for a demonstration of the 'doubling-up' technique.

- For **coarse powders** a minimum quantity of cream should be placed in the centre of the tile and used to levigate the powders. A considerable lateral shearing force should be applied to avoid a gritty product. The powder/fatty base mixture may then either be returned to the evaporating basin with the remaining cream and stirred until cold or the remaining cream in the evaporating basin may be allowed to cool and triturated with the powder/cream mixture on the tile.
- **Fine powders** may be triturated into the otherwise finished cream on an ointment tile. Small amounts of powder should be added to an equal amount of cream (i.e. using the 'doubling-up' technique). These should be well triturated.

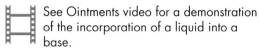 See Ointments video for a demonstration of the incorporation of a powder into a base.

Incorporation of liquids into a cream base

- **Non-volatile, miscible liquids** may be mixed with the molten cream in the evaporating basin. Alternatively, if a pre-prepared base is used, then incorporate as for volatile or immiscible liquids.
- **Volatile or immiscible liquids** (e.g. coal tar solutions) should be triturated with the cream on the ointment tile. A very small amount of the cream should be placed on the tile and a 'well' made in the centre. Traditionally, small quantities of liquid should be gently folded in to avoid splashing. An alternative method is to spread a small amount of the cream on the tile and then 'score' it with a spatula. Then add small quantities of the liquid and fold into the base gently. If using coal tar or other volatile ingredients, these should not be weighed until immediately before use and the beaker in which it has been weighed should be covered with a watch glass to prevent evaporation.

See Ointments video for a demonstration of the incorporation of a liquid into a base.

9.4 Worked examples

Example 9.1 Preparation of 20 g Cetrimide Cream BP

Product formula (British Pharmacopoeia 1988, page 653):

	1000 g	100 g	10 g	30 g
Cetrimide BP	5 g	500 mg	50 mg	150 mg
Cetostearyl Alcohol BP	50 g	5 g	500 mg	1.5 g
Liquid Paraffin BP	500 g	50 g	5 g	15 g
Freshly boiled and cooled purified water	445 g	44.5 g	4.45 g	13.35 g

Point of clarity – Product formula
The exact quantity cannot be prepared for a cream as losses will be encountered on transfer. Therefore, a suitable overage must be produced in order to dispense the required final amount. Note that all liquid ingredients (including the Liquid Paraffin BP) must be weighed.

Melting points and solubilities of the ingredients:

Melting point:	Cetostearyl Alcohol BP	49–56 °C
Solubilities:	Cetostearyl Alcohol BP	Practically insoluble in water
		When melted, miscible with liquid paraffin
	Cetrimide BP	Soluble in 2 parts water
	Liquid Paraffin BP	Practically insoluble in water
		Slightly soluble in alcohol
		Miscible with hydrocarbons

Method to prepare 30 g of Cetrimide Cream BP from the formula above:
1. Weigh 1.5 g Cetostearyl Alcohol BP on a Class II or electronic balance.
2. Weigh 15 g of Liquid Paraffin BP on a Class II or electronic balance.
3. Weigh 13.35 g of freshly boiled and cooled purified water on a Class II or electronic balance.
4. Weigh 150 mg of Cetrimide BP on a Class II or electronic balance.
5. Melt the Cetostearyl Alcohol BP in an evaporating basin over a water bath to a temperature no higher than 60 °C.
6. Add the Liquid Paraffin BP to the molten Cetostearyl Alcohol BP and remove from the heat.
7. Stir to form the OILY phase.
8. Transfer the freshly boiled and cooled purified water to a beaker and heat to 60 °C.
9. Add the Cetrimide BP to the freshly boiled and cooled purified water and remove from the heat.
10. Stir to form the AQUEOUS phase.
11. When the oily phase and the aqueous phase are both at about 60 °C, add the aqueous phase to the oily phase with constant, not too vigorous stirring.

> *Point of clarity – Step 11*
> Stirring is constant and not too vigorous to ensure that there are no 'cold spots' within the cream as these would hasten cooling in discrete areas and result in a lumpy cream.

12. Stir until cool enough to pack.
13. Weigh 20 g of the product and pack into an amber glass jar; label and dispense.

 See Creams video for a demonstration of the preparation of a cream from first principles.

Example 9.2 Preparation of 20 g of Salicylic Acid and Sulphur Cream BP

Product formula (British Pharmacopoeia 1980, page 548):

	1000 g	100 g	10 g	30 g
Salicylic Acid BP	20 g	2 g	200 mg	600 mg
Precipitated Sulphur BP	20 g	2 g	200 mg	600 mg
Aqueous Cream BP	960 g	96 g	9.6 g	28.8 g

Method to prepare 30 g of Salicylic Acid and Sulphur Cream BP from the formula above:

1. Weigh 600 mg Salicylic Acid BP on a Class II or electronic balance.
2. Transfer to a glass mortar and grind with a pestle.
3. Weigh 600 mg Precipitated Sulphur BP on a Class II or electronic balance.
4. Add to the Salicylic Acid BP in the glass mortar and continue mixing with a pestle until a smooth, well mixed powder is formed.
5. Transfer the powder to a glass tile.
6. Weigh 28.8 g Aqueous Cream BP on a Class II or electronic balance.
7. Transfer the Aqueous Cream BP to the glass tile and triturate with the powders to produce a smooth product.

   Point of clarity – Step 7
   Note: a vulcanite spatula would be the spatula of choice as traditional stainless steel spatulas may react with acids, tannins, iodine and mercury salts, etc. Vulcanite (also called ebonite) is a hard, usually black rubber, produced by vulcanizing natural rubber with sulphur. Such spatulas are used for making ointments containing corrosive substances or substances that react with steel.

8. Weigh 20 g of the product and pack into an amber glass jar. Label and dispense.

Example 9.3 Preparation of 50 g of Dermovate Cream 25%

Product formula (i.e. the diluent to use) must be decided by the compounder. Refer to a diluent directory, which in this case states that although the dilution of the product is not recommended by the manufacturer, in cases where it is insisted upon, the following may be used:

- Aqueous Cream BP – Only stable if less than 50% of the resultant cream. Therefore unsuitable for this formulation.
- Buffered Cream BP – May be used but can raise the pH of the resulting cream.
- Cetomacrogol Cream (Formula A) BPC – No problems with dilution recorded.

Therefore in this instance the diluent of choice would be Cetomacrogol Cream (Formula A) BPC.

Point of clarity – sources of information
Suitable sources to provide information on the dilution of creams and ointments would be:

- NPA Diluent Directory
- Product data sheet (Summary of Product Characteristics – SPC)
- Reports in the pharmaceutical literature
- Personal contact with product manufacturer.

Product formula:

	Master formula	100 g	10 g	60 g
Dermovate Cream	25%	25 g	2.5 g	15 g
Cetomacrogol Cream (Formula A) BPC	75%	75 g	7.5 g	45 g

Method to prepare 60 g of Dermovate Cream 25% from the formula above:
1. Weigh 15 g Dermovate Cream on Class II or electronic balance.
2. Transfer to a glass tile.
3. Weigh 45 g Cetomacrogol Cream (Formula A) BPC on as Class II or electronic balance.
4. Transfer to the glass tile.
5. Triturate the Dermovate Cream with the Cetomacrogol Cream (Formula A) BPC using a spatula.

Point of clarity – Step 5
When triturating the creams together remember the principle of 'doubling-up' in order to achieve an adequate mix of the active Dermovate Cream and the base cream.

6. Weigh 50 g of the final cream on a Class II or electronic balance.
7. Pack into an amber glass jar, label and dispense to the patient.

9.5 Summary of essential principles relating to creams

This section will recap the main principles relating to creams that have been covered in other sections of the book. To assist compounders in understanding the extemporaneous preparation of creams, this section contains the following:

- Further notes on the packaging of extemporaneously prepared creams.
- Specific points relevant to the expiry of extemporaneously prepared creams.
- Additional key points relating to the labelling of pharmaceutical creams.

9.5.1 Packaging

The packaging of extemporaneous preparations has been covered in Section 5.7. An overview of the main considerations for the packaging of creams will be given here. As all pharmaceutical creams are intended for external use, a suitable container would be either an amber wide-necked ointment jar or a metal collapsible tube.

Pharmaceutical ointment jars come in a variety of different sizes and it is important to choose a suitably sized container to match the volume of preparation to be dispensed. This is best done by eye. Obviously it is important not to use a size of container that is too large for the volume of preparation to be dispensed, for both cost and appearance reasons. Do not be fooled by the size marked on the bottom of the jar: the value refers to the weight of water that the container will hold. As ointments are less dense than water, 100 g of ointment will not fit in a 100 g ointment jar.

Amber glass jars are preferable to clear glass jars as they protect the preparation from degradation by light. More recently, plastic ointment jars have become available and although cheaper than glass jars, are less preferable because of an increased likelihood of the products reacting with the container (e.g. as can occur with preparations containing coal tar).

When packaging a cream into an ointment jar, ensure that the cream is packed well and that no air pockets are visible. This will produce a product with a professional appearance.

 See Creams video for a demonstration of the packaging of a cream.

9.5.2 Discard dates

Some official texts may give a suggested discard date for certain extemporaneously prepared creams. In the absence of any guide, it is suggested that creams are given a four-week discard date. This is significantly shorter than the suggested discard date for extemporaneously prepared ointments (which is three months) because of their susceptibility for microbial contamination (see Section 10.6.2).

Diluted creams (see Example 9.3) would normally be given a two-week discard date.

Remember that as patients frequently misunderstand the term 'expiry' it is suggested that a preferred method of indicating shelf life on the label of extemporaneously compounded products is to apply the term 'Discard after' followed by a definite date and/or time.

Further guidance on expiry dates for pharmaceutical preparations can be found in Section 5.6.1.

9.5.3 Labelling

The labelling of pharmaceutical creams has been covered in Section 5.6.2. An overview of the main considerations for the labelling of creams will be given here.

In addition to the standard requirements for the labelling of extemporaneous preparations, the following points need to be taken into consideration:

- **'For external use only'** – This warning must be added to the label of all extemporaneously prepared creams as all creams are for external use only.

Further guidance on auxiliary labelling can be found in Section 5.6.1, Table 5.10.

10

Ointments, pastes and gels

10.1 Introduction and overview

This chapter will focus on three common dosage forms: ointments, pastes and gels.

10.2 Ointments

Ointments are preparations for external application but differ from creams in that they have greasy bases. The base is usually anhydrous and immiscible with skin secretions. Ointments usually contain a medicament or a mixture of medicaments dissolved or dispersed in the base.

According to the British Pharmacopoeia (BP):

Ointments are formulated to provide preparations that are immiscible, miscible or emulsifiable with the skin secretion. Hydrophobic ointments and water-emulsifying ointments are intended to be applied to the skin or certain mucous membranes for emollient, protective, therapeutic or prophylactic purposes where a degree of occlusion is desired. Hydrophilic ointments are miscible with the skin secretion and are less emollient as a consequence.

10.2.1 Ointment bases

The base of a traditional ointment consists of a mixture of waxes, fats and oils:

- **Waxes** – Solid and hard at room temperature.
- **Fats** – Semi-solid, soft at room temperature.
- **Oils** – Liquid at room temperature.

A change in temperature can affect the physical state of a base (e.g. coconut oil is solid in winter but is more likely to be liquid in summer).

The addition of a wax to an ointment makes the preparation smoother and lighter in consistency. Altering the proportions of oil, fat and wax in the ointment may vary the consistency. For example, extra wax will make the ointment stiffer; extra oil will make the ointment less viscous. The proportions used may vary depending on storage or the climatic conditions (e.g. whether the product is intended for use in the Tropics or in the Arctic).

Different types of ointment bases are available (see below and also Section 5.5.3).

Hydrocarbon bases

These bases are immiscible with water and are not absorbed by the skin. They usually consist of soft paraffin or mixtures of soft paraffin with hard paraffin or liquid paraffin. The paraffins form a greasy waterproof film on the skin. This inhibits water loss from the skin, thereby improving the hydration of the skin, which is particularly important in the treatment of dry scaly conditions (see also Section 5.5.3).

Absorption bases

Absorption bases are good emollients and are less occlusive and easier to apply than hydrocarbon bases (see also Section 5.5.3). Absorption bases can be divided into non-emulsified bases and water-in-oil emulsions:

- **Non-emulsified** – These bases absorb water to form water-in-oil emulsions. Generally they consist of a hydrocarbon base combined with a water-in-oil emulsifier such as Wool Alcohols BP or Wool Fat BP.

Emulsifying agent	Ointment
Wool Alcohols BP	Wool Alcohols Ointment BP
Wool Fat BP	Simple Ointment BP

- **Water-in-oil emulsions** – These are similar to non-emulsified bases but are capable of absorbing more water. The constituents of emulsified bases include Hydrous Wool Fat BP (lanolin) and Oily Cream BP (Hydrous Ointment BP).

Water-miscible/emulsifying bases

These are anhydrous bases that contain oil-in-water emulsifying agents, which makes them miscible with water and therefore washable and easily removed after use. The following three emulsifying ointments are used as water-miscible bases:

- Emulsifying Ointment BP (anionic)
- Cetrimide Emulsifying Ointment BP (cationic)
- Cetomacrogol Emulsifying Ointment BPC (non-ionic).

As the bases mix readily with the aqueous secretions of the skin and therefore wash out easily, they are particularly suitable for use on the scalp (see also Section 5.5.3).

Hydrophilic bases

These have been developed from polyethylene glycols (macrogols). They are non-occlusive, mix readily with skin secretions and are easily removed by washing (e.g. Macrogol Ointment BP). Macrogol bases are commonly used with local anaesthetics such as Lidocaine BP (see also Section 5.5.3).

10.2.2 General method for ointment preparation

This section contains information on the preparation of ointments by fusion and the incorporation of both solids and liquids into ointment bases. An explanation of the terminology used in ointment preparation can be found in Section 9.2 and a summary of the methods for incorporating solids and liquids into cream or ointment bases can be found in Table 9.1.

Fusion

This involves melting together the bases over a water bath before incorporating any other ingredients. The ointment base may include a mixture of waxes, fats and oils, of which some are solid at room temperature and others are liquid:

- **Hard** – Paraffin BP, Beeswax BP, Cetostearyl Alcohol BP
- **Soft** – Yellow and White Soft Paraffin BP, Wool Fat BP
- **Liquid** – Liquid Paraffin BP and vegetable oils.

General method (fusion):

1. Always make excess as transference losses will always occur.
2. Determine the melting points of the fatty bases and then melt together. Starting with the base with the highest melting point, each base should be melted at the lowest possible temperature as the mixture progressively cools.
3. Add the ingredients to an evaporating basin over a water bath to avoid overheating – use a thermometer to check the temperature regularly.
4. As the first base cools add the ingredients with decreasing melting points at the respective temperatures, stirring continuously to ensure a homogeneous mix before leaving to set. It is important to stir gently to avoid incorporating excess air, which could result in localised cooling and a lumpy product.

 See Ointments video for a demonstration of the fusion method.

General method for incorporating powders into an ointment base

Soluble solids

Soluble solids should be added to the molten fatty bases at the lowest possible temperature and the mixture stirred until cold. Alternatively, if using a pre-prepared base, soluble solids may be incorporated using the method employed for insoluble solids.

Insoluble solids

Insoluble solids should be incorporated using an ointment tile and spatula. If there is more than one powder to be added these should be mixed in a mortar using the 'doubling-up' method.

 See Powders video for a demonstration of the 'doubling-up' technique.

- **Coarse powders** – A minimum quantity of molten fatty base should be placed in the centre of the tile and used to levigate the powders. A considerable shearing force should be applied to avoid a gritty product. The powder/fatty base mixture may then either be returned to the evaporating basin with the

remaining fatty base and stirred until cold, or the remaining fatty base in the evaporating basin may be allowed to cool and triturated with the powder/fatty base mixture on the tile.

- **Fine powders** may be triturated into the otherwise finished ointment on an ointment tile. Small amounts of powder should be added to an equal amount of ointment (i.e. using the 'doubling-up' technique). These should be well triturated to incorporate all of the ointment base. Alternatively, a small amount of powder may be levigated with some molten ointment base on a tile and the resulting mixture returned to the remaining molten mass and stirred to achieve a homogeneous product.

 See Ointments video for a demonstration of the incorporation of a powder into a base.

General method for incorporating liquids into an ointment base

Non-volatile, miscible liquids

Non-volatile, miscible liquids may be mixed with the molten fat in the evaporating basin. Alternatively, if a pre-prepared base is used, then incorporate as for volatile or immiscible liquids.

Volatile or immiscible liquids

Volatile or immiscible liquids (e.g. coal tar solutions) should be triturated with the ointment on the ointment tile. A very small amount of the ointment should be placed on the tile and a 'well' made in the centre. Traditionally, small quantities of liquid should be gently folded in to avoid splashing. An alternative method is to spread a small amount of the ointment on the tile and then 'score' it with a spatula. Then add small quantities of the liquid and fold into the base gently.

If using coal tar or other volatile ingredients, these should not be weighed until immediately before use and the beaker in which it has been weighed should be covered with a watch glass to prevent evaporation.

See Ointments video for a demonstration of the incorporation of a liquid into an ointment.

10.3 Pastes

Pastes are semi-solid preparations for external use. They consist of finely powdered medicaments combined with White Soft Paraffin BP or Liquid Paraffin BP or with a non-greasy base made from glycerol, mucilages or soaps. Pastes contain a high proportion of powdered ingredients and therefore are normally very stiff. Because pastes are stiff they do not spread easily and therefore this localises drug delivery. This is particularly important if the ingredient to be applied to the skin is corrosive, such as dithranol, coal tar or salicylic acid. It is easier to apply a paste to a discrete skin area such as a particular lesion or plaque, and thereby not compromising the integrity of healthy skin.

Pastes are also useful for absorbing harmful chemicals, such as the ammonia that is released by bacterial action on urine, and so are often used in nappy products. Also because of their high powder content, they are often used to absorb wound exudates.

Because pastes are so thick they can form an unbroken layer over the skin which is opaque and can act as a sun filter. This makes them suitable for use for skiers as they prevent excessive dehydration of the skin (wind burn) in addition to sun blocking.

The principal use of pastes traditionally was as an antiseptic, protective or soothing dressing. Often before application the paste was applied to lint and applied as a dressing.

10.4 Gels

Pharmaceutical gels are often simple-phase, transparent semi-solid systems that are being increasingly used as pharmaceutical topical formulations. The liquid phase of the gel may be retained within a three-dimensional polymer

Example 10.1 Compound Aluminium Paste BPC (also known as Baltimore Paste) (BPC 1973, page 767)

Formula:

Aluminium Powder BP	200 g
Zinc Oxide BP	400 g
Liquid Paraffin BP	400 g

Method:
1. Sieve the Aluminium Powder BP and the Zinc Oxide BP.
2. Mix the powders using the 'doubling-up' technique.
3. Mix the combined powders with the Liquid Paraffin BP, stirring until a smooth product is formed.

This was what was originally used to protect the skin and prevent maceration around colostomies and ileostomies.

Example 10.2 Zinc and Coal Tar Paste BP (also known as White's Tar Paste) (BP 1988, page 868)

Formula:

Zinc Oxide BP (finely sifted)	60 g
Coal Tar BP	60 g
Emulsifying Wax BP	50 g
Starch BP	380 g
Yellow Soft Paraffin BP	450 g

Method:
1. Melt the Yellow Soft Paraffin BP and Emulsifying Wax BP at the lowest possible temperature.
2. Mix well and stir until just setting.
3. Mix the powders using the 'doubling-up' technique.
4. Levigate the semi-molten base with the powders on a warmed tile.
5. Finally incorporate the Coal Tar BP.

The emulsifying wax is added to help with the dispersal of the coal tar through the product. The method outlined is designed to reduce the amount of heat to which the coal tar is exposed as the constituents of coal tar tend to precipitate out quickly on heating.

This is used as an antipruritic preparation.

Example 10.3 Zinc Gelatin BPC (also known as Unna's Paste) (BPC 1968, page 1097)

Formula:

Zinc Oxide BP (finely sifted)	150 g
Gelatin BP	150 g
Glycerol BP	350 g
Water	350 g
	(or sufficient quantity)

Method:

1. Heat the water to boiling.
2. Remove from the heat and add the gelatin.
3. Stir gently until dissolved.
4. Add the glycerol which has previously been heated to 100 °C (no higher).
5. Stir gently to prevent incorporation of air bubbles until solution is complete.
6. Maintain the base at 100 °C for 1 hour to remove any contaminant microorganisms.
7. Adjust the base to weight by evaporation or adding hot water as required.
8. Sift the Zinc Oxide BP and add in small amounts of molten base.
9. Continue stirring until the preparation is viscous enough to support the powder but is still pourable.
10. Pour into a shallow tray and allow to set. This is usually cut up into cubes which are weighed out and dispensed.

The preparation is designed to be re-melted before application as a dressing for varicose ulcers. The gel reforms on cooling and the zinc oxide acts as an absorbent and mild astringent.

Re-melting is achieved by standing the container of Unna's Paste in hot water. By cutting the paste into cubes this reduces the tendency of the zinc oxide to sediment out. Usually this is dispensed in portions of appropriate size intended for single use by the patient or nurse.

matrix. Drugs can be suspended in the matrix or dissolved in the liquid phase.

The advantages of gels are that:

- They are stable over long periods of time.
- They have a good appearance.

- They are suitable vehicles for applying medicaments to skin and mucous membranes, giving high rates of release of the medicament and rapid absorption.

Gels are usually translucent or transparent and have a number of uses:

- Anaesthetic gels
- Coal tar gels for use in treatment of psoriasis or eczema
- Lubricant gels
- Spermicidal gels.

10.4.1 Gelling agents

The consistency of gels can vary widely depending on the gelling agent used in their preparation. Common gelling agent used in aqueous gels are discussed below. Generally the medication in a gel is released quite freely provided the medicament does not bind with the polymer or clay used in its formation.

Tragacanth

- Concentrations of 2–5% of tragacanth are used to produce different viscosities.
- Tragacanth is a natural product and is therefore liable to microbial contamination.
- The gum tends to form lumps when added to water and therefore most formulae will include a wetting agent such as ethanol, glycerol or propylene glycol. By pre-wetting the tragacanth, the problems of a lumpy product should be minimised, and should lumps develop they will disperse easily on standing.

Alginates

- The viscosity of alginate gels is more standardised than those of tragacanth.
- Alginate concentrations of 1.5% produce fluid gels.
- Alginate concentrations of 5–10% produce dermatological grade gels suitable for topical application.
- Wetting agents (such as glycerol) need to be employed to prevent production of a lumpy product.

Example 10.4 A typical tragacanth gel formula

Formula:

Tragacanth BP	3% w/w
Glycerol BP	20% w/w
Alcohol BP	2.5% w/w
Methylparahydroxybenzoate BP	0.2% w/w
Water	to 100%

Method:

1. Mix together the Tragacanth BP and the Methylparahydroxybenzoate BP (the preservative) in a mortar.
2. Place the Alcohol BP and a small amount of Glycerol BP in a beaker.
3. Add the powder slowly.
4. Stir to form a smooth-flowing liquid.
5. Add any remaining glycerol.
6. Add all the water in one addition and stir (not too rapidly to avoid incorporation of air bubbles).

As a general rule, any powdered ingredients to be added to a gel, such as the crystalline Methylparahydroxybenzoate BP, should be admixed with the Tragacanth BP powder prior to wetting.

Example 10.5 A typical alginate gel formula

Formula:

Sodium Alginate BP	7% w/w
Glycerol BP	7% w/w
Methylparahydroxybenzoate BP	0.2% w/w
Water	to 100%

Method:

1. Mix together the Sodium Alginate BP and the Methylparahydroxybenzoate BP (the preservative) in a mortar.
2. Place the Glycerol BP in a beaker.
3. Add the powder slowly.
4. Stir to form a smooth-flowing liquid.
5. Add all the water in one addition and stir (not too rapidly to avoid incorporation of air bubbles).

Pectin

- Pectin is suitable for acid products.
- It is prone to microbial contamination.
- It is prone to water loss and therefore necessitates the addition of a humectant (e.g. glycerol, propylene glycol or sorbitol).

Gelatin

Gelatin is rarely used as the sole gelling agent in dermatological preparations. It is usually combined with other ingredients such as pectin or carmellose sodium.

Cellulose derivatives

- Cellulose derivatives are widely used and form neutral, stable gels.
- They exhibit good resistance to microbial attack.
- They form clear gels with good film strength when dried on the skin.
- Methylcellulose 450 is used in strengths of 3–5% to produce gels.
- Carmellose sodium (sodium carboxymethylcellulose) is used in concentrations of 1.5–5% to make lubricating gels. In higher concentrations it is used to make dermatological gels.

Carbomer

- Carbomer is useful in production of clear gels (provided too much air is not incorporated in the gel production).
- In concentrations of 0.3–1%, carbomer acts as a lubricant.
- Carbomer is used in dermatological preparations in concentrations of 0.5–5%.

Polyvinyl alcohol

- Polyvinyl alcohol is useful for preparing quick-drying gels.
- It leaves a residual film that is strong and plastic.
- It provides gels that have good skin contact and therefore ensures the medicament has good skin contact.
- Differing viscosities are achieved depending

on the concentration of polyvinyl alcohol used (normally 10–20%) and the grade of polyvinyl alcohol employed.

Clays

- Bentonite is used in concentrations of 7–20% to formulate dermatological bases.
- The resultant gel is opalescent, therefore less attractive to the patient.
- On drying, the gel leaves a powdery residue on the skin.

10.4.2 Other additives for gels

Other additives for gels include humectants and preservatives.

Humectants

Loss of water from a gel results in a skin forming. The addition of a humectant can minimise this.

Examples of additives that may be added to help retain water include:

- Glycerol in concentrations of up to 30%.
- Propylene glycol in concentrations of approximately 15%.
- Sorbitol in concentrations of 3–15%.

Preservatives

Gels have a higher water content than either ointments or pastes and this makes them susceptible to microbial contamination. Choice of preservative is determined by the gelling agent employed (Table 10.1).

10.4.3 General method of manufacture for gels

1. Heat all components of the gel (with the exception of water) to approximately 90 °C.
2. Heat water to approximately 90 °C.
3. Add water to oil, stirring continuously. Avoid vigorous stirring as this will introduce bubbles.

Table 10.1 Choice of preservative to be used in a gel

Preservative	Gelling agent
Benzalkonium chloride (0.01% w/v)	Hypromellose Methylcellulose
Benzoic acid (0.2%)	Alginates Pectin (provided the product is acidic in nature)
Chlorhexidine acetate (0.02%)	Polyvinyl alcohols
Chlorocresol (0.1–0.2%)	Alginates Pectin (provided the product is acidic in nature)

Methyl/propyl hydroxybenzoates (0.02–0.3%)
  Activity is increased if used in combination.
  Propylene glycol (10%) has been shown to
  potentiate the antimicrobial activity
	Carbomer
	Carmellose sodium
	Hypromellose
	Pectin
	Sodium alginate
	Tragacanth

Phenylmercuric nitrate (0.001%)	Methylcellulose

10.5 Worked examples

 Example 10.6 Preparation of 30 g of Simple Ointment BP

Product formula (British Pharmacopoeia 1988, page 713):

	1000 g	100 g	10 g	40 g
Cetostearyl Alcohol BP	50 g	5 g	0.5 g	2 g
Hard Paraffin BP	50 g	5 g	0.5 g	2 g
Wool Fat BP	50 g	5 g	0.5 g	2 g
White/Yellow Soft Paraffin BP	850 g	85 g	8.5 g	34 g

Point of clarity – Product formula
The exact quantity cannot be prepared for an ointment, and so a suitable overage must be produced in order to dispense the required amount.

   Yellow or White Soft Paraffin BP may be used when making this ointment, which is often used as a base for other ointments. As a general rule if it is to be used as a base and the ingredients to be added are coloured (e.g. Coal Tar Solution BP) Yellow Soft Paraffin BP would be used. If the ingredients to be added are white or pale in colour (e.g. Zinc Oxide BP or Calamine BP) White Soft Paraffin BP would be used to produce a more pharmaceutically elegant product.

Method to prepare 40 g of Simple Ointment BP from the formula above: Note that the melting points of the ingredients are as follows:

Cetostearyl Alcohol BP	49–56 °C
Hard Paraffin BP	50–61 °C
White/Yellow Soft Paraffin BP	38–56 °C
Wool fat BP	38–44 °C

1. Weigh 2 g Hard Paraffin BP on a Class II or electronic balance.
2. Weigh 2 g Cetostearyl Alcohol BP on a class II or electronic balance.
3. Weigh 2 g Wool Fat BP on a Class II or electronic balance.
4. Weigh 34 g Yellow/White Soft Paraffin BP on a Class II or electronic balance.
5. Place the Hard Paraffin BP into an evaporating dish and melt over a water bath.
6. Remove from the heat and add the other ingredients in descending order of melting point until all are melted in (return to the heat if necessary to ensure even melting, but take care not to overheat).
7. Stir until cold.
8. Weigh 30 g and pack into an amber glass jar. Label and dispense.

 See Ointments video for a demonstration of the preparation of an ointment by the fusion method.

Example 10.7 Preparation of 20 g Calamine and Coal Tar Ointment BP

Product formula (British Pharmacopoeia 1988, page 706):

	1000 g	100 g	10 g	30 g
Calamine BP	125 g	12.5 g	1.25 g	3.75 g
Strong Coal Tar Solution BP	25 g	2.5 g	0.25 g	0.75 g
Zinc Oxide BP	125 g	12.5 g	1.25 g	3.75 g
Hydrous Wool Fat BP	250 g	25 g	2.5 g	7.5 g
White Soft Paraffin BP	475 g	47.5 g	4.75 g	14.25 g

Point of clarity – Product formula
The exact quantity cannot be prepared for an ointment, and so a suitable overage must be produced in order to dispense the required amount. Note that the quantity of Strong Coal Tar Solution BP is in grams and so must be weighed.

Method to prepare 30 g of Calamine and Coal Tar Ointment BP from the formula above: Note that the melting points of the ingredients are as follows:

Hydrous Wool Fat BP   38–44 °C
White/Yellow Soft Paraffin BP   38–56 °C

1. Weigh 3.75 g Calamine BP on a Class II or electronic balance.
2. Weigh 3.75 g Zinc Oxide BP on a Class II or electronic balance.
3. Transfer the Calamine BP and the Zinc Oxide BP to a porcelain mortar and triturate together with a pestle.
4. Weigh 14.25 g White Soft Paraffin BP on a Class II or electronic balance.
5. Weigh 7.5 g Hydrous Wool Fat BP on a Class II or electronic balance.
6. Place the White Soft Paraffin BP into an evaporating dish and melt over a water bath.
7. Remove from the heat and add the Hydrous Wool Fat BP, stir until melted to ensure an even, well mixed base.
8. Transfer the powders to a glass tile and levigate with some of the molten base.
9. Transfer the powder/base mix to the rest of the molten base and stir until homogeneous.
10. Weigh 0.75 g Strong Coal Tar Solution BP on a Class II or electronic balance.
11. Allow the base/powder mixture to cool and add the Strong Coal Tar Solution BP and stir until homogeneous.

Point of clarity – Step 11
The Strong Coal Tar Solution BP cannot be added until the bases are quite cool (less than 40 °C) as it is a volatile preparation. This method would also avoid heating the Strong Coal Tar Solution BP and therefore reduce the volatilisation of some of the coal tar constituents and reduce the risk of sedimentation (see Method section, Example 10.2).

See Ointments video for a demonstration
of the preparation of an ointment.

Example 10.8 Preparation of 20 g of Zinc Ointment BP

Product formula (British Pharmacopoeia 1988, page 715):

	1000 g	100 g	10 g	30 g
Zinc Oxide BP	150 g	15 g	1.5 g	4.5 g
Simple Ointment BP	850 g	85 g	8.5 g	25.5 g

Point of clarity – Product formula
The exact quantity cannot be prepared for an ointment as losses will be experienced on transfer. Therefore, a suitable overage must be produced in order to dispense the required amount.

Method to prepare 30 g of Zinc Ointment BP from the formula above:
1. Weigh 4.5 g Zinc Oxide BP on a Class II or electronic balance.
2. Transfer to a porcelain mortar and sir with a pestle.

   Point of clarity – Step 2
   The Zinc Oxide BP is transferred to a mortar so that the size of any lumps can be reduced, enabling a smooth product to be made.

3. Transfer the Zinc Oxide BP to a glass tile.
4. Weigh 25.5 g Simple Ointment BP on a Class II or electronic balance.
5. Transfer the Simple Ointment BP to the glass tile.
6. Triturate the Zinc Oxide BP with the Simple Ointment BP until a smooth product is formed.

   Point of clarity – Step 6
   To triturate means to mix. A smooth product will be produced if the Zinc Oxide BP is finely sifted and then just mixed with the base. The particle size reduction of the Zinc Oxide BP in this example has only been achieved by mixing in a mortar, rather than sifting with a sieve. In order to achieve a smooth product, considerably more shear force will need to be applied to the powder and we suggest that the process employed would be more akin to levigation (wet grinding), but in this case using a semi-solid base rather than a molten base.

7. Weigh 20 g of the product and pack into an amber glass jar. Label and dispense.

See Ointments video for a demonstration of the preparation of an ointment.

Example 10.9 Unofficial ointment request from local doctor to prepare 20 g of CCS & S Ointment

The local dermatology clinic has a formulary which gives the following formula:

Salicylic Acid BP	3%
Camphor BP	3%
Sulphur BP	3%
Phenol BP	3%
White Soft Paraffin BP	to 100%

Product formula:

	100 g	10 g	30 g
Salicylic Acid BP	3 g	300 mg	900 mg
Camphor BP	3 g	300 mg	900 mg
Sulphur BP	3 g	300 mg	900 mg
Phenol BP	3 g	300 mg	900 mg
White Soft Paraffin BP	88 g	8.8 g	26.4 g

Method to prepare 30 g of CCS & S Ointment from the formula above: Note that when phenol is combined with camphor, a liquid mixture results.

1. Weigh 900 mg Salicylic Acid BP on a Class II or electronic balance.
2. Weigh 900 mg Sulphur BP on a Class II or electronic balance.
3. Transfer the Salicylic Acid BP to a glass mortar and grind with a pestle to reduce particle size.
4. Add the Sulphur BP and continue mixing.
5. Transfer the mixed powders to a glass tile.
6. Weigh 26.4 g White Soft Paraffin BP on a Class II or electronic balance
7. Transfer the White Soft Paraffin BP to the glass tile.
8. Triturate the powders with the White Soft Paraffin BP until a smooth product is formed.
9. Weigh 900 mg Camphor BP on a Class II or electronic balance.
10. Transfer to a clean dry glass mortar.
11. Weigh 900 mg of Phenol BP on a Class II or electronic balance.
12. Add the Phenol BP to the Camphor BP and mix together with a pestle.
13. Make a well in the ointment mass and add the liquid mixture.

> *Point of clarity – Step 13*
> The Camphor BP and Phenol BP are weighed and mixed at the final stage of preparation of the product as both are volatile ingredients.

14. Triturate until all the liquid is incorporated and a homogeneous product is formed.
15. Weigh 20 g of product and pack into an amber glass jar and label.

 See Ointments video for a demonstration of the preparation of an ointment.

Example 10.10 Unofficial ointment request from local doctor for 40 g of Salicylic Acid BP 2% in Betnovate Ointment

The suitability of the product formula must be decided by the compounder. Refer to a diluent directory, which in this case states that up to 5% of Salicylic Acid BP can be added to Betnovate Ointment. Had the formula requested Betnovate Cream this would have been unsuitable as the Salicylic Acid BP causes the cream to crack.

Note: Suitable sources to provide information on the dilution of creams and ointments would be:

• NPA Diluent Directory
• Product data sheet (Summary of Product Characteristics – SPC)
• Reports in the pharmaceutical literature
• Personal contact with product manufacturer.

Product formula:

	Master formula	100 g	10 g	50 g
Salicylic Acid BP	2%	2 g	200 mg	1 g
Betnovate Ointment	98%	98 g	9.8 g	49 g

Method to prepare 50 g of Salicylic Acid BP 2% in Betnovate Ointment from the formula above:

1. Weigh 1 g Salicylic Acid BP on a Class II or electronic balance.
2. Transfer to a glass mortar and grind with a pestle to reduce any lumps in the powder.
3. Transfer the powder to a glass tile.
4. Weigh 49 g Betnovate Ointment.
5. Transfer to the tile.
6. Triturate the Salicylic Acid BP and the Betnovate Ointment together, remembering the 'doubling-up' technique for adequate mixing.
7. Weigh 40 g of the resultant ointment, pack in an amber glass jar, label and dispense.

See Ointments video for a demonstration of the preparation of an ointment.

Example 10.11 Preparation of 20 g Compound Zinc Paste BP

Product formula (British Pharmacopoeia 1988, page 868):

	1000 g	100 g	10 g	30 g
Zinc Oxide BP	250 g	25 g	2.5 g	7.5 g
Starch BP	250 g	25 g	2.5 g	7.5 g
White Soft Paraffin BP	500 g	50 g	5 g	15 g

Point of clarity – Product formula
The exact quantity cannot be prepared for an ointment as losses will be experienced on transfer. Therefore, a suitable overage must be produced in order to dispense the required amount.

Method to prepare 30 g of Compound Zinc Paste BP from the formula above: Note that the melting point of the base is as follows:

White/Yellow Soft Paraffin BP   38–56 °C

1. Weigh 7.5 g Zinc Oxide BP on a Class II or electronic balance.
2. Weigh 7.5 g Starch BP on a Class II or electronic balance.
3. Weigh 15 g White Soft Paraffin BP on a Class II or electronic balance.
4. Transfer the Zinc Oxide BP to a porcelain mortar.
5. Add the Starch BP to the mortar and triturate with the pestle to form an evenly mixed powder.

   Point of clarity – Step 5
   A porcelain mortar is used because of the volume of powder involved.

6. Transfer the powder to a glass tile.
7. Transfer the White Soft Paraffin BP to the glass tile.
8. Mix the powders with the White Soft Paraffin BP using a metal spatula and remembering the principle of 'doubling-up' when mixing.
9. Triturate until a smooth product is formed.
10. Weigh 30 g and pack into an amber glass jar. Label and dispense.

    Point of clarity – Method
    An alternative way to prepare this paste would involve melting the base then combining the powders with the molten base and stirring until cooled.

 See Ointments video for a demonstration
of the preparation of an ointment.

Example 10.12 Preparation of 20 g Zinc and Coal Tar Paste BP

Product formula (British Pharmacopoeia 1988, page 868):

	1000 g	100 g	10 g	30 g
Emulsifying Wax BP	50 g	5 g	500 mg	1.5 g
Coal Tar BP	60 g	6 g	600 mg	1.8 g
Zinc Oxide BP	60 g	6 g	600 mg	1.8 g
Starch BP	380 g	38 g	3.8 g	11.4 g
Yellow Soft Paraffin BP	450 g	45 g	4.5 g	13.5 g

Point of clarity – Product formula
The exact quantity cannot be prepared for an ointment as losses will be experienced on transfer. Therefore, a suitable overage must be produced in order to dispense the required amount.

Method to prepare 30 g of Zinc and Coal Tar Paste BP from the formula above: Note the melting points of the ingredients:

Emulsifying Wax BP	52 °C
White/Yellow Soft Paraffin BP	38–56 °C

1. Weigh 1.8 g Zinc Oxide BP on a Class II or electronic balance.
2. Transfer to a porcelain mortar.
3. Weigh 11.4 g Starch BP on a Class II or electronic balance.
4. Add the Starch BP to the Zinc Oxide BP in the porcelain mortar and stir with the pestle.

   Point of clarity – Step 4
   The powders must be mixed remembering the principle of 'doubling-up' in order to ensure even mixing of the powders.

5. Weigh 1.5 g Emulsifying Wax BP on a Class II or electronic balance.
6. Weigh 1.8 g Coal Tar BP on a Class II or electronic balance.
7. Weigh 13.5 g Yellow Soft Paraffin BP on a Class II or electronic balance.
8. Place the Emulsifying Wax BP into an evaporating dish and melt over a water bath at 70 °C.
9. Add the Coal Tar BP and half of the Yellow Soft Paraffin BP to the evaporating basin.
10. Stir at 70 °C until melted.
11. Add the remaining Yellow Soft Paraffin BP stir until melted.
12. Cool to approximately 30 °C and add the powders and stir constantly until cold.
13. Weigh 20 g of the paste transfer to an amber glass jar, dispense and label.

   Point of clarity – Method
   The above method is as recommended by the British Pharmacopoeia. An alternative method would be:

   1. Melt the Yellow Soft Paraffin BP and Emulsifying Wax BP together at the lowest possible temperature, stirring until cool to make a homogeneous product.
   2. Mix the powders as before but transfer them to a glass tile and incorporate the powders using a spatula.
   3. Finally, using a spatula (preferably ebonite), incorporate the Coal Tar BP.

Example 10.12 Continued

This method may be preferred because of the possible problem of toxicity associated with Coal Tar BP. This method would avoid heating the Coal Tar BP and therefore reduce the volatilisation of some of the coal tar constituents and reduce the risk of sedimentation (see Method section, Example 10.2).

 See Ointments video for a demonstration of the preparation of an ointment.

 Example 10.13 Preparation of 40 g of Dithranol Paste BP 0.1%

Note: the strength of dithranol paste can vary between 0.1% and 1%.

Product formula (British Pharmacopoeia 1988, page 866):

	1000 g	100 g	10 g	50 g
Dithranol BP	1 g	100 mg	10 mg	50 mg
Zinc and Salicylic Acid Paste BP	999 g	99.9 g	9.99 g	49.95 g

Point of clarity – Product formula
The exact quantity cannot be prepared for an ointment as losses will be experienced on transfer. Therefore, a suitable overage must be produced in order to dispense the required amount.

Method to prepare 50 g of Dithranol paste BP 0.1% from the formula above:

1. Weigh 50 mg Dithranol BP on a sensitive electronic balance.
2. Transfer to a glass tile.
3. Weigh 49.95 g Zinc and Salicylic Acid Paste BP on a Class II or electronic balance.
4. Transfer the Zinc and Salicylic Acid Paste BP to the glass tile.
5. Triturate Dithranol BP with the Zinc and Salicylic Acid paste BP, remembering the principle of 'doubling-up' until a smooth product is formed.

   Point of clarity – Steps 1–5
   Dithranol BP is extremely irritant and care should be taken when handling. If large quantities are to be made anecdotal evidence suggests using Liquid Paraffin BP to dissolve the powder prior to addition to the paste because this reduces the likelihood of dispersal of the powder when admixing with the paste. If used, the formula would need to be adjusted slightly to allow for the weight of Liquid Paraffin BP used.

6. Weigh 40 g of the product and pack into an amber glass jar. Label and dispense.

 See Ointments video for a demonstration of the preparation of an ointment.

10.6 Summary of essential principles relating to ointments, pastes and gels

This section will recap the main principles relating to ointments, pastes and gels that have been covered in other sections of the book. To assist compounders in understanding the extemporaneous preparation of ointments, pastes and gels, this section contains the following:

- Further notes on the packaging of extemporaneously prepared ointments, pastes and gels.
- Specific points relevant to the expiry of extemporaneously prepared ointments, pastes and gels.
- Additional key points relating to the labelling of pharmaceutical ointments, pastes and gels.

10.6.1 Packaging

The packaging of extemporaneous preparations has been covered previously in Section 5.7. An overview of the main considerations for the packaging of ointments, pastes and gels will be given here.

As all pharmaceutical ointments, pastes and gels are intended for external use, a suitable container would be either an amber wide-necked ointment jar or metal collapsible tube. Pharmaceutical ointment jars come in a variety of different sizes and it is important to choose a suitably sized container to match the volume of preparation to be dispensed. Obviously it is important not to use a size of container that is too large for the volume of preparation to be dispensed for both cost and appearance issues.

Amber glass jars are preferable to clear glass jars as they protect the preparation from degradation by light. More recently, plastic ointment jars have become available and although cheaper than glass jars, are less preferable because of an increased likelihood of the products reacting with the container (e.g. as can occur in preparations containing coal tar).

When packaging a pharmaceutical product into an ointment jar, ensure that the product is packed well and that no air pockets are visible. This will produce a final product with a professional appearance.

 See Creams video for a demonstration of the packaging of an ointment.

10.6.2 Discard dates

Some official texts may give a suggested discard date for extemporaneously prepared ointments, pastes and gels. In the absence of any guide, it is suggested that ointments and pastes are given a three-month discard date. This is significantly longer than the suggested discard date for extemporaneously prepared creams (which is four weeks) owing to fact that ointments are less susceptible to microbial contamination (see Section 9.5.2).

Diluted ointments (see Example 10.10) would normally be given a two-week discard date.

Gels, which have a higher water content, will attract a shorter discard date. In the absence of any official guidance, it is suggested that gels are given a four-week expiry date.

Remember that as patients frequently misunderstand the term 'expiry' it is suggested that a preferred method of indicating shelf life on the label of extemporaneously compounded products is to apply the term 'Discard after' followed by a definite date and/or time.

Further guidance on expiry dates to pharmaceutical preparations can be found in Section 5.6.1.

10.6.3 Labelling

The labelling of pharmaceutical ointments, pastes and gels has been covered in Section 5.6.2. An overview of the main considerations for the labelling of ointments, pastes and gels will be given here.

In addition to the standard requirements for the labelling of extemporaneous preparations, the following points need to be taken into consideration:

- **'For external use only'** – This warning must be added to the label of all extemporaneously prepared ointments pastes and gels as all are for external use only.
- **'Store below 15 °C'** – Depending on the temperature of the environment, it may be

advisable to place a storage temperature warning on the label. This would not normally be necessary in the UK (depending on the ingredients within the preparation) but may be advisable if the patient is travelling to a location with a warmer climate.

Further guidance on auxiliary labelling can be found in Section 5.6.1, Table 5.10.

11

Suppositories and pessaries

11.1 Introduction and overview

11.1.1 Suppositories

Suppositories are solid unit dosage forms suitably shaped for insertion into the rectum. The bases used either melt when warmed to body temperature or dissolve or disperse when in contact with mucous secretions. Suppositories may contain medicaments, dissolved or dispersed in the base, which are intended to exert a systemic effect. Alternatively the medicaments or the base itself may be intended to exert a local action. Suppositories are prepared extemporaneously by incorporating the medicaments into the base and the molten mass is then poured at a suitable temperature into moulds and allowed to cool until set.

The British Pharmacopoeia (BP) definition is as follows:

Suppositories are solid, single-dose preparations.

The shape, volume and consistency of suppositories are suitable for rectal administration.

They contain one or more active substances dispersed or dissolved in a suitable basis which may be soluble or dispersible in water or may melt at body temperature. Excipients such as diluents, adsorbents, surface-active agents, lubricants, antimicrobial preservatives and colouring matter, authorised by the competent authority, may be added if necessary.

The advantages of suppositories as dosage forms are that:

- They can be used to exert a local effect on the rectal mucosa (e.g. anaesthetic etc.).
- They can be used to promote evacuation of the bowel.
- If a particular drug causes irritation of the gastrointestinal tract this can be avoided by rectal administration.
- They can be used for patients who are unconscious, fitting or vomiting, etc.

173

• Systemic absorption can be achieved by rectal delivery and has the added advantage of avoiding first-pass metabolism by the liver.

The disadvantages of suppositories as dosage forms are that:

• They may be unacceptable to certain patients/cultures.
• They may be difficult to self-administer by arthritic or physically compromised patients.
• They have unpredictable and variable absorption *in vivo*.

The advantages and disadvantages of suppositories as dosage forms are summarised in Box 11.1.

11.1.2 Pessaries

Pessaries are a type of suppository intended for vaginal use. The larger size moulds are usually used in the preparation of pessaries, such as 4 g and 8 g moulds. Pessaries are used almost exclusively for local medication, the exception being prostaglandin pessaries that do exert a systemic effect.

Common ingredients for inclusion in pessaries for local action include:

• Antiseptics
• Contraceptive agents
• Local anaesthetics
• Various therapeutic agents to treat trichomonal, bacterial and monilial infections.

The British Pharmacopoeia (BP) definition is as follows:

> Pessaries are solid, single-dose preparations. They have various shapes, usually ovoid, with a volume and consistency suitable for insertion into the vagina. They contain one or more active substances dispersed or dissolved in a suitable basis that may be soluble or dispersible in water or may melt at body temperature. Excipients such as diluents, adsorbents, surface-active agents, lubricants, antimicrobial preservatives and colouring matter authorised by the competent authority may be added, if necessary.

11.2 General principles of suppository and pessary preparation

The methods used in the preparation of pessaries are the same as those for suppositories. In this chapter, points relating to suppositories can also apply to pessaries. For further details on suppository and pessary bases, see Section 5.5.4.

The preparation of suppositories invariably involves some wastage and therefore it is recommended that calculations are made for excess. For example, if you are required to dispense six suppositories, to include a suitable excess calculate for 10.

Box 11.1   Advantages and disadvantages of suppositories as dosage forms

Advantages

Can exert local effect on rectal mucosa
Used to promote evacuation of bowel
Avoids any gastrointestinal irritation
Can be used in unconscious patients (e.g. during fitting)
Can be used for systemic absorption of drugs and avoids first-pass metabolism

Disadvantages

May be unacceptable to certain patients
May be difficult to self-administer by arthritic or physically compromised patients
Unpredictable and variable absorption *in vivo*

11.2.1 Suppository mould calibration

Suppository moulds are calibrated in terms of the weight of Theobroma Oil BP each will contain. Typical sizes are 1 g, 2 g or 4 g. Because the moulds are filled volumetrically, use of a base other than Theobroma Oil BP will require recalibration of the moulds. Many synthetic fats have been formulated to match the specific gravity of Theobroma Oil BP and therefore the mould sizing will be the same and not require recalibration. However, this is not the case for all synthetic bases.

To recalibrate a suppository mould, the compounder needs to prepare a number (e.g. five) of (perfectly formed) suppositories containing only the base. These can then be weighed and the total weight divided by the number of suppositories present to find the mould calibration value.

11.2.2 Displacement values

Problems also arise when medicaments are added to the base, where the density of the medicament differs from that of the base and a specific quantity of ingredient is required to be incorporated into each suppository. The amount of base displaced will depend on the densities of the ingredients and the base. For ease of calculation this is expressed in terms of a series of displacement values, where the displacement value of an ingredient is defined as the number of parts by weight of the ingredient that displaces one part of Theobroma Oil BP (or other fatty base, e.g. Hard Fat BP). Displacement values are given in standard texts, e.g. (British) Pharmaceutical Codex twelfth edition, page 174 (also see Table 11.1).

The displacement value is defined as the quantity of medicament that displaces one part of the base. For example, Hydrocortisone BP has a displacement value of 1.5.

This means that 1.5 g Hydrocortisone BP displaces 1 g of the suppository base (Theobroma Oil BP or Hard Fat BP).

A summary of some common displacement values can be found in Table 11.1.

 Example 11.1 Calibrate a 1 g mould with a synthetic base

1. The synthetic base is melted in an evaporating basin over a water bath until around two-thirds of the base has melted.
2. The evaporating basin is then removed from the heat and stirred, using the residual heat to melt the remaining synthetic base.
3. When the base has cooled to close to its melting point, it is poured into the mould and allowed to overfill slightly.
4. After around 5 minutes, trim the tops and then leave the suppositories to set completely.
5. Weigh all the perfect suppositories (i.e. avoiding any chipped suppositories) and divide the total weight by the number of suppositories weighed. This will give the value that should be used for this particular mould with this base.

Table 11.1   Displacement values of some common drugs incorporated into suppositories

Medicament	Displacement value
Aminophylline BP	1.3
Aspirin BP	1.1
Bismuth Subgallate BP	2.7
Castor Oil BP	1.0
Chloral Hydrate BP	1.4
Codeine Phosphate BP	1.1
Diphenhydramine Hydrochloride BP	1.3
Hydrocortisone BP	1.5
Metronidazole BP	1.7
Morphine Hydrochloride BP	1.6
Morphine Sulphate BP	1.6
Paracetamol BP	1.5
Phenobarbital BP	1.1
Phenobarbital Sodium BP	1.2
Resorcinal BP	1.5
Sulphur BP	1.6
Theophylline Sodium Acetate BP	1.7
Zinc Oxide BP	4.7
Zinc Sulphate BP	2.4

11.2.3 Calculations using displacement values

If the active ingredient in a suppository is expressed in terms of weight then a calculation based on displacement values will need to be made in order to determine the amount of Hard Fat BP required.

 Example 11.2 Prepare six codeine phosphate suppositories 60 mg

	For one suppository	For 10 suppositories
Codeine Phosphate BP	60 mg	600 mg
Hard Fat BP	sufficient to fill 1 × 1 g size mould	sufficient to fill 10 × 1 g size moulds

Displacement value for codeine phosphate is 1.1. Hence 1.1 g of codeine phosphate displaces 1 g of base. Therefore 0.6 g displaces (1 × 0.6 g) ÷ 1.1 = 0.55 g of base. Therefore the amount of fatty base needed is 10 − 0.55 g = **9.45 g**.

11.2.4 Formulae requiring percentage calculations

If the active ingredient in a suppository is expressed in terms of a % w/w then a calculation based on displacement value *will not be required*. The drug is present in the suppository as a proportion. Therefore, simply subtract the total weight of the medicament from the total weight of the fat to determine the amount of fat required.

11.2.5 Calculations using percentage calculations

 Example 11.3 Prepare five suppositories each containing 6% copper sulphate w/w

	For one suppository	For 10 suppositories
Copper Sulphate BP	60 mg	600 mg
Hard Fat BP	to 1 g = 940 mg	to 10 g = 9.4 g

11.3 General method for suppository preparation

1. Most moulds prepare six suppositories, but it is necessary to calculate to include an excess (usually a multiple of 10).
2. Choose a suppository mould to provide the suppositories of the required size (usually a 1 g size). Check that the two halves of the mould are matched (numbers are etched on the sides).
3. Check that the mould is clean and assemble the mould but do not over-tighten the screw.
4. For some suppository bases it is necessary to lubricate the mould (e.g. use Liquid Paraffin BP), but this is not required when using Hard Fat BP.
5. If the suppository is to contain insoluble, coarse powders these must be ground down in a glass mortar before incorporation.
6. It is important not to overheat the base, which may change its physical characteristics. Find the melting point of the base and heat it to about 5–10 °C less than the melting point. (There should still be *some* solid base present.) Hold the evaporating basin in the palm of your hand and stir (do not use the thermometer to stir) to complete the melting process.
7. Immiscible liquids and insoluble solids should be incorporated into the fatty base by

levigation (wet grinding). The substance should be rubbed into the minimum quantity of molten base on a tile using a spatula. The 'shearing' effect will not be obtained if too much base is used, resulting in a gritty product.

8. The paste obtained in Step 7 above should be returned to the evaporating basin with the remainder of the base, stirring constantly.

9. The molten mass should be poured into the mould when it is just about to solidify. (This is usually judged by experience. Look for a slight sheen on the surface of the mass, similar to a skin forming on custard as it cools.)

10. Pour the mass into the mould uniformly in one movement.

11. Allow the mixture to overfill slightly but not to run down the sides of the mould (if this happens, it is likely to be due to the mixture still being too hot).

12. When the suppositories have contracted, but before they have set completely, trim off the excess Hard Fat BP. This can easily be achieved by rubbing the flat blade of the spatula over the top of the mould.

13. After further cooling, when the suppositories have set, loosen the screw and tap once sharply on the bench. Remove the suppositories carefully (avoid overhandling or damaging the suppositories with your nails).

14. Pack the required number of suppositories individually in foil and place in an amber wide-necked jar.

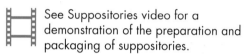 See Suppositories video for a demonstration of the preparation and packaging of suppositories.

11.4 Worked examples

Example 11.4 Preparation of six child-size Glycerol Suppositories BP

Product formula (British Pharmacopoeia 1988, page 889):

	Master formula	100 g	10 g	5 g	25 g
Gelatin BP	14 %	14 g	1.4 g	0.7 g	3.5 g
Glycerol BP	70 %	70 g	7 g	3.5 g	17.5 g
Purified water	to 100 %	16 g	1.6 g	0.8 g	4 g

Point of clarity – Product formula
The choice of suppository mould for a child's glycerol suppository is traditionally 2 g (a 1 g mould is usually used for an infant's glycerol suppository, a 2 g mould for a child's glycerol suppository and a 4 g mould for an adult's glycerol suppository).

   The mould will have been calibrated for use with Theobroma Oil BP or Hard Fat BP. The glycero-gelatin base has a greater density, therefore the nominal weight required to fill the moulds will be greater than with the other two bases. To calculate correctly the quantities required the amount that would be required to fill the nominal weight will need to multiplied by a factor of 1.2.

Calculations: Six suppositories are required; however, an overage will need to be prepared to successfully prepare this quantity. Calculations are therefore based on the amounts required to prepare 10 suppositories.

   The mass of base that would be needed to prepare 10 child-size (2 g suppositories) is $10 \times 2 \times 1.2 = 24$ g

For ease of calculation and weighing etc., sufficient quantities of ingredients to prepare 25 g of base are used.

Method:
1. Prepare the mould by lubricating it with either Arachis Oil BP or Liquid Paraffin BP.

   Point of clarity – Step 1
   Care should be taken when using Arachis Oil BP to ensure that the patient does not have any nut allergies. If this is not known, it would be safest to use Liquid Paraffin BP.

2. Weigh approximately 10 g of purified water and place in a previously weighed evaporating basin.

   Point of clarity – Step 2
   The weight of the evaporating basin will be needed for the final adjustment of the weight of the product. An excess of water is used to allow for evaporation and in addition, the use of excess water aids the dissolution of the Gelatin BP.

3. Weigh 17.5 g of Glycerol BP on a Class II or electronic balance and place in an evaporating basin.
4. Heat the Glycerol BP over a water bath to 100 °C.
5. Weigh 3.5 g Gelatin BP on a Class II or electronic balance.
6. Heat the water to boiling point.
7. Remove from the heat (to prevent excess evaporation).
8. Add the Gelatin BP powder to the water and stir to dissolve.

Example 11.4 Continued

9. Add the hot Glycerol BP to the solution and stir until homogeneous.

   Point of clarity – Step 9
   Stir gently and not too vigorously to prevent the incorporation of air bubbles.

10. Adjust the weight by adding sufficient hot water or by evaporation of any excess water.
11. Pour the mass into the mould, taking care not to overfill as the base does not contract upon cooling.
12. Leave to cool then remove from the mould, wrap, pack and label.

   Point of clarity – Product
   • This glycero-gelatin base is used as a carrier base for other medicaments in some instances.

   Water-soluble thermolabile ingredients are dissolved in a little water before being added to the molten mass.

   • Insoluble substances are rubbed down on the tile with a little of the Glycerol BP (Glycerol BP and not the base is used as it is difficult to re-melt solidified base).
   • Gelatin BP may be contaminated with pathogenic microorganisms because of its origin. Pharmaceutical grade gelatin should be pathogen free, but as an added precaution when used for pessaries the base may be heat treated by steam at a temperature of 100 °C for 1 hour (this is prior to making up to weight and prior to the addition of any thermolabile ingredients).
   • Patients with strict religious beliefs and vegetarians may object to the use of animal gelatin (although non-animal gelatin may be available).

    See Suppositories video for a demonstration of the preparation and packaging of suppositories.

Example 11.5 Preparation of three 8 g Ichthammol BP Pessaries 5%

Product formula:

	Master formula	100 g	10 g	50 g
Ichthammol BP	5 %	5 g	0.5 g	2.5 g
Glycero-gelatin base	95 %	95 g	9.5 g	47.5 g

Calculations: Three pessaries are required, but an overage will need to be prepared to successfully prepare this quantity. Calculations are therefore based on the amounts required to prepare five pessaries.

The mass of base that would be needed to prepare five pessaries is $5 \times 8 \times 1.2 = 48$ g

Point of clarity – Calculations
The glycero-gelatin base has a greater density, therefore the nominal weight required to fill the moulds will be greater than with the other two bases (Theobroma Oil BP and Hard Fat BP). To calculate the quantities required correctly the amount that would be required to fill the nominal weight will need to multiplied by a factor of 1.2.

For ease of calculation and weighing etc., sufficient quantities to prepare 50 g are as follows:

	Master formula	100 g	50 g
Gelatin BP	14%	14 g	7 g
Glycerol BP	70%	70 g	35 g
Purified water	to 100%	16 g	8 g

Point of clarity – Formula
The British Pharmacopoeia states that purified gelatin can be produced by two different methods:

• Partial acid hydrolysis (type A [anionic] gelatin)
• Partial alkaline hydrolysis (type B [cationic] gelatin).

Because the active ingredient to be incorporated in these pessaries is Ichthammol BP, type B should be used to avoid incompatibilities.

Method:
1. Prepare the mould by lubricating it with either Arachis Oil BP or Liquid Paraffin BP.

   Point of clarity – Step 1
   Care should be taken when using Arachis Oil BP to ensure that the patient does not have any nut allergies. If this is not known, it would be safest to use Liquid Paraffin BP.

2. Prepare the base as in Example 11.4 above.
3. Weigh 2.5 g of Ichthammol BP on a Class II or electronic balance.

Example 11.5 Continued

4. Weigh 47.5 g of base.

   Point of clarity – Step 4
   Because the base was prepared in a tared container, it is easier to remove any excess base rather than try to weigh the amount of base required and transfer to another vessel.
   Note: 2.5 g of the base needs to be replaced by Ichthammol BP. This amount of base needs to be removed. It would not be correct to adjust the base weight by evaporation as this would mean that the Ichthammol BP was replacing water not base.

5. Remove the base from the heat and add the Ichthammol BP.
6. Stir until homogeneous and then pour into the lubricated mould.
7. Leave the pessaries to cool, remove from the mould, wrap, pack and label.

Example 11.6 Preparation of six Compound Bismuth Subgallate Suppositories BP

Product Formula (British Pharmacopoeia 1980, page 723):

	1 suppository	10 suppositories
Bismuth Subgallate BP	200 mg	2 g
Resorcinol BP	60 mg	600 mg
Zinc Oxide BP	120 mg	1.2 g
Castor Oil BP	60 mg	600 mg
Base	qs	qs

Point of clarity – Product formula

Hard Fat BP is a suitable base to use. The quantity to be used must be calculated using displacement values. A nominal 1 g mould is used.

Calculations: Prepare for 10 suppositories to allow for losses during preparation.

Displacement values:

Bismuth Subgallate BP	2.7
Resorcinol BP	1.5
Zinc Oxide BP	4.7
Castor Oil BP	1.0

Bismuth Subgallate BP displaces $2 \div 2.7$ g Hard Fat BP = 0.74 g
Resorcinol BP displaces $0.6 \div 1.5$ g Hard Fat BP = 0.4 g
Zinc Oxide BP displaces $1.2 \div 4.7$ g Hard Fat BP = 0.26 g
Castor Oil BP displaces $0.6 \div 1$ g Hard Fat BP = 0.6 g
The amount of base required = $(10 \times 1$ g$) - (0.74 + 0.4 + 0.26 + 0.6)$
= 10 – 2.00
= 8.00 g

Working formula:

	10 suppositories
Bismuth Subgallate BP	2 g
Resorcinol BP	600 mg
Zinc Oxide BP	1.2 g
Castor Oil BP	600 mg
Hard Fat BP	8 g

Method:
1. Weigh 8 g of Hard Fat BP on a Class II or electronic balance.
2. Transfer to an evaporating basin and melt over a water bath.
3. Weigh 2 g of Bismuth Subgallate BP on a Class II or electronic balance.
4. Weigh 600 mg Resorcinol BP on a Class II or electronic balance.
5. Weigh 1.2 g Zinc Oxide BP on a Class II or electronic balance.

Example 11.6 Continued

6. Weigh 600 mg Castor Oil BP on a Class II or electronic balance.

   Point of clarity – Step 6
   Any liquid ingredients to be added to suppositories must be weighed NOT measured.

7. Mix the powders together in a mortar using the 'doubling-up' technique and transfer to a warmed tile.
8. Levigate the powders with the Castor Oil BP and a little molten base.
9. Return the resultant mix to the molten mass and stir.
10. Stir until almost set then transfer to a clean, dry matched suppository mould and allow to set.
11. Trim the tops and remove from the mould.
12. Wrap individually in foil and transfer to an amber glass jar and label.

See Suppositories video for a demonstration of the preparation and packaging of suppositories.

11.5 Summary of essential principles relating to suppositories and pessaries

This section will recap the main principles relating to suppositories and pessaries that have been covered in other sections of the book. To assist compounders in understanding the extemporaneous preparation of suppositories and pessaries, this section contains the following:

- Further notes on the packaging of extemporaneously prepared suppositories and pessaries.
- Specific points relevant to the expiry of extemporaneously prepared suppositories and pessaries.
- Additional key points related to the labelling of pharmaceutical suppositories and pessaries.

11.5.1 Packaging

The packaging of extemporaneous preparations has been covered in Section 5.7. An overview of the main considerations for the packaging of suppositories and pessaries will be given here.

Suppositories and pessaries that have been manufactured in metal moulds should be removed from the mould carefully and individually wrapped in suitably sized pieces of aluminium foil. Once wrapped, the suppositories can be placed in an ointment jar or cardboard carton and labelled.

Suppositories that have been manufactured in a disposable mould are often dispensed to the patient in the mould. It is important to ensure that the patient will be able to release each suppository from the mould and that the label is placed on a suitable part of the mould. Sometimes, it will be necessary to remove the suppositories from the disposable mould and wrap and package as for those prepared in metal moulds.

See Suppositories video for a demonstration of the packaging of suppositories.

11.5.2 Discard dates

In practical terms it is suggested that an expiry date of three months is given to suppositories and pessaries in the absence of any official guidance.

Remember that because patients frequently misunderstand the term 'expiry' it is suggested that a preferred method of indicating shelf life on the label of extemporaneously compounded products is to apply the term 'Discard after' followed by a definite date and/or time.

Further guidance on expiry dates to pharmaceutical preparations can be found in Section 5.6.1.

11.5.3 Labelling

The labelling of pharmaceutical suppositories and pessaries has been covered in Section 5.6.2. An overview of the main considerations for the labelling of suppositories and pessaries will be given here.

In addition to the standard requirements for the labelling of extemporaneous preparations, the following points need to be taken into consideration:

- '**For rectal use only**' – This warning must be added to the label of any suppositories.
- '**For vaginal use only**' – This warning must be added to the label of any pessaries.
- '**Store below 15 °C**' – This warning must be added to the label of all suppositories and pessaries.

Further guidance on auxiliary labelling can be found in Section 5.6.1, Table 5.10.

12

Powders and capsules

12.1 Introduction and overview

This section will include solid preparations intended for both internal and external use. The following types of preparation will be considered:

- Bulk powders for external use – termed dusting powders
- Bulk oral powders
- Individual unit dose powders
- Unit dose capsules.

12.2 Bulk powders for external use

These are dry, free-flowing preparations consisting of one or a mixture of finely powdered substances and intended for external application.

The advantages of dusting powders as pharmaceutical products are that:

- They are easy to apply.
- They are pleasant to use.
- They absorb skin moisture, which leads to reduced friction between skin surfaces, discourages bacterial growth and has a cooling effect.

The disadvantages of dusting powders as pharmaceutical products are that:

- They may block pores, causing irritation, or if applied to parietal surfaces, granulomas, fibrosis or adhesions.
- There is a possibility of contamination:
    - Starch, although an excellent dusting powder, is organic and can support microbial growth.
    - Talc, despite being an inert compound, can be contaminated with microorganisms and must therefore always be sterilised prior to incorporation into a dusting powder.
- Light fluffy powders may be inhaled by infants, causing breathing difficulties.
- They are not suitable for application to broken skin.

Box 12.1   Advantages and disadvantages of dusting powders as dosage forms

Advantages	**Disadvantages**
Easy to apply	May block pores causing irritation
Pleasant to use	Possibility of contamination
Absorbs skin moisture	Light fluffy powders may be inhaled by infants leading to breathing difficulties
Decreasing skin friction	Not suitable for application to broken skin
Discouraging bacterial growth	
Drying action gives cooling effect	

The advantages and disadvantages of dusting powders as dosage forms are summarised in Box 12.1.

12.2.1 Formulation

Some commonly used ingredients such as talc, kaolin and other natural mineral substances are liable to be heavily contaminated with bacteria, including *Clostridium tetani*, *Clostridium welchii* and *Bacillus anthracis*, which can cause tetanus and gangrene. Therefore, such ingredients must have been sterilised before use.

Dusting powders are applied to the skin for a surface effect such as drying or lubrication. Some dusting powders incorporate medicaments, giving them antibacterial or antifungal action. Examples include:

- Talc Dusting Powder BP – Used as a lubricant to prevent chafing.
- Chlorhexidine Dusting Powder BP – Used for its antibacterial effect.
- Tinaderm Powder – A proprietary product used for the treatment of fungal infections (e.g. *Tinea* infections such as athlete's foot).

Common ingredients included in dusting powders and the properties they contribute are listed in Table 12.1.

12.2.2 General method for preparing dusting powders

The method for mixing powders in the formulation of a dusting powder is the standard 'doubling-up' technique (see Key Skill 7.1).

See Powders video for a demonstration of the 'doubling-up' technique.

12.3 Bulk oral powders

Bulk oral powders resemble dusting powders (see Section 12.2) with the exception that they are intended for oral administration. The dose to be taken is measured with a 5 mL spoon, stirred into a quantity of water and then swallowed. Unfortunately, this method of measurement creates considerable problems with regard to the expected standards of precision of dosage.

Preparations in this group are formulated on the basis of dose-weights, whereas the dose is actually measured by volume. The measure of volume used is a heaped 5 mL spoonful, which is considered to be the equivalent of 5 g of powder. It is obvious that both the accuracy and precision of the dosage will be significantly influenced by a large number of varying factors. These include the density of the powders used, the interpretation of 'heaped' 5 mL spoon by the patient, etc. Consequently, this formulation is restricted to use in preparations consisting of relatively non-potent medicaments such as Kaolin BP and

Table 12.1   Common ingredients included in dusting powders and their properties

Properties	Ingredients
Absorbent	Bentonite BP
	Kaolin BP
	Starch BP
	Talc BP
Dispersing and lubricating for ease of application	Starch BP
	Talc BP
Adhesives that help the powder to stick to the skin	Aluminium Stearate BP
	Magnesium Stearate BP
	Zinc Stearate BP
Increase 'lightness and fluffiness'	Prepared Chalk BP
	Zinc Stearate BP
White, with good covering properties	Talc BP
	Zinc Oxide BP
Miscellaneous ingredients added to dusting powders:	
Antibiotics	Boric Acid BP (not used in modern preparations)
	Sulphur BP
Astringents	Aluminium Chloride BP
	Tannic Acid BP
Cooling antipruritic ingredients	Camphor BP
	Menthol BP
	Thymol BP

Magnesium Trisilicate BP, where such products are intended for the symptomatic relief of minor ailments.

Bulk powders may be a single powder (e.g. Magnesium Trisilicate Powder BP) or a mix of several powders (e.g. Calcium Carbonate Compound Powder BPC 1973).

Common proprietary products include Actonorm Powder, Andrews Salts, Bisodol Indigestion Relief Powder and Eno Powder.

The advantages of bulk oral powders as pharmaceutical products are that:

- Dry powders may be more stable than their liquid equivalent.
- Large doses of bulky powders may be administered with relative ease (e.g. indigestion powders).
- Absorption from the gastrointestinal tract will be quicker than with capsules or tablets.

The disadvantages of bulk oral powders as pharmaceutical products are that:

- The accuracy of dosage is not guaranteed,

therefore it is not a suitable dosage form for potent medication.
- The large size container means that they may be inconvenient to carry.
- It is difficult to mask any unpleasant taste.

The advantages and disadvantages of bulk oral powders as dosage forms are summarised in Box 12.2.

The method used in the manufacture of bulk oral powders is the same as that for dusting powders (see Section 12.2.2).

12.4 Individual unit dose powders

The sole difference between individual unit dose powders and bulk oral powders is that the dosage problem is overcome by providing the patient with a set of separate doses, each of which has been individually wrapped.

Single-dose powders usually consist of one or more powdered active medicaments, together

---

Box 12.2   Advantages and disadvantages of bulk oral powders as dosage forms

Advantages	Disadvantages
May be more stable than liquid equivalent	Variable dose accuracy
Administered with relative ease	Bulky and inconvenient to carry
Absorption quicker than capsules or tablets	Difficult to mask unpleasant tastes

---

with an inert diluent, and wrapped as single doses in white demy paper, folded to a uniform shape and size. The weight of each powder should be 200 mg, our recommended weight, for ease of handling by the patient. This weight is chosen because:

- 200 mg can be weighed on a Class II balance (or electronic equivalent) (i.e. 200 mg is greater than the minimum weighable quantity of the balance).
- 200 mg is an easy figure to use in pharmaceutical calculations (it is easy to undertake calculations using multiples or divisions of 200).
- 200 mg is the amount of powder that will fit into a size 3 capsule and, for ease, it would make sense to use the same calculations for both powders and capsules (see Section 12.5).

The diluent used is normally Lactose BP as it is colourless, soluble and harmless and therefore shows the ideal properties of an inert diluent. Starch BP is an alternative diluent if the patient is lactose intolerant.

Powders are useful for administration to children who cannot swallow tablets. They may be taken by pouring onto the back of the tongue and swallowing, or alternatively they may be added to a small amount of water and swallowed. There are a number of proprietary brands of individual powders of prescription-only medicines (POM) (e.g. Paramax Powders (paracetamol and metoclopramide), Stemetil Powders (prochlorperazine)) and powders readily available as over the counter (OTC) medicines include Beechams Powders, oral rehydration sachets (Dioralyte), Fennings Children's Cooling Powders and Resolve. Powders that have been commercially manufactured are often packed in sealed sachets. This is particularly true if they contain ingredients intended to produce effervescence, to protect the contents from moisture.

The advantages of unit dose powders as pharmaceutical products are that:

- They show greater stability than liquid dosage forms as the rate of reaction between drugs in a dosage form in atmospheric conditions is slower than the rate of reaction in a liquid medium.
- Accurate dosage is possible.
- They are easy to administer. Powders are relatively easy to swallow and may be mixed with food or drink in order to assist administration.
- The small particle size leads to more rapid absorption from the gastrointestinal tract compared with tablets. This in turn leads to reduced local irritation of the gastrointestinal tract which may be caused by local concentration of a drug, as encountered when taking an equivalent tablet.
- They are well accepted by patients, attractive to patients and convenient to carry.

The disadvantages of unit dose powders as pharmaceutical products are that:

- They may be difficult to swallow.
- Unpleasant flavours, bitter or nauseous, are difficult to mask when in powder form.

The advantages and disadvantages of unit dose powders as dosage forms are summarised in Box 12.3.

Box 12.3   Advantages and disadvantages of unit dose powders as dosage forms

---

Advantages	**Disadvantages**
More stable than liquid dosage forms	May be difficult to swallow
Accurate dosing	Hard to mask unpleasant flavours
Easy to administer	
Small particle size of drug	
Acceptable to patients	

12.4.1 Calculations for powders

There are two main calculations for powders, the choice being dependent on the quantity of active ingredient to be incorporated into each powder and the total number of unit doses (or excess) to be made. The two different calculations are termed single dilution and double dilution (or serial dilution).

Single dilution

Write out the formula for one powder based on a final weighing of 200 mg. Then write out the formula for the total number of powders. Remember to always make an excess.

For example, if the prescription is for five Furosemide 25 mg powders, including a suitable excess, calculate for 10 powders:

	For one powder	for 10 powders
Furosemide BP	25 mg	250 mg
Lactose BP	to 200 mg	to 2000 mg
	(i.e. 175 mg)	(i.e. 1750 mg)

So long as the final quantities to be weighed are above the minimum weighable quantity of the balance (see Section 4.1.2 and Key Skill 4.2), single dilution can be used. In this case, 250 mg is the smallest amount to be weighed. This is greater than the minimum weighable quantity of the balance and so single dilution will be suitable. If, however, the amount of active ingredient to be weighed is below the minimum weighable quantity of the balance, double dilution must be used.

Double dilution (serial dilution)

When dosages of very potent drugs are required, the active ingredient will be present in very low concentrations. By simply multiplying the quantities of the ingredients up to weighable quantities, owing to the small amount of active ingredient that would be present, it would be difficult to ensure that a uniform mix of active ingredient and diluent would be obtained. This might result in 'clumping' of the active ingredient, which could have potentially fatal consequences for the patient.

The dosage at which serial, rather than single, dilution would be required is to a certain extent arbitrary and really a matter of professional judgement. Our suggested limit is that **concentrations of active ingredient below 15 mg require serial dilution.** This limit is based on an initial mix (including an excess) for 10 powders. If each powder contains 15 mg of active ingredient, the total for 10 powders will be 150 mg of active ingredient ($10 \times 15 = 150$). This (150 mg) is equal to the accepted usual minimum weighable quantity of a Class II balance (see Section 4.1.2). Any smaller quantity would be less than the minimum weighable quantity of the balance and therefore require double dilution.

For example, if a prescription is for five Bromocriptine powders 1 mg, a total for 10 powders should be made:

	For one powder	for 10 powders
Bromocriptine BP	1 mg	10 mg
Lactose BP	to 200 mg	to 2000 mg

However, the minimum recommended weight achievable on a Class II balance for potent substances is 150 mg. This is 15 times more than the 10 mg required so single dilution would not be suitable. Therefore, dilution with lactose is required, usually based on multiples of 200 mg (see Section 12.4). Therefore if one part of bromocriptine = 200 mg then 200 mg is 19 times greater than the 10 mg required:

19 parts of lactose = 19 × 200 mg = 3800 mg

Let's call this concentrate Mix X.
  Mix X is:

Bromocriptine BP	200 mg
Lactose BP	3800 mg

It is known that 200 mg of Mix X will contain the 10 mg of Bromocriptine BP required for the master formula.
  Master formula for 10 powders:

Bromocriptine BP 10 mg		= Mix X 200 mg
Lactose BP	to 2000 mg	= to 2000 mg
	(i.e. 1990 mg)	(i.e. 1800 mg)

This will provide 10 powders each containing 10 mg of Bromocriptine BP.

12.4.2 General method for producing unit dose powders

1. Remember, for ease of handling, the minimum weight of powder in a unit dose paper is 200 mg.
2. Calculate to make an excess of the number of powders requested.
3. Determine whether a single or double dilution of the active ingredient is required (see Section 12.4.1).
4. Mix the active ingredient and the diluent (Lactose BP unless there is a reason not to use Lactose BP, for example if the patient is intolerant to lactose, or due to instability of the ingredients) in a mortar using the 'doubling-up' technique (see Key Skill 7.1).

 See Powders video for a demonstration of the 'doubling-up' technique.

5. Work on a clean dry glass tile, select a suitable size of paper (e.g. 10 cm × 10 cm), and turn in one edge and fold down approximately half an inch (1 cm). Repeat for the required number of powders.
6. Place the papers on the glass tile, with the folded edge away from the compounder, and each slightly overlapping, next to the balance pan to be used for weighing.
7. Weigh out the individual powder from the bulk powder, and transfer to the centre of the paper (if placed too near the fold, the powder will fall out during opening).
8. Fold the bottom of the powder paper up to, and underneath, the flap folded originally.
9. Fold down the top of the paper until it covers about two-thirds of the width of the paper. This top edge of this fold should help to hold the contents in the centre of the paper.
10. Fold the two ends under, so that the loose ends slightly overlap, and then tuck one flap inside the other.

    Historically, a powder trestle was used to assist the compounder with step 10 above. The paper containing the powder was placed centrally, on the top of the trestle, and then the sides bent underneath using the edges of the trestle to form neat creases. The use of a powder trestle ensured that all the powders would be of a uniform size.

📷 See Picture 29

11. Wrap each powder in turn, making sure they are all the same size.
12. Stack the powders, in pairs, flap to flap.
13. Tie together with a rubber band (not too tightly).
14. Place in a rigid cardboard box.
15. The label should be placed on the outer pack such that when the patient opens the box they do not destroy the label.

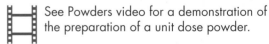 See Powders video for a demonstration of the preparation of a unit dose powder.

12.5 Unit dose capsules

Capsules are a further development from unit dose powders in that each dose of powder is enclosed in an edible container, which is swallowed whole with a draught of water (about 30–60 mL). The powder is not released from its container until it is in the stomach. This type of presentation is more convenient for the patient, and is particularly useful for medicaments which have an unpleasant taste.

The advantages and disadvantages of unit dose capsules are similar to those of unit dose powders (see Section 12.4). The advantages of unit dose capsules as pharmaceutical products are that:

- They are stable. Powders show greater stability than liquid dosage forms as the rate of reaction between drugs in a dosage form in atmospheric conditions is slower than the rate of reaction in a liquid medium.
- Accurate dosage is possible.
- They are easy to administer – capsules are relatively easy to swallow (suitable shape and slippery when moistened).
- Unpleasant tastes can be easily masked.
- The release characteristics of the drugs can be controlled.
- They can be made light resistant using opaque capsules.
- The smaller particle size of powdered drugs leads to more rapid absorption from the gastrointestinal tract compared to tablets. This

in turn leads to reduced local irritation of the gastrointestinal tract which may be caused by local concentration of a drug as encountered when taking an equivalent tablet.
- They are well accepted by patients, attractive to patients and convenient to carry.

The disadvantages of unit dose capsules as pharmaceutical products are that:

- They may be difficult to swallow.
- Capsules are unsuitable for very small children.
- Patients with strict religious beliefs and vegetarians may object to the use of animal gelatin (although non-animal gelatin capsules may be available).

The advantages and disadvantages of unit dose capsules as dosage forms are summarised in Box 12.4.

There are two main basic types of capsule:

- **Soft gelatin capsules** – These are flexible capsules and may be spherical, ovoid or cylindrical in shape. They are usually used in manufacturing when they are formed, filled and sealed in one operation. Examples of this type of capsule include Atromid S, Efamast, Epogam and nifedipine capsules (they tend to be used mainly for oils, gels, etc.).
- **Hard capsules** – These are made of hard gelatin and formed in two halves. The medicament is inserted into the longer portion and the second half fitted. Patients should be

---

Box 12.4   Advantages and disadvantages of unit dose capsules as dosage forms

Advantages

More stable than liquid dosage forms
Accurate dosing
Easy to administer
Unpleasant tastes easily masked
Release characteristics can be controlled
Can be made light resistant
Small particle size of drug
Acceptable to patients

Disadvantages

May be difficult to swallow
Unsuitable for very small children
Possible problems with the use of animal gelatin

Table 12.2   Approximate capacities of capsules

Size of capsule	Contents (mg)
000	950
00	650
0	450
1	300
2	250
3	200
4	150
5	100

instructed to swallow the capsules whole and NOT to open them. Hard gelatin capsules are available in a variety of different sizes (Table 12.2).

12.5.1 General method of preparation of capsules

1. Choose an appropriate size capsule for the powder bulk. Normally a size 3 capsule would be chosen and so work on the basis of filling each capsule with 200 mg of powder (Table 12.2).
2. Calculate quantities required and make an excess, as with the manufacture of individual unit dose powders (see Section 12.4).
3. Mix using the 'doubling-up' technique (see Key Skill 7.1).

 See Powders video for a demonstration of the 'doubling-up' technique.

4. Handle the capsules as little as possible as powder fill weights will be inaccurate as a result of contamination with grease, moisture, etc., and also for reasons of hygiene. Fill powder into the longer half of the capsule.
5. There are at least three methods of filling capsules manually. Always work on a clean tile: remember these capsules are to be swallowed by a patient.

   a. Place some powder onto a piece of weighing paper. Hold the capsule with one hand and lift the paper with the other and scoop the powder into the capsule.
   b. Place some powder onto a piece of weighing paper and fill the capsule using a chemical spatula.
   c. Weigh approximately 200 mg of powder onto a piece of weighing paper, which has been folded in half. Use the weighing paper to pour the powder into the capsule.

6. Ensure capsule outer surface is powder free. Check weight of the filled capsule. Remember to tare with an empty capsule of the same size so you are only weighing the contents of the capsule (and not including the weight of the capsule itself).

 See Powders video for a demonstration of the preparation of a capsule.

12.6 Worked examples

Example 12.1 Preparation of 100 g of Zinc Starch and Talc Dusting Powder BPC

Product formula (British Pharmaceutical Codex 1973, page 664):

	1000 g	100 g
Zinc Oxide BP	250 g	25 g
Starch BP	250 g	25 g
Purified Talc BP	500 g	50 g

Method:

1. Weigh 25 g Zinc Oxide BP using a Class II or electronic balance.
2. Weigh 25 g Starch BP using a Class II or electronic balance.
3. Weigh 50 g Purified Talc BP using a Class II or electronic balance.
4. Transfer the Starch BP to a porcelain mortar.
5. Add the Zinc Oxide BP to the Starch BP in the mortar and mix using a pestle.

   Point of clarity – Step 5
   The powders are admixed in order of volume, remembering the 'doubling-up' technique (see Key Skill 7.1).

6. Add the Purified Talc BP to the powders in the mortar and continue mixing.
7. Transfer the mixed powder to a 'powder shaker' container or an amber glass jar.
8. Label and dispense to the patient.

 See Powders video for a demonstration of the preparation of a dusting powder.

Example 12.2 Preparation of 100 g of Compound Magnesium Trisilicate Oral Powder BP

Product formula (British Pharmacopoeia 1988, page 873):

	1000 g	100 g
Magnesium Trisilicate BP	250 g	25 g
Chalk (powdered) BP	250 g	25 g
Heavy Magnesium Carbonate BP	250 g	25 g
Sodium Bicarbonate BP	250 g	25 g

Method:
1. Weigh 25 g Magnesium Trisilicate BP using a Class II or electronic balance.
2. Weigh 25 g Chalk BP using a Class II or electronic balance.
3. Weigh 25 g Heavy Magnesium Carbonate BP using a Class II or electronic balance.
4. Weigh 25 g Sodium Bicarbonate BP using a Class II or electronic balance.
5. Mix the powders in a porcelain mortar in order of bulk volume.

   Point of clarity – Step 5
   The suggested order is Sodium Bicarbonate BP first, then add Chalk BP, Heavy Magnesium Carbonate BP and finally Magnesium Trisilicate BP. The Sodium Bicarbonate BP is noticeably smallest volume and also the most likely to suffer clumping and be lumpy in appearance.

6. Transfer to an amber glass jar, label and dispense to the patient.

 See Powders video for a demonstration of the preparation of an oral powder.

Example 12.3 Preparation of five individual dose powders of Codeine Phosphate BP 10 mg

Product formula:

	1 powder	10 powders
Codeine Phosphate BP	10 mg	100 mg
Lactose BP	to 200 mg	to 2000 mg

Point of clarity – Product formula
The final weight of individual powders that we recommend for ease of calculation and administration is 200 mg. An excess is made to allow for losses during preparation.

Calculation: The quantity of Codeine Phosphate BP required for the 10 powders is 100 mg, which is below the minimum weighable quantity for a Class II balance, therefore it is recommended to follow the double (serial) dilution process.

A concentrated powder (Mix X), each 200 mg of which contains 100 mg Codeine Phosphate BP, needs to be prepared. As 100 mg cannot be accurately weighed, the quantities in Mix X need to be adjusted. To keep Mix X the same concentration, both parts of the concentration ratio must be multiplied by the same factors, i.e.

2 × 100 mg = 200 mg
2 × 200 mg = 400 mg

Therefore Mix X must have a concentration 200 mg/400 mg (200 mg Codeine Phosphate BP per 400 mg of Mix X).
As we must have exact weights the quantities for Mix X are:

Codeine Phosphate BP	200 mg
Lactose BP	200 mg (i.e. to 400 mg)

Therefore the final formula for preparation for the 10 powders, Mix Y, will be:

Mix X	200 mg (containing 100 mg Codeine Phosphate BP)
Lactose BP	to 2000 mg (1800 mg)

Method for preparing Codeine Phosphate 10 mg unit dose powders using the above formula:
1. Weigh 200 mg Codeine Phosphate BP using a Class II or electronic balance.
2. Transfer to a porcelain mortar.
3. Weigh 200 mg Lactose BP using a Class II or electronic balance.
4. Add the Lactose BP to the Codeine Phosphate BP in the mortar using the 'doubling-up' technique.
5. This is Mix X.
6. Weigh 200 mg Mix X using a Class II or electronic balance and transfer to a clean dry mortar.
7. Weigh 1800 mg Lactose BP using a Class II or electronic balance.
8. Add the Lactose BP to the Mix X in the mortar using the 'doubling-up' technique.
9. This is Mix Y.
10. Weigh 200 mg aliquots of the Mix Y and wrap as individual dose powders.
11. Pack the powders flap to flap end enclose with a rubber band.
12. Pack into a cardboard box and label.

 See Powders video for a demonstration
of the preparation of a unit dose powder.

12.7 Summary of essential principles relating to powders and capsules

This section will recap the main principles relating to powders and capsules that have been covered in other sections of the book. To assist compounders in understanding the extemporaneous preparation of powders and capsules, this section contains the following:

- Further notes on the packaging of extemporaneously prepared powders and capsules.
- Specific points relevant to the expiry of extemporaneously prepared powders and capsules.
- Additional key points related to the labelling of pharmaceutical powders and capsules.

12.7.1 Packaging

The packaging of powders and capsules is dependent on the formulation.

Bulk powders for external use

Bulk powders for external use are either packaged as for bulk oral powders or in a powder shaker with a sifter top.

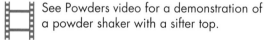

See Powders video for a demonstration of a powder shaker with a sifter top.

Bulk oral powders

Bulk oral powders are usually packaged in an airtight glass or plastic jar. It is important that the preparation is not exposed to moisture as this will result in clumping of the product and may encourage microbial growth.

Individual unit dose powders

Once made, individual unit dose powders are placed flap to flap and secured together by a rubber band. The whole set of powders is then placed in a rigid cardboard container and the label is placed on the container before the preparation is dispensed to the patient.

Preparations containing effervescent or deliquescent ingredients need to be packed in a sealed container (e.g. an ointment jar).

Unit dose capsules

Unit dose capsules are dispensed in a glass or plastic tablet bottle with a child-resistant closure.

12.7.2 Discard dates

Proprietary powders and capsules are manufactured in special environments and usually attract a long shelf life. When dealing with extemporaneously prepared preparations, the compounder must take a number of considerations into mind when deciding the length of expiry to give a product, such as the stability of the ingredients within the preparation and the susceptibility of the preparation to microbial contamination. As a general rule, an expiry of up to three months may be given to any of the preparations in this chapter, although consideration must be given to each individual formulation.

Remember that as patients frequently misunderstand the term 'expiry' it is suggested that a preferred method of indicating shelf life on the label of extemporaneously compounded products is to apply the term 'Discard after' followed by a definite date and/or time.

Further guidance on expiry dates for pharmaceutical preparations can be found in Section 5.6.1.

12.7.3 Labelling

The labelling of extemporaneous preparations has been covered in Section 5.6.2. An overview of the main considerations for the labelling of powders and capsules will be given here.

In addition to the standard requirements for the labelling of extemporaneous preparations, the following points need to be taken into consideration:

- Bulk oral powders, individual unit dose powders and bulk powders for external use are all susceptible to moisture. For this reason, it is necessary to include the caution '**Store in a**

dry place' on the label of any of these preparations.

- Dusting powders will also attract the caution 'Not to be applied to open wounds or raw weeping surfaces'.
- In addition, any preparation intended for external use (i.e. bulk powders for external use) would attract the additional caution 'For external use only'.

Further guidance on auxiliary labelling can be found in Section 5.6.1, Table 5.10.

In addition to labels about storage, labels for individual powders and capsules containing potent ingredients may also require British National Formulary additional caution labels. These can all be found in Appendix 9 of the current edition of the British National Formulary.

13

Specialised formulation issues

13.1 Introduction and overview

Many items that are dispensed extemporaneously are unlicensed medicines. The purpose of licensing medicines in the UK is to ensure that they are examined for their safety, efficacy and quality. During the extemporaneous dispensing process, 'one-off' medication for a particular patient is often prepared and there is no licence and no stability or safety data available. The main areas where ad hoc formulations are prepared are in paediatric medicine and dermatology, where extemporaneous dispensing is widespread.

13.2 Posology

Posology (derived from the Greek *posos*, how much, and *logos*, science) is the branch of medicine/pharmacy dealing with doses. Doses cannot be rigidly fixed. In many cases, allowances may need to be made for:

- The age of the patient
- The weight of the patient
- The condition being treated and its severity
- The route of administration
- The frequency of administration
- Any co-existing disease(s) or condition(s), such as renal failure, liver failure or pregnancy

- Any acquired tolerance. For example:

  - Drug addicts can, over a long period of time, acquire the ability to take with comparative safety large doses of certain drugs which, in normal patients, would produce harmful or fatal effects.
  - Terminally ill patients can also show the same type of tolerance to high doses of opioid pain killers (e.g. morphine, diamorphine, etc.) and the British National Formulary gives some guidelines with regard to doses used in palliative care.

Scrupulous checking of the dose and frequency of all drugs intended for internal use is essential. When an unusual dose appears to have been prescribed it is the responsibility of the **pharmacist** to satisfy themselves that the prescriber's intention has been correctly interpreted. Similarly, the concentration of active constituents in products for external use must be checked.

13.2.1 Paediatric formulations

Some medicines are either specifically marketed for children or have a product licence for use in both children and adults. In these situations, recommended doses for paediatric use may be given in monographs of individual drugs by age. Other terms that may be used instead of age include the following recommended by the Royal College of Paediatrics and Child Health:

- **Preterm newborn infant** – Born at less than 37 weeks' gestation.
- **Term newborn infant neonate** – 0 to 27 days.
- **Infants and toddlers** – 28 days to 23 months.
- **Children** – 2 to 11 years.
- **Adolescents** – 12 to 18 years.

Although, as highlighted above, some medicines are specifically designed for paediatric use, many medicines are licensed for use solely in adults and are therefore routinely made in formulations that are most appropriate for use by adults, usually tablets or capsules. However, medicinal agents licensed for adults are frequently used in children in a so-called 'off-label' manner. This means that the product licence for the medication was issued for use in adults and that use in children has not been examined and the product is therefore not licensed. Alternatively, a product can be licensed for use in a particular paediatric condition and then subsequently found to be efficacious in another. If the medicine is used to treat the latter condition, it is also termed being used 'off label'.

When considering formulations for children, the child should not be considered to be a 'mini adult'. The drug-handling capabilities of the body change markedly from birth to adulthood. Doses cannot be just determined by comparison of adult and child weights – age-related differences in drug handling and drug sensitivity prevent this from being accurate. The use of body surface area is a more accurate way to determine doses in individual paediatric situations. These principles also apply in geriatric medicine.

Most 'one-off' extemporaneous preparations originate in hospitals. Since current healthcare strategies are to shift therapy from secondary to primary care, it is important that two-way communication between hospital pharmacy and community pharmacy is encouraged, in order to provide seamless care. This is particularly important in the case of extemporaneously prepared medicines, as the formulation given may affect the bioavailability of the drug. It is, therefore, imperative that formulations should remain unchanged.

Dose checking for paediatric preparations can be extremely difficult and may involve a lengthy search for information. In the primary care situation, if normal reference sources found in the pharmacy fail to confirm the safety of a particular preparation with regard to dose of active ingredient, the local hospital from where the formula originated is often the next best source of information, although there are also other information sources, for example:

- DIAL (Drug Information Advisory Line) – a national unit providing paediatric medicines information. Tel: (0151) 252 5837, Fax: (0151) 220 3885, e-mail: info@dial.org.uk, Web: www.dial.org.uk.
- Drug information centres and local hospitals – contact details for Regional and District Medicines Information Services can be found in the current edition of the British National Formulary (BNF) or British National Formulary for Children.
- The current edition of the British National Formulary for Children (www.bnfc.org).
- The Royal College of Paediatrics and Child Health (RCPCH) (http://www.rcpch.ac.uk/).
- The Neonatal and Paediatric Pharmacists Group (NPPG) (http://www.nppg.org.uk/).

When using formulae from sources such as the local hospital, it must be remembered that the compounder is still responsible for checking that the product formula is safe and suitable for use. It must not be assumed that as the formula originated from a hospital (or other healthcare environment) it is safe for the patient.

Formulation considerations for extemporaneous preparations for children

- Source of drug
  a. Adult dosage form (tablet or capsule)
  b. Chemical ingredient
- Route of administration
  a. Topical
  b. Parenteral
    i. Intramuscular (painful, therefore less acceptable)
    ii. Intravenous (higher risk associated with calculation errors)

c. Rectal – acceptability to the parent or patient (if child rather than infant)

d. Oral

Types of oral formulation to consider are:

- Powders
- Segments from tablets (uniformity of dose is limited by accuracy of tablet splitting)
- Liquid

    a. Formulation – solution, suspension etc.
    b. Palatability, taste and texture
    c. Stability.

Powders

Smaller or tailored doses of drugs that are available in tablet or capsule form can be made by crushing the required number of tablets in a mortar and mixing with a diluent such as Starch BP or Lactose BP, or combining the contents of the required number of capsules with a suitable diluent. This is a good method to use if there are issues concerning the stability of a drug in aqueous solution. Obvious exceptions to suitability for conversion of a tablet or capsule to this dosage form include:

- Enteric coated tablets or other coated tablets.
- Sustained-release (SR) or modified-release (MR) tablets or capsules.
- Dispersible tablets which may lend themselves to the production of a liquid formulation.

Factors influencing drug therapy in paediatric patients

When checking paediatric doses we need to be aware of the factors that influence drug therapy in children. These factors include absorption, distribution, metabolism and excretion.

Absorption

- **Oral absorption** – This can be affected by variable gastric and intestinal transit times. In young infants the gastric emptying time may be prolonged, but by six months of age it will be approaching adult rates. Although the extent of drug absorption is not normally affected, the rate of absorption can be. Therefore, sustained-release preparations need to be used with caution in young children.

Oral absorption is also affected by increased gastric pH. Before the age of two years the output of gastric acid is reduced and therefore gastric pH is not comparable to adult levels. This can cause, for example, increased absorption of acid-labile medicines such as penicillin because of reduced drug breakdown, or slowed or reduced absorption of acidic medicines such as phenytoin or phenobarbital because of changes in ionisation state.

- **Topical absorption** – Neonates have a greater body surface area to weight ratio than adults. In addition, the stratum corneum of the neonate is thinner. Therefore, there is greater potential for systemic absorption and resultant side effects after topical application in the neonate. This is particularly so when potent agents are applied, when application is to broken or inflamed skin, or when occlusive coverings are applied. This can cause, for example, neurotoxicity and death following hexochlorophene absorption. Topical corticosteroids may be absorbed systemically and produce significant adrenal suppression.
- **Rectal absorption** – Absorption via the rectal route can be erratic and variable in children and is not one favoured by parents. However, it is useful if the child is vomiting or is disinclined or unable to take medicine orally. Certain drugs should never be administered to children rectally. These are usually ones with narrow therapeutic indices, where predicting the absorption is important, for example in the case of theophylline, where the absorption from the rectum can be erratic. Other drugs are employed rectally because of the rapid absorption through the rectal mucosa and their rapid onset of action. For example, diazepam solution stops seizures rapidly and can be administered rectally in an emergency.

Distribution

- **Increased total body water** – During infancy, the percentage body weight contributed by water is appreciably higher than in older children and adults. Therefore, on a dose to body weight basis, larger doses of water-soluble drugs are often required than would otherwise be expected.
- **Decreased plasma protein binding** – Because

neonates have relatively high levels of bilirubin, which protein binds, significant competition between the bilirubin and highly protein-bound drugs can occur. For example, phenytoin, furosemide and indometacin are appreciably less protein bound in a neonate than in an adult. This results in higher levels of free drug and therefore it may be necessary to give larger loading doses of highly protein-bound drugs in neonates.

- **Blood–brain barrier** – The blood–brain barrier is poorly developed in neonates and drugs that would not normally penetrate the central nervous system may do so. This can be used to advantage, for example where gentamicin is used to treat central sepsis and meningitis in neonates.

Metabolism

- Enzyme systems mature at different times and may be absent at birth. Hepatic oxidation and glucuronidation are reduced in the neonate, but demethylation and sulphation are little affected. Oxidised drugs, such as lidocaine, phenobarbital, phenytoin and diazepam, have prolonged half-lives and tend to accumulate in neonates. Similarly, drugs that undergo glucuronidation, such as chloramphenicol, have longer half-lives.
- Altered metabolic pathways may exist for some drugs. Paracetamol is metabolised by sulphation in the neonate, rather than by glucuronidation as in adults. This is because the latter metabolic route takes several months to become fully mature.
- Metabolic rate increases dramatically in children and in some cases is greater than in adults. Therefore, children may require more frequent dosing or higher doses on a mg/kg basis. Hepatic microsomal oxidation is more rapid in children (1–10 years) than in adults. Drugs such as carbamazepine, ethosuximide, phenobarbital, phenytoin and theophylline all have significantly shorter half-lives in children than they do in adults. Consequently, children need higher doses of anticonvulsants per kilogram bodyweight than adults.

Excretion

Renal excretory capacity is reduced in neonates, reaching adult values at 6–12 months of age. Therefore, any drugs that will be excreted by this route will require dose reduction. This is especially true of the aminoglycosides, cephalosporins, digoxin and penicillins, all of which have prolonged half-lives during the first week of life.

Dose calculations

There are a number of factors that need to be taken into consideration when calculating a dose for a paediatric patient:

- **Body surface area** – This is the most accurate way to calculate a dose for a child. This is because the surface area reflects cardiac output, fluid requirements and renal function better than weight-based dosing. In practice, however, this method is of limited use as the surface area can increase by 1–2% per day in a young child and therefore any dose would need frequent readjustment. It can also be difficult to ascertain the height of a child accurately, especially in small children.
- **Weight** – Weight-based calculations are the most commonly used, with tables to guide percentage calculations being available in the British National Formulary.
- **Age** – Doses based on age range are mainly used for drugs with a wide therapeutic index.

The British National Formulary gives guidance on the relationship between ideal body weight, height and body surface area (Table 13.1) and a number of specialist paediatric formularies are available.

13.2.2 Extemporaneous formulations for geriatric patients

Just as there are differences in doses recommended for children because of the pharmacokinetic differences between adults and children, this also applies to the elderly population (generally accepted as the over-65s). An awareness of the differences in drug handling presented by the elderly is significant if you consider that the over-65s constitute about 18% of the UK population but receive 39% of the prescribed drugs (twice as many as younger people).

Table 13.1 Relationship between ideal body weight, height and body surface area for children of different ages and adults (adapted from the British National Formulary, 48th edition)

Age	Ideal body weight		Height		Body surface
	kg	lb	cm	inch	m^2
Newborn[a]	3.5	7.7	50	20	0.23
1 month[a]	4.2	9	55	22	0.26
3 months[a]	5.6	12	59	23	0.32
6 months	7.7	17	67	26	0.40
1 year	10	22	76	30	0.47
3 years	15	33	94	37	0.62
5 years	18	40	108	42	0.73
7 years	23	51	120	47	0.88
12 years	39	86	148	58	1.25
Adult					
Male	68	150	173	68	1.80
Female	56	123	163	64	1.60

[a]The figures relate to full-term and not preterm infants, who may need reduced dosage according to their clinical condition.

Factors influencing drug therapy in geriatric patients

When checking geriatric doses, the following need to be taken into consideration:

- **Absorption** – Age differences are of little clinical value but consideration must be given to the rate of gastric emptying, the effect of food and any disease of the small intestine.
- **Distribution**
  a. Body fat – Geriatric patients tend to have lean body mass and consequently there tends to be an increased volume of distribution of lipophilic drugs (e.g. benzodiazepines).
  b. Decrease in body water which results in a decreased volume of distribution of water-soluble drugs.
  c. Protein binding does not significantly change with age. It is more likely to change because of an existing disease state.
- **Metabolism** – Hepatic metabolism is affected by the reduced liver blood flow that occurs with age. This means that there is reduced clearance of drugs that undergo extensive first-pass metabolism (e.g. propranolol, verapamil, warfarin).
- **Excretion** – Renal excretion is heavily reliant on the glomerular filtration rate of the kidney, which usually declines with age. If renal function is impaired, water-soluble drugs, especially those with a narrow therapeutic index (e.g. digoxin), should be given in reduced dosages.

13.2.3 The dose check

Is the formula safe?

Products for internal route of administration
If the formula is official, then it should be safe. If the formula is unofficial, then it must be checked. The easiest way to check the formula is to find a **similar official product** and then look at the ingredients that differ and determine whether they are within safe limits (e.g. compare the amounts in other products with similar uses).

If there is no similar official formula then **all the ingredients** must be checked individually (i.e. compare the contents of products with similar uses, or find information on safe dose ranges for each individual ingredient).

Products for external application

Checks should be used similar to those outlined above. In addition it should be borne in mind that too high a concentration of an active ingredient could potentially cause serious damage to the skin and also introduce the possibility of systemic absorption. Too low a concentration could render the product ineffective.

Is the dose safe?

Products for internal administration

- **What is the dose?** The dose is the quantity to be administered at one time (e.g. if two tablets are to be taken three times a day, **two** would be the dose; If two 5 mL spoonfuls are to be given three times a day, 10 mL would be the dose).
- **Is the dose frequency safe?** In older references the dose frequency may not be specified. Note that if the dose of an oral liquid is specified as 5 mL or 10 mL, the dose regimen would be 5 mL or 10 mL **three or four times daily** by convention.

Dose checks that do not concur with the literature should be queried with the prescriber. This includes doses/quantities that appear to be **LOWER** than those in the literature as well as those that appear to be **HIGHER.**

When querying a dose it is also advisable to have a suggested alternative to offer that would be acceptable; however, always take into consideration that, whatever dose is suggested, it must be suitable for administration to the patient in the given pharmaceutical form. For example, it would be of little use working out a dose that would mean a patient had to administer/measure 3.642 mL of a solution to obtain the appropriate dose as this would not be measurable in the primary care environment, where the accepted dosage measure is a 5 mL spoon or an oral syringe.

Remember that underdosing can be as serious as overdosing. Underdosing can result in:

- Reduced or no therapeutic effect.
- Loss of control of a medical condition with possible progression of the disease.

- Symptoms suffered unnecessarily.
- Discontinuation of treatment by the patient as they perceive no benefit.

Overdosing can result in:

- Adverse effects to patient that may be temporary or long term.
- Possible fatal consequences.
- Possibility of hospital admission, which can be inconvenient to the patient and have high cost implications.
- Increased likelihood of side effects associated with the medication.
- Reduced patient compliance because of increased side effects (e.g. drowsiness).
- New medical problems being encountered that have been precipitated by the overdose.

13.2.4 Incompatibilities

When formulating extemporaneous products care must be taken to avoid incompatibilities between ingredients that might result in the production of an unsatisfactory product. Incompatibilities can be therapeutic, physical or chemical.

Therapeutic

This is normally the responsibility of the prescriber and is more akin to the drug interactions we are aware of in modern dispensing. A classic example of an extemporaneously prepared therapeutic incompatibility would be the formulation of a cough medicine containing both an expectorant and a cough suppressant.

Physical

Immiscibility

- Oils and water. This can be overcome using emulsifying agents.
- Insoluble powders that are difficult to wet (e.g. sulphur) and some corticosteroids that are difficult to wet with water. This problem is solved by the addition of wetting agents.

Insolubility

- Liquid preparations containing an indiffusible powder such as chalk require a suspending agent or thickening agent to ensure an even dose delivery.

• Resinous tinctures produce precipitates when diluted with an aqueous vehicle. Once again the addition of a suspending agent will ensure even dose delivery.

• A potent insoluble drug may be replaced with a soluble salt in some cases to prevent uneven dosing owing to insufficient shaking of a suspension. Failure to do this can result in possibly fatal overdose in the overly concentrated last few doses. For example, it may be better to replace an insoluble alkaloid with a soluble alkaloidal salt.

Chemical

When practitioners regularly made their own formulae there was always concern that a combination of prescribed substances could result in the formation of a harmful or dangerous product.

13.3 Dermatological extemporaneous formulation

Extemporaneous formulation of products for topical application is probably the most common form of extemporaneous dispensing seen in the primary care setting. In addition, many specialist hospital units have their own dermatological formulary, which will consist of formulae ranging from the preparation of creams and ointments from first principles to diluting or combining proprietary products.

Advantages of extemporaneously prepared products, including combining different proprietary brands within the same formulation, include:

• Two or more active ingredients combined in one preparation may have a synergistic effect.
• Ease of administration leading to better patient compliance.
• May lead to reduction in course of treatment because of 1 and 2 above.
• Ability to prepare a formulation when no suitable/equivalent proprietary preparation is available.

Problems that may be encountered include:

• Unpredictable interactions may occur.
• There may be decreased stability of the active ingredients, either rendering them virtually inactive or converting the active form of the drug into a less active form.
• Any preservative present may have its activity reduced as a result of varying combinations of products.

Dilutions of topical steroids have been popular for some time and have even led to manufacturers producing ready-made dilutions of their products (e.g. Betnovate and Betnovate-RD preparations, Synalar and Synalar 1 in 10 Dilution and Synalar 1 in 4 Dilution).

Dilution of a topical steroid allows the prescriber to change the strength of product based on the observed clinical response. However, there may be a problem in that dilution of the product does not necessarily result in a proportional dilution of potency. In addition there is a risk of incompatibility between the complex proprietary formulations and the simple bases used for dilution. This issue was addressed to a certain extent by the introduction of diluent directories, which recommended the diluent to use if dilution, although not recommended by the manufacturer, was insisted upon.

In addition to the dilution of topical steroid a number of other ingredients form part of the standard formulary in many specialist units. These include:

• **Coal Tar BP** – Used in the treatment of psoriasis, eczema and other skin conditions. Ointments containing coal tar or an alcoholic solution of coal should be prepared without heating. There is concern over the potential carcinogenic effects of coal tar and therefore gloves must be worn when preparing a product.
• **Dithranol BP** – Used to treat psoriasis, where it has the advantage of penetrating the psoriatic lesions more speedily than normal skin. One problem is that dithranol is subject to oxidative degradation, and therefore an antioxidant added to the formulation would be an advantage. Salicylic acid does this in ointment formulations such as dithranol in

Lassar's paste. In cream preparations the addition of ascorbic acid or oxalic acid as an antioxidant has been found to be helpful.

Dithranol is extremely irritant and therefore precautions must be taken when preparing extemporaneous formulations, such as wearing goggles, gloves and a mask. As the powder is so irritant it is advised that during trituration a solvent is used to dissolve the powder initially. Liquid Paraffin BP or chloroform have been used successfully.

- **Ichthammol BP** – This has slight bacteriostatic properties and is used topically for a wide range of skin disorders. In ointment preparations the strength usually employed is 10–50%.
- **Salicylic Acid BP** – This is used in varying strengths depending on the condition treated. Ointments for the treatment of chronic ulcers, dandruff, eczema or psoriasis usually contain 1–5%, collodion paints for warts and corns 10–12%, and plasters for the destruction of warts and corns 20–50%.

Bases regularly used for extemporaneous preparation of ointments/creams or the dilution of ointments/creams include:

- Aqueous Cream BP
- Buffered Cream BP
- Cetomacrogol Cream (Formula A) BP
- Cetomacrogol Cream (Formula B) BP
- Emulsifying Ointment BP
- Unguentum Merck
- Yellow Soft Paraffin BP and White Soft Paraffin BP.

Both the vehicle (base) and the active ingredients are important in the treatment of skin conditions. The vehicle itself has a greater effect than just a placebo or carrier, and the choice of vehicle is of importance in terms of:

- Suitability for intended use (for example, White Soft Paraffin BP would not be a suitable base for a preparation intended for use a as a pomade or shampoo).
- Any solubility characteristics of the active ingredient.
- Cosmetic and general acceptability to the patient.
- The safety and stability of the final preparation.

Further reading

It is beyond the scope of this book to go into detail on the science behind the different formulations described in the various chapters. The texts listed below will be of use to compounders who wish to learn more about the science behind the formulations.

Aulton M E (ed) 1988, *Pharmaceutics – The Science of Dosage For Design*. Churchill Livingstone, Edinburgh.

Banker G S, Rhodes C T (ed) 2002, *Modern Pharmaceutics*. Marcel Dekker, New York, USA.

Collett D M, Aulton M E (ed) 1990, *Pharmaceutical Practice*. Churchill Livingstone, Edinburgh.

Florence A T, Attwood D 1998, *Physicochemical Principles of Pharmacy*. Palgrave, Hampshire.

Ghosh T K, Jasti B R (ed) 2005, *Theory and Practice of Contemporary Pharmaceutics*. CRC Press, Florida, USA.

Martin A N 1993, *Physical Pharmacy*. Lippincott, Williams & Wilkins, Baltimore, Maryland, USA.

In addition, the following text will be of use to compounders wishing to practise and further understand pharmaceutical calculations.

Rees J A, Smith I, Smith B 2001, *Introduction to Pharmaceutical Calculations*. Pharmaceutical Press, London.

Finally, the following text would be of interest to those compounders wishing to find out more about the history behind the formulations.

Anderson S (ed) 2005, *Making Medicines: A Brief History of Pharmacy and Pharmaceuticals*. Pharmaceutical Press, London.

Part 3

Product formulae

Preface

As a result of recent changes in pharmaceutical practice it is becoming less common for pharmacists, especially within a primary care setting, to compound extemporaneous products for patients. This has resulted in a comparable decline in the inclusion of extemporaneous formulae in modern official text books.

To assist the compounder in their choice of formulation for an extemporaneous product, this part of the book contains a selection of extemporaneous formulae. These are a mixture of old formulae that are now rarely used but which still have a place in therapeutics along with some formulae that have been derived from old texts.

Formulae contents

The following index lists, in alphabetical order, product formulae contained in all three parts of the book. The source of each formula is included with its entry.

14

Creams

14.1 Cetrimide Cream BP (Cremor Cetrimidi) (BP 1988, page 653)

Ingredients	Quantities
Liquid Paraffin BP	500 g
Cetostearyl Alcohol BP	50 g
Cetrimide BP	5 g
Freshly boiled and cooled purified water	445 g

Dose: Apply when required (but do not apply repeatedly).

Use: Used as an antiseptic cream.

14.2 Dimethicone Cream BPC (Cremor Dimethiconi) (BPC 1973, page 657)

Ingredients	Quantities
Liquid Paraffin BP	400 g
Dimethicone 350 BP	100 g
Cetostearyl Alcohol BP	50 g
Cetrimide BP	5 g
Chlorocresol BP	1 g
Freshly boiled and cooled purified water	444 g

Dose: Apply when required.

Use: Used as a barrier cream, for example for the prevention of napkin rash or pressure sores.

14.3 Salicylic Acid and Sulphur Cream BP (Cremor Acidi Salicylici et Sulphuris) (BP 1980, page 548)

Ingredients	Quantities
Aqueous Cream BP	960 g
Salicylic Acid BP	20 g
Sulphur BP	20 g

Dose: Apply twice a day.
    Use: Used to treat mild acne.

14.4 Zinc and Ichthammol Cream BP (Cremor Zinci et Ichthammolis) (BP 1988, page 666)

Ingredients	Quantities
Zinc Cream BP	820 g
Wool Fat BP	100 g
Ichthammol BP	50 g
Cetostearyl Alcohol BP	30 g

Dose: Apply twice daily.
    Use: Used to treat psoriasis and eczema. Ichthammol is milder than coal tar and is used to treat less acute forms of eczema.

14.5 Calamine Cream Aqueous BPC (Cremor Calaminae Aquosus) (BPC, 1973, page 656)

Ingredients	Quantities
Calamine BP	40 g
Zinc Oxide BP	30 g
Arachis Oil BP	300 g
Emulsifying Wax BP	60 g
Freshly boiled and cooled purified water	570 g

Dose: Apply when required.
    Use: Used to relieve itching.

14.6 Buffered Cream BP (Cremor Normalis) (BP 1988, page 652)

Ingredients	Quantities
Sodium Phosphate BP	25 g
Citric Acid BP	5 g
Chlorocresol BP	1 g
Emulsifying Ointment BP	300 g
Freshly boiled and cooled purified water	669 g

Use: Emollient cream used as a base carrier of other active ingredients.

14.7 Aqueous Cream BP (Cremor Cerae Aquos – also known as Simple Cream) (BP 1988, page 650)

Ingredients	Quantities
Emulsifying Ointment BP	300 g
Phenoxyethanol BP	10 g
Freshly boiled and cooled purified water	690 g

Phenoxyethanol is used as a preservative. Earlier formulae use 0.1% chlorocresol as a preservative.
    Use: Emollient cream used as a base carrier of other active ingredients.

14.8 Zinc Cream BP (BP 1988, page 665)

Ingredients	Quantities
Zinc Oxide BP	320 g
Calcium Hydroxide BP	0.45 g
Oleic Acid BP	5 mL
Arachis Oil BP	320 mL
Wool Fat BP	80 g
Freshly boiled and cooled purified water	to 1000 g

Use: Used as a mild astringent for the skin and as a soothing and protective application in eczema.

14.9 Cetomacrogol Cream BP
(BP 1988, page 653)

Formula A:

Ingredients	Quantities
Cetomacrogol Emulsifying Ointment BP	300 g
Chlorocresol BP	1 g
Purified water freshly boiled and cooled	to 1000 g

Formula B:

Ingredients	Quantities
Cetomacrogol Emulsifying Ointment BP	300 g
Benzyl Alcohol BP	15 g
Propyl Hydroxybenzoate BP	0.8 g
Methyl Hydroxybenzoate BP	1.5 g
Purified water freshly boiled and cooled	to 1000 g

The difference between Formulae A and B is that they contain different preservatives.

A better product is produced if the Cetomacrogol Emulsifying Ointment BP is replaced by the appropriate quantities of ingredients (i.e. Liquid Paraffin BP, White Soft Paraffin BP and Cetomacrogol Emulsifying Wax BP; see Chapter 18 for formula).

Use: Rarely used in its own right as an emollient; usually used as a diluent for other creams (see NPA diluent directory).

14.10 Chlorhexidine Cream BPC (Cremor Chlorhexidinae) (BPC 1973, page 657)

Ingredients	Quantities
Chlorhexidine Gluconate Solution BP	50 mL
Cetomacrogol Emulsifying Wax BP	250 g
Liquid Paraffin BP	100 g
Purified water freshly boiled and cooled	to 1000 g

Use: Antiseptic cream.

14.11 Clioquinol Cream BPC
(BPC 1973, page 658)

Ingredients	Quantities
Clioquinol BP	30 g
Chlorocresol BP	1 g
Cetomacrogol Emulsifying Ointment BP	300 g
Purified water freshly boiled and cooled	669 g

Caution: Clioquinol may stain clothing or discolour fair hair.

Use: Treat skin infections.

14.12 Hydrocortisone Cream BPC (Cremor Hydrocortisoni) (BPC 1973, page 659)

Ingredients	Quantities
Hydrocortisone BP or Hydrocortisone Acetate BP	10 g
Chlorocresol BP	1 g
Cetomacrogol Emulsifying Ointment BP	300 g
Purified water freshly boiled and cooled	689 g

Use: Used to treat eczema.

15

Dusting powders

15.1 Chlorhexidine Dusting Powder BPC (BPC 1973, page 662)

Ingredients	Quantities
Chlorhexidine Hydrochloride BP	5 g
Maize Starch BP	995 g

Use: Disinfectant powder.

15.2 Hexachlorophane Dusting Powder BPC (BPC 1973, page 663)

Ingredients	Quantities
Hexachlorophane	3 g
Zinc Oxide BP	30 g
Maize Starch BP	967 g

Use: Disinfectant powder with bacteriostatic activity against *Staphylococcus aureus*. Used to apply to the umbilicus of babies.

15.3 Talc Dusting Powder BP (Conspersus Talci) (BP 1988, page 668)

Ingredients	Quantities
Purified Talc BP	900 g
Maize Starch BP	100 g

Use: A dusting powder to relieve irritation and prevent chafing.

15.4 Zinc, Starch and Talc Dusting Powder BPC (Conspersus Zinci, Amyli et Talci) (BPC 1973, page 664)

Ingredients	Quantities
Purified Talc BP	500 g
Starch BP	250 g
Zinc Oxide BP	250 g

Use: Absorbent dusting powder.

16

Internal mixtures

16.1 Saline Mixture BPC (Mistura Diaphoretica) (BPC 1968, page 1185)

Ingredients	Quantities
Sodium Citrate BP	50 g
Sodium Nitrite BP	3 g
Strong Ammonium Acetate Solution BP	50 mL
Concentrated Camphor Water BP	25 mL
Water	to 1000 mL

Dose: 10–20 mL.

This product would need to be Freshly Prepared as there is no preservative and hence would attract a two-week discard date.

Use: This product was used as an expectorant.

16.2 Belladonna Mixture Paediatric BPC (Mistura Belladonna pro Infantibus) (BPC 1973, page 737)

Ingredients	Quantities
Belladonna Tincture BP	30 mL
Syrup BP	200 mL
Glycerol BP	100 mL
Benzoic Acid Solution BP	20 mL
Compound Orange Spirit BP	2 mL
Water	to 1000 mL

Dose: Child up to 1 year – 5 mL; 1–5 years – 10 mL.

This product would be Recently Prepared as Benzoic Acid BP acts as a preservatives and therefore would attract a four-week discard date.

Use: This product was used to treat colic.

16.3 Gentian and Rhubarb Mixture BPC (Mistura Gentianae cum Rheo) (BPC 1973, page 744)

Ingredients	Quantities
Sodium Bicarbonate BP	50 g
Concentrated Compound Gentian Infusion BP	50 mL
Compound Rhubarb Tincture BP	100 mL
Concentrated Peppermint Emulsion BP	25 mL
Double Strength Chloroform Water BP	500 mL
Water	to 1000 mL

Dose: 10–20 mL.

This product would be Recently Prepared as Double Strength Chloroform Water BP acts as a preservative and therefore would attract a four-week discard date.

Use: This product was used to stimulate appetite. The gentian acts as a bitter. Although known for its purgative action in low doses, the astringent action of the rhubarb predominates. Rhubarb is therefore used as an astringent bitter in products such as this.

16.4 Magnesium Carbonate Mixture BPC (Mistura Magnesii Carbonatis) (BPC 1973, page 746)

Ingredients	Quantities
Light Magnesium Carbonate BP	50 g
Sodium Bicarbonate BP	80 g
Concentrated Peppermint Emulsion BP	25 mL
Double Strength Chloroform Water BP	500 mL
Water	to 1000 mL

Dose: 10–20 mL.

This product would be Recently Prepared as Double Strength Chloroform Water BP acts as a preservative and therefore would attract a four-week discard date.

Use: This product was used as an antacid.

16.5 Aromatic Magnesium Carbonate Mixture BPC (Mistura Carminativa) (BPC 1973, page 746)

Ingredients	Quantities
Light Magnesium Carbonate BP	30 g
Sodium Bicarbonate BP	50 g
Aromatic Cardamom Tincture BP	30 mL
Double Strength Chloroform Water BP	500 mL
Water	to 1000 mL

Dose: 10–20 mL.

This product would be Recently Prepared as Double Strength Chloroform Water BP acts as a preservative and therefore would attract a four-week discard date.

Use: This product was used as an antacid.

16.6 Magnesium Sulphate Mixture BPC (Mistura Alba) (BPC 1973, page 747)

Ingredients	Quantities
Magnesium Sulphate BP	400 g
Light Magnesium Carbonate BP	50 g
Concentrated Peppermint Emulsion BP	25 mL
Double Strength Chloroform Water BP	300 mL
Water	to 1000 mL

Dose: 10–20 mL.

This product would be Recently Prepared as Double Strength Chloroform Water BP acts as a preservative and therefore would attract a four-week discard date.

The taste of this preparation is unpalatable and it was suggested that the taste may further be disguised by the addition of syrup, fruit syrups, ginger syrup or liquorice.

Use: This product was used as a laxative because of the purgative action of the Magnesium Sulphate BP.

16.7 Potassium Citrate Mixture BP (Mistura Potassii Citratis) (BP 1988, page 748)

Ingredients	Quantities
Potassium Citrate BP	300 g
Citric Acid BP	50 g
Syrup BP	250 mL
Quillaia Tincture BP	10 mL
Lemon Spirit BP	5 mL
Double Strength Chloroform Water BP	300 mL
Water	to 1000 mL

Dose: 10 mL well diluted with water.

This product would be Recently Prepared as Double Strength Chloroform Water BP acts as a preservative and therefore would attract a four-week discard date.

Use: This product was used to treat inflammatory conditions of the bladder (e.g. cystitis). Potassium Citrate BP makes the urine less acidic and causes a mild diuresis.

16.8 Paediatric Chalk Mixture BP (Mistura Cretae pro Infantibus) (BP 1988, page 724)

Ingredients	Quantities
Chalk BP	20 g
Tragacanth BP	2 g
Syrup BP	100 mL
Concentrated Cinnamon Water BP	4 mL
Double Strength Chloroform Water	500 mL
Water	to 1000 mL

Dose: Child up to 1 year – 5 mL; 1–5 years – 10 mL.

This product would be Recently Prepared as Double Strength Chloroform Water BP acts as a preservative and therefore would attract a four-week discard date.

Use: This product was used in the treatment of diarrhoea as Chalk BP acts as an adsorbent.

16.9 Ammonia and Ipecacuanha Mixture BP (Mistura Expectorans) (BP 1988, page 719)

Ingredients	Quantities
Ammonium Bicarbonate BP	20 g
Liquorice Liquid Extract BP	50 mL
Ipecacuanha Tincture BP	30 mL
Concentrated Camphor Water BP	10 mL
Concentrated Anise Water BP	5 mL
Double Strength Chloroform Water	500 mL
Water	to 1000 mL

Dose: 10–20 mL.

This product would be Recently Prepared as Double Strength Chloroform Water BP acts as a preservative and therefore would attract a four-week discard date.

Use: This product was used as an expectorant. The Ammonium Bicarbonate BP is irritant to mucous membranes and is used in small doses as a reflex expectorant.

16.10 Ferrous Sulphate Mixture Paediatric BP (Mistura Ferri Sulphatis pro Infantibus) (BP 1988, page 734)

Ingredients	Quantities
Ferrous Sulphate BP	12 g
Ascorbic Acid BP	2 g
Orange Syrup BP	100 mL
Double Strength Chloroform Water BP	500 mL
Freshly boiled and cooled purified water	to 1000 mL

Dose: Child. Well diluted with water: up to 1 year – 5 mL; 1–5 years – 10 mL.

Freshly boiled and cooled purified water is used in this preparation to help prevent discoloration. This product would be Recently Prepared as Double Strength Chloroform Water BP acts as a preservative and therefore would attract a four-week discard date. However, consideration must be given to the tendency of the ferrous ion to oxidise the ferric ion, which will cause discoloration, and guidance to discard the product should discoloration occur would be advisable.

Use: This product was used to treat iron-deficiency anaemia.

16.11 Aluminium Hydroxide and Belladonna Mixture BPC (BPC 1973, page 735)

Ingredients	Quantities
Belladonna Tincture BP	100 mL
Chloroform Spirit BP	50 mL
Aluminium Hydroxide Gel BP	to 1000 mL

Dose: 5 mL suitably diluted.

This product would be Recently Prepared and would attract a four-week discard date.

Use: Used to treat indigestion and colic.

16.12 Compound Calcium Carbonate Mixture Paediatric BPC (Mistura Calcii Carbonatis Composita pro Infantibus) (BPC 1968, page 1158)

Ingredients	Quantities
Calcium Carbonate BP	10 g
Light Magnesium Carbonate BP	10 g
Sodium Bicarbonate BP	10 g
Aromatic Cardamom Tincture BP	10 mL
Syrup BP	100 mL
Chloroform Water BP	to 1000 mL

Dose: Up to 1 year – 5 mL, 1–5 years – 10 mL.

This product would be Recently Prepared and would attract a four-week discard date.

Use: For diarrhoea.

16.13 Cascara and Belladonna Mixture BPC (Mistura Cascarae et Belladonnae) (BPC 1973, page 738)

Ingredients	Quantities
Cascara Elixir BP	200 mL
Belladonna Tincture BP	50 mL
Double Strength Chloroform Water BP	500 mL
Water	to 1000 mL

Dose: 10–20 mL.

This product would be Recently Prepared and attract a four-week discard date

Use: Constipation.

16.14 Colchicum and Sodium Salicylate Mixture BPC (Mistura Colchici et Sodii Salicylate) (BPC 1973, page 740)

Ingredients	Quantities
Colchicum Tincture BP	100 mL
Sodium Salicylate BP	100 g
Potassium Bicarbonate BP	100 g
Liquid Liquorice Extract BP	30 mL
Double Strength Chloroform Water BP	500 mL
Water	to 1000 mL

Dose: 10–20 mL.

This product would be Recently Prepared and attract a four-week discard date.

Use: Pain in gout.

16.15 Gelsemium and Hyoscyamus Mixture Compound BPC (Mistura Gelsemii et Hyoscyami Composita)
(BPC 1973, page 743)

Ingredients	Quantities
Gelsemium Tincture BP	30 mL
Hyoscyamus Tincture BP	100 mL
Potassium Bromide BP	50 g
Double Strength Chloroform Water BP	500 mL
Water	to 1000 mL

Dose: 10–20 mL.

This product would be Recently Prepared and would attract a four-week discard date.

Use: To treat trigeminal neuralgia and migraine.

16.16 Gentian Acid Mixture with Nux Vomica BPC (Mistura Gentianae Acida cum Nuce Vomica)
(BPC 1973, page 743)

Ingredients	Quantities
Nux Vomica Tincture BP	50 mL
Acid Gentian Mixture BP	to 1000 mL

Dose: 10–20 mL.

This product would be Recently Prepared and would attract a four-week discard date.

Use: Because of the bitter taste of the nux vomica this was also a tonic.

16.17 Gentian Alkaline Mixture with Nux Vomica BPC (Mistura Gentianae Alkalina cum Nuce Vomica)
(BPC 1973, page 744)

Ingredients	Quantities
Nux Vomica Tincture BP	50 mL
Alkaline Gentian Mixture BP	to 1000 mL

Dose: 10–20 mL.

This product would be Recently Prepared and would attract a four-week discard date.

Use: Because of the bitter taste of the nux vomica this was also a tonic.

16.18 Alkaline Gentian Mixture with Phenobarbitone BPC (Mistura Gentianae Alkalina cum Phenobarbitono)
(BPC 1973, page 744)

Ingredients	Quantities
Phenobarbitone Sodium BP	1.5 g
Alkaline Gentian Mixture BP	to 1000 mL

Dose: 10–20 mL.

This product must be Freshly Prepared and will therefore attract a two-week discard date.

Use: As a sedative.

16.19 Ipecacuanha and Squill Linctus Paediatric BPC (Mist Tussi Rubra pro Inf)
(BPC 1973, page 723)

Ingredients	Quantities
Ipecacuanha Tincture BP	20 mL
Squill Tincture BP	30 mL
Compound Orange Spirit BP	1.5 mL
Blackcurrant Syrup BP	500 mL
Syrup BP	to 1000 mL

Dose: 5 mL.

This product would be Recently Prepared and would attract a four-week discard date.

Use: Expectorant.

16.20 Ipecacuanha Mixture Paediatric BPC (Mistura Ipecacuanha pro Infantibus)
(BPC 1973, page 744)

Ingredients	Quantities
Ipecacuanha Tincture BP	20 mL
Sodium Bicarbonate BP	20 g
Tolu Syrup BP	200 mL
Double Strength Chloroform Water BP	500 mL
Water	to 1000 mL

Dose: up to 1 year – 5 mL; 1–5 years – 10 mL.

This product would be Recently Prepared and would attract a four-week discard date.

Use: Cough mixture.

16.21 Paediatric Opiate Ipecacuanha Mixture BPC (BPC 1973, page 744)

Ingredients	Quantities
Ipecacuanha Tincture BP	20 mL
Camphorated Opium Tincture BP	30 mL
Sodium Bicarbonate BP	20 g
Tolu Syrup BP	200 mL
Double Strength Chloroform Water BP	500 mL
Water	to 1000 mL

Dose: up to 1 year – 5 mL; 1–5 years – 10 mL.

This product would be Recently Prepared and would attract a four-week discard date.

Use: Cough mixture.

16.22 Ipecacuanha and Ammonia Mixture Paediatric BPC (Mistura Ipecacuanhae et Ammoniae pro Infantibus) (BPC 1973, page 745)

Ingredients	Quantities
Ipecacuanha Tincture BP	20 mL
Ammonium Bicarbonate BP	6 g
Sodium Bicarbonate BP	20 g
Tolu Syrup BP	100 mL
Double Strength Chloroform Water BP	500 mL
Water	to 1000 mL

Dose: up to 1 year – 5 mL; 1–5 years – 10 mL.

This product would be Recently Prepared and would attract a four-week discard date.

Use: Expectorant cough mixture.

16.23 Lobelia and Stramonium Mixture Compound BPC (Mistura Lobeliae et Stramonii Composta)
(BPC 1973, page 746)

Ingredients	Quantities
Lobelia Etheral Tincture BP	50 mL
Stramonium Tincture BP	100 mL
Potassium Iodide BP	20 g
Tragacanth Mucilage	100 mL
Double Strength Chloroform Water BP	500 mL
Water	to 1000 mL

Dose: 10 mL.

This product would be Recently Prepared and would attract a four-week discard date.

Use: To treat asthma.

16.24 Nux Vomica Mixture Acid BPC (Mistura Nucis Vomicae Acida)
(BPC 1973, page 748)

Ingredients	Quantities
Nux Vomica Tincture BP	50 mL
Dilute Hydrochloric Acid BP	50 mL
Double Strength Chloroform Water BP	500 mL
Water	to 1000 mL

Dose: 10–20 mL.

This product would be Recently Prepared and would attract a four-week discard date.

Use: Bitter to stimulate appetite.

16.25 Nux Vomica Mixture Alkaline BPC (Mistura Nucis Vomicae Alkalina) (BPC 1973, page 749)

Ingredients	Quantities
Nux Vomica Tincture BP	50 mL
Sodium Bicarbonate BP	50 g
Double Strength Chloroform Water BP	500 mL
Water	to 1000 mL

Dose: 10–20 mL.

This product would be Recently Prepared and would attract a four-week discard date.

Use: Bitter to stimulate appetite.

16.26 Compound Camphorated Opium Mixture BPC (Mistura Opii Camphorata Composita) (BPC 1973, page 749)

Ingredients	Quantities
Camphorated Opium Tincture BP	100 mL
Ammonium Bicarbonate BP	10 g
Strong Ammonium Acetate Solution	100 mL
Water	to 1000 mL

Dose: 10–20 mL

This product would be Recently Prepared and would attract a four-week discard date.

Use: Expectorant cough mixture.

16.27 Potassium Citrate and Hyoscyamus Mixture BPC (Mistura Potassii Citratis et Hyoscyamus)
(BPC 1973, page 751)

Ingredients	Quantities
Potassium Citrate BP	300 g
Hyoscyamus Tincture BP	200 mL
Citric Acid BP	50 g
Lemon Spirit BP	5 mL
Quillaia Tincture BP	10 mL
Syrup BP	250 mL
Double Strength Chloroform Water BP	200 mL
Water	to 1000 mL

Dose: 10 mL well diluted with water.

This product would be Recently Prepared and would attract a four-week discard date.

Use: Treatment of cystitis.

16.28 Ammoniated Potassium Iodide Mixture BPC (Mistura Potassii Iodide Ammoniata)
(BPC 1973, page 751)

Ingredients	Quantities
Potassium Iodide BP	15 g
Ammoniuim Bicarbonate BP	15 g
Liquorice Liquid Extract BP	100 mL
Double Strength Chloroform Water BP	500 mL
Water	to 1000 mL

Dose: 10–20 mL.

This product would be Recently Prepared and would attract a four-week discard date.

Use: Expectorant.

16.29 Compound Rhubarb Mixture BPC (Mistura Rhei Composita)
(BPC 1973, page 752)

Ingredients	Quantities
Compound Rhubarb Tincture BP	100 mL
Light Magnesium Carbonate BP	50 g
Sodium Bicarbonate BP	50 g
Strong Ginger Tincture BP	30 mL
Double Strength Chloroform Water BP	500 mL
Water	to 1000 mL

Dose: 10–20 mL.

This product would be Recently Prepared and would attract a four-week discard date.

Use: To treat constipation.

16.30 Compound Rhubarb Mixture Paediatric BPC (Mistura Rhei Composita pro Infantibus) (BPC 1973, page 752)

Ingredients	Quantities
Compound Rhubarb Tincture BP	60 mL
Light Magnesium Carbonate BP	15 g
Sodium Bicarbonate BP	15 g
Ginger Syrup BP	100 mL
Double Strength Chloroform Water BP	500 mL
Water	to 1000 mL

Dose: Up to 1 year – 5 mL; 1–5 years – 10 mL.

This product would be Recently Prepared and would attract a four-week discard date.

Use: To treat constipation.

16.31 Ammoniated Rhubarb and Soda Mixture BPC (Mistura Rhei Ammoniate et Sodae) (BPC 1973, page 752)

Ingredients	Quantities
Rhubarb Powder BP	25 g
Sodium Bicarbonate BP	80 g
Ammonium Bicarbonate BP	20 g
Conc Peppermint Emulsion BP	25 mL
Double Strength Chloroform Water BP	500 mL
Water	to 1000 mL

Dose: 10–20 mL.

This product would be Recently Prepared and would attract a four-week discard date.

Use: Laxative.

16.32 Compound Sodium Chloride Mixture BPC (Mistura Sodii Chloridi Composita) (BPC 1973, page 753)

Ingredients	Quantities
Sodium Chloride BP	20 g
Sodium Bicarbonate BP	50 g
Double Strength Chloroform Water BP	500 mL
Water	to 1000 mL

Dose: 10–20 mL in a tumblerful of hot water, sipped slowly twice daily.

This product would be Recently Prepared and would attract a four-week discard date.

Use: Emetic.

16.33 Sodium Citrate Mixture BPC (Mistura Sodium Citratis) (BPC 1973, page 753)

Ingredients	Quantities
Sodium Citrate BP	300 g
Citric Acid BP	50 g
Lemon Spirit BP	5 mL
Quillaia Tincture BP	10 mL
Syrup BP	250 mL
Double Strength Chloroform Water BP	300 mL
Water	to 1000 mL

Dose: 10 mL well diluted with water.

This product would be Recently Prepared and would attract a four-week discard date.

Use: Treatment of cystitis.

16.34 Sodium Salicylate Mixture BPC (Mistura Sodii Salicylatis) (BPC 1973, page 753)

Ingredients	Quantities
Sodium Salicylate BP	50 g
Sodium Metabisulphite BP	1 g
Concentrated Orange peel infusion BP	50 mL
Double Strength Chloroform Water BP	500 mL
Water	to 1000 mL

Dose: 10–20 mL.

This product would be Recently Prepared and would attract a four-week discard date.

Use: Analgesic.

16.35 Stramonium and Potassium Iodide Mixture BPC (Mistura Stramonii et Potassii Iodidi) (BPC 1973, page 753)

Ingredients	Quantities
Stramonium Tincture BP	125 mL
Potassium Iodide BP	20 g
Double Strength Chloroform Water BP	500 mL
Water	to 1000 mL

Dose: 10 mL.

This product would be Recently Prepared and would attract a four-week discard date.

Use: Asthma.

16.36 Gentian Alkaline Mixture BP (Mistura Gentianae cum Soda) (BP 1988, page 736)

Ingredients	Quantities
Concentrated Compound Gentian Infusion BP	100 mL
Sodium Bicarbonate BP	50 g
Double Strength Chloroform Water BP	500 mL
Water	to 1000 mL

Dose: 10–20 mL.

This product would be Recently Prepared as Double Strength Chloroform Water BP acts as a preservative and therefore would attract a four-week discard date.

Use: This product was used to stimulate appetite. The gentian acts as a bitter.

16.37 Gentian Acid Mixture BPC (Mistura Gentianae Acida) (BPC 1973, page 743)

Ingredients	Quantities
Concentrated Compound Gentian Infusion BP	100 mL
Dilute Hydrochloric Acid BP	50 mL
Double Strength Chloroform Water BP	500 mL
Water	to 1000 mL

Dose: 10–20 mL.

This product would be Recently Prepared as Double Strength Chloroform Water BP acts as a preservative and therefore would attract a four-week discard date.

Use: This product was used to stimulate appetite. The gentian acts as a bitter.

16.38 Magnesium Trisilicate Mixture BP (Mistura Magnesii Trisilicatis) (BP 1988, page 740)

Ingredients	Quantities
Magnesium Trisilicate BP	50 g
Light Magnesium Carbonate BP	50 g
Sodium Bicarbonate BP	50 g
Concentrated Peppermint Emulsion BP	25 mL
Double Strength Chloroform Water BP	500 mL
Water	to 1000 mL

Dose: 10–20 mL.

This product would be Recently Prepared as Double Strength Chloroform Water BP acts as a preservative and therefore would attract a four-week discard date.

Use: This product was used to treat indigestion/dyspepsia.

16.39 Sodium Salicylate Mixture Strong BP (Mistura Sodii Salicylatis Fortis) (BP 1988, page 751)

Ingredients	Quantities
Sodium Salicylate BP	100 g
Sodium Metabisulphite BP	1 g
Concentrated Peppermint Emulsion BP	25 mL
Double Strength Chloroform Water BP	500 mL
Water	to 1000 mL

Dose: 10–20 mL.

This product would be Recently Prepared as Double Strength Chloroform Water BP acts as a preservative and therefore would attract a four-week discard date.

Use: This product was used to treat pain and inflammation, as sodium salicylate has analgesic, anti-inflammatory and antipyretic actions.

16.40 Ammonium Chloride Mixture BP (Mistura Ammonii Chloridi) (BP 1988, page 720)

Ingredients	Quantities
Ammonium Chloride BP	100 g
Liquorice Liquid Extract BP	100 mL
Aromatic Ammonia Solution BP	50 mL
Water	to 1000 mL

Dose: 10–20 mL.

This product would be Recently Prepared and therefore would attract a four-week discard date.

Use: This product was used as an expectorant cough mixture.

16.41 Kaolin Mixture BP (Mistura Kaolini) (BP 1988, page 738)

Ingredients	Quantities
Light Kaolin BP	200 g
Light Magnesium Carbonate BP	50 g
Sodium Bicarbonate BP	50 g
Concentrated Peppermint Emulsion BP	25 mL
Double Strength Chloroform Water BP	500 mL
Water	to 1000 mL

Dose: 10 mL.

This product would be Recently Prepared as Double Strength Chloroform Water BP acts as a preservative and therefore would attract a four-week discard date.

Use: This product was used to treat colitis, enteritis, dysentery and diarrhoea associated with food poisoning.

16.42 Kaolin Mixture Paediatric BP (Mistura Kaolini pro Infantibus) (BP 1980, page 691)

Ingredients	Quantities
Light Kaolin BP	200 g
Raspberry Syrup BP	200 mL
Benzoic Acid Solution BP	20 mL
Amaranth Solution BP	10 mL
Double Strength Chloroform Water BP	500 mL
Water	to 1000 mL

Dose: Child up to 1 year – 5 mL; 1–5 years – 10 mL.

This product would be Recently Prepared as Double Strength Chloroform Water BP acts as a preservative and therefore would attract a four-week discard date.

Use: This was used for the treatment of diarrhoea in children.

16.43 Belladonna and Ephedrine Mixture Paediatric BPC (Mistura Belladonnae et Ephedrinae pro Infantibus) (BPC 1973, page 737)

Ingredients	Quantities
Belladonna Tincture BP	30 mL
Potassium Iodide BP	10 g
Ephedrine Hydrochloride BP	1.5 g
Syrup BP	100 mL
Liquorice Liquid Extract BP	30 mL
Concentrated Anise Water BP	20 mL
Benzoic Acid Solution BP	20 mL
Water	to 1000 mL

Dose: Child up to 1 year – 5 mL; 1–5 years – 10 mL.

This product would be Recently Prepared as benzoic acid acts as a preservative and therefore would attract a four-week discard date.

Use: This product would have been used to treat asthma or whooping cough.

16.44 Belladonna and Ipecacuanha Mixture Paediatric BPC (BPC 1973, page 738)

Ingredients	Quantities
Belladonna Tincture BP	30 mL
Ipecacuahna Tincture BP	20 mL
Sodium Bicarbonate BP	20 g
Tolu Syrup BP	200 mL
Double Strength Chloroform Water BP	500 mL
Water	to 1000 mL

Dose: Child up to 1 year – 5 mL; 1–5 years – 10 mL.

This product would need to be Freshly Prepared and therefore would attract a two-week discard date. Two weeks would be suitable because although the product contains Double Strength Chloroform Water BP as a preservative the high vegetable content in the form of tinctures makes it more liable to microbial contamination.

Use: This product would have been used to treat asthma or whooping cough.

16.45 Ammonium Chloride and Morphine Mixture BP (Mistura Tussi Sedativa) (BP 1988, page 720)

Ingredients	Quantities
Ammonium Chloride BP	30 g
Ammonium Bicarbonate BP	20 g
Liquorice Liquid Extract BP	50 mL
Chloroform and Morphine Tincture BP	30 mL
Water	to 1000 mL

Dose: 10–20 mL.

This product would be Recently Prepared and therefore would attract a four-week discard date.

Use: This product was used as an expectorant.

16.46 Chalk with Opium Mixture Aromatic BPC (Mistura Cretae Aromatica cum Opio) (BPC 1973, page 739)

Ingredients	Quantities
Aromatic Chalk Powder BP	130 g
Tragacanth Powder BP	2 g
Aromatic Ammonia Solution BP	50 mL
Compound Cardamom Tincture BP	50 mL
Catechu Tincture BP	50 mL
Opium Tincture BP	50 mL
Double Strength Chloroform Water BP	500 mL
Water	to 1000 mL

Dose: Adult 10–20 mL. Child up to 1 year – 5 mL; 1–5 years – 10 mL.

This product would be Recently Prepared as Double Strength Chloroform Water BP acts as a preservative and therefore would attract a four-week discard date.

Use: This product was used to treat diarrhoea.

16.47 Chloral Mixture BP (Mist Chloral) (BP 1988, page 725)

Ingredients	Quantities
Chloral Hydrate BP	100 g
Syrup BP	200 mL
Water	to 1000 mL

Dose: Adult 5–20 mL at bedtime. Child 1–5 years – 2.5–5 mL at bedtime; 6–12 years – 5–10 mL at bedtime. Each dose should be taken well diluted with water because of the possible irritant action of the chloral hydrate.

This product would be Recently Prepared and therefore would attract a four-week discard date.

Use: This product was used as a hypnotic and sedative.

16.48 Ferric Ammonium Citrate Mixture BPC (Mist Ferr et Ammon Cit) (BPC 1973, page 741)

Ingredients	Quantities
Ferric Ammonium Citrate BP	200 g
Double Strength Chloroform Water BP	500 mL
Water	to 1000 mL

Dose: 10 mL.

This product would be Recently Prepared as Double Strength Chloroform Water BP acts as a preservative and therefore would attract a four-week discard date.

Use: This product was used to treat iron-deficiency anaemia.

16.49 Ferric Ammonium Citrate Mixture Paediatric BPC (Mistura Ferri et Ammonii Citratis pro Infantibus) (BPC 1973, page 742)

Ingredients	Quantities
Ferric Ammonium Citrate BP	80 g
Compound Orange Spirit BP	2 mL
Syrup BP	100 mL
Double Strength Chloroform Water BP	500 mL
Water	to 1000 mL

Dose: Child up to 1 year – 5 mL; 1–5 years – 10 mL. The dose should be taken well diluted with water.

This product would be Recently Prepared as Double Strength Chloroform Water BP acts as a preservative and therefore would attract a four-week discard date.

Use: This product was used to treat iron-deficiency anaemia in children.

16.50 Ferrous Sulphate Mixture BPC (Mistura Ferri Sulphatis) (BPC 1973, page 742)

Ingredients	Quantities
Ferrous Sulphate BP	30 g
Ascorbic Acid BP	1 g
Orange Syrup BP	50 mL
Double Strength Chloroform Water BP	500 mL
Freshly boiled and cooled purified water	to 1000 mL

Dose: 10 mL well diluted with water.

Freshly boiled and cooled purified water is used in this preparation to help prevent discoloration. This product would be Recently Prepared as Double Strength Chloroform Water BP acts as a preservative and therefore would attract a four-week discard date. However, consideration must be given to the tendency of the ferrous ion to oxidise to the ferric ion, which will cause the discoloration, and guidance to discard the product should discoloration occur would be advisable.

Use: This product was used to treat iron-deficiency anaemia.

16.51 Ipecacuanha and Morphine Mixture BPC (Mistura Tussi Nigra) (BPC 1973, page 745)

Ingredients	Quantities
Liquorice Liquid Extract BP	100 mL
Chloroform and Morphine Tincture BP	40 mL
Ipecacuanha Tincture BP	20 mL
Water	to 1000 mL

Dose: 10 mL.

This product would be Recently Prepared and therefore would attract a four-week discard date.

Use: This product was used as an expectorant.

16.52 Kaolin and Morphine Mixture BP (Mistura Kaolini Sedativa) (BP 1988, page 738)

Ingredients	Quantities
Light Kaolin BP	200 g
Sodium Bicarbonate BP	50 g
Chloroform and Morphine Tincture BP	40 mL
Water	to 1000 mL

Dose: 10 mL.

This product would be Recently Prepared and therefore would attract a four-week discard date.

Use: This product is used to treat diarrhoea.

16.53 Magnesium Trisilicate and Belladonna Mixture BPC (Mist Mag Trisil et Bellad) (BPC 1973, page 747)

Ingredients	Quantities
Magnesium Trisilicate BP	50 g
Light Magnesium Carbonate BP	50 g
Sodium Bicarbonate BP	50 g
Belladonna Tincture BP	50 mL
Concentrated Peppermint Emulsion BP	25 mL
Double Strength Chloroform Water BP	500 mL

Dose: 10–20 mL.

This product would be Recently Prepared as Double Strength Chloroform Water BP acts as a preservative and therefore would attract a four-week discard date.

Use: This product was used as an antacid. The atropine and hyoscine were adsorbed on to the magnesium trisilicate and only released at pH less than 2 – a level that was unlikely to be achieved in this preparation.

16.54 Sodium Bicarbonate Paediatric Mixture BPC (Mist Sod Bicarb pro Inf) (BPC 1973, page 752)

Ingredients	Quantities
Sodium Bicarbonate BP	10 g
Syrup BP	370 mL
Concentrated Dill Water BP	20 mL
Weak Ginger Tincture BP	10 mL
Double Strength Chloroform Water BP	500 mL
Water	to 1000 mL

Dose: Child up to 1 year – 5 mL; 1–5 years – 10 mL.

This product would be Recently Prepared as Double Strength Chloroform Water BP acts as a preservative and therefore would attract a four-week discard date.

Use: This product was used to treat flatulence and vomiting in children. It was the official 'Gripe Mixture'.

16.55 Chloral Elixir Paediatric BPC (Elixir Chloralis pro Infantibus) (BPC 1973, page 668)

Ingredients	Quantities
Chloral Hydrate BP	40 g
Water	20 mL
Blackcurrant Syrup BP	200 mL
Syrup BP	to 1000 mL

Dose: Child up to 1 year – 5 mL.

Use: Short-term treatment of insomnia.

16.56 Codeine Linctus BPC (Linctus Codeinae) (BPC 1973, page 722)

Ingredients	Quantities
Codeine Phosphate BP	3 g
Compound Tartrazine Solution BP	10 mL
Benzoic Acid Solution BP	20 mL
Chloroform Spirit BP	20 mL
Water	20 mL
Lemon Syrup BP	200 mL
Syrup BP	to 1000 mL

Dose: 5 mL.

Use: Cough suppressant.

16.57 Codeine Linctus Paediatric BPC (BPC 1973, page 722)

Ingredients	Quantities
Codeine Linctus BP	200 mL
Syrup BP	to 1000 mL

Dose: Child up to 1 year – 5 mL; 1–5 years – 10 mL.

Discard date: Two weeks as it should be Freshly Prepared.

Use: Cough suppressant.

16.58 Diamorphine and Cocaine Elixir BPC (BPC 1973, page 669)

Ingredients	Quantities
Diamorphine Hydrochloride BP	1 g
Cocaine Hydrochloride BP	1 g
Alcohol (90%) BP	125 mL
Syrup BP	250 mL
Chloroform Water	to 1000 mL

Dose: As determined by physician in accordance with the needs of the patient. The quantities of diamorphine and cocaine can be altered in accordance with doctor's instruction.

Discard date: Two weeks as it should be Freshly Prepared.

Use: Pain in terminal illness.

Note: The alcohol used quite often was the alcohol of preference to the patient (e.g. gin, whisky, brandy, etc.).

16.59 Diamorphine, Cocaine and Chlorpromazine Elixir BPC (BPC 1973, page 669)

Ingredients	Quantities
Diamorphine Hydrochloride BP	1 g
Cocaine Hydrochloride BP	1 g
Alcohol (90%) BP	125 mL
Chlorpromazine Elixir BP	250 mL
Chloroform Water BP	to 1000 mL

Dose: As determined by physician in accordance with the needs of the patient. The quantities of diamorphine and cocaine can be altered in accordance with doctor's instruction.

Discard date: Two weeks as it should be Freshly Prepared.

Use: Pain in terminal illness.

Note: The alcohol used quite often was the alcohol of preference to the patient (e.g. gin, whisky, brandy, etc.).

16.60 Morphine and Cocaine Elixir BPC (BPC 1973, page 669)

Ingredients	Quantities
Morphine Hydrochloride BP	1 g
Cocaine Hydrochloride BP	1 g
Alcohol (90%) BP	125 mL
Syrup BP	250 mL
Chloroform Water BP	to 1000 mL

Dose: As determined by physician in accordance with the needs of the patient. The quantities of morphine and cocaine can be altered in accordance with doctor's instruction.

Discard date: Two weeks as it should be Freshly Prepared.

Use: Pain in terminal illness.

Note: The alcohol used quite often was the alcohol of preference to the patient (e.g. gin, whisky, brandy, etc.).

16.61 Ephedrine Elixir BPC (Elixir Ephedrinae) (BPC 1973, page 671)

Ingredients	Quantities
Ephedrine Hydrochloride BP	3 g
Lemon Spirit BP	0.2 mL
Compound Tartrazine Solution BP	10 mL
Chloroform Spirit BP	40 mL
Water	60 mL
Alcohol (90%) BP	100 mL
Invert Syrup BP	200 mL
Glycerol BP	200 mL
Syrup BP	to 1000 mL

Dose: Adult 5–10 mL. Child up to 1 year – 2.5 mL; 1–5 years – 5 mL;

6–12 years – 10 mL.

Use: Bronchodilator.

16.62 Paracetamol Elixir Paediatric BPC (Elixir Paracetamolis pro Infantibus) (BPC 1973, page 674)

Ingredients	Quantities
Paracetamol BP	24 g
Amaranth Solution BP	2 mL
Chloroform Spirit BP	20 mL
Concentrated Raspberry Juice BP	25 mL
Alcohol (95%) BP	100 mL
Propylene Glycol BP	100 mL
Invert Syrup BP	275 mL
Glycerol BP	to 1000 mL

Dose: Child up to 1 year – 5 mL; 1–5 years – 10 mL.

The elixir should not be diluted.

Use: Analgesia.

16.63 Isoniazid Elixir BPC
(BPC 1973, page 672)

Ingredients	Quantities
Isoniazid BP	10 g
Citric Acid BP	2.5 g
Sodium Citrate BP	12 g
Concentrated Anise Water BP	10 mL
Compound Tartrazine Solution BP	10 mL
Glycerol BP	200 mL
Double Strength Chloroform Water BP	400 mL
Water	to 1000 mL

Dose: Child twice daily. Up to 1 year – 2.5–5 mL; 1–5 years – 5–10 mL.

This product would be Recently Prepared and therefore would attract a four-week discard date.

If dilution is necessary, chloroform water is the diluent of choice. Syrup should not be used as isoniazid is unstable in the presence of sugars.

Use: Treatment of pulmonary tuberculosis.

16.64 Phenobarbitone Elixir BPC (Elixir Phenobarbitoni) (BPC 1973, page 675)

Ingredients	Quantities
Phenobarbitone BP	3 g
Compound Tartrazine Solution BP	10 mL
Compound Orange Spirit BP	24 mL
Alcohol (90%) BP	400 mL
Glycerol BP	400 mL
Water	to 1000 mL

Dose: Adult 5–10 mL. Child up to 5 years – 5 mL tds increased to 10 mL tds.

Use: Sedative to control epileptic seizures and as long-acting barbiturate used to aid sleep as a night-time dose. Anticonvulsant.

16.65 Diamorphine Linctus BPC (Linctus Diamorphinae) (BPC 1973, page 723)

Ingredients	Quantities
Diamorphine Hydrochloride BP	0.6 g
Compound Tartrazine solution BP	12 mL
Glycerol BP	250 mL
Oxymel BP	250 mL
Syrup BP	to 1000 mL

Dose: 2.5–10 mL.

This product would be Recently Prepared and therefore would attract a four-week discard date.

Use: To treat terminal cough.

16.66 Methadone Linctus BPC (Linctus Methadoni) (BPC 1973, page 723)

Ingredients	Quantities
Methadone Hydrochloride BP	0.4 g
Compound Tartrazine Solution BP	8 mL
Water	120 mL
Glycerol BP	250 mL
Tolu Syrup BP	to 1000 mL

Dose: 5 mL.

This product would be Recently Prepared and therefore would attract a four-week discard date.

Use: To treat terminal cough.

16.67 Pholcodine Linctus Strong BPC (Linctus Pholcodinae Fortis) (BPC 1973, page 724)

Ingredients	Quantities
Pholcodine BP	2 g
Citric acid BP	20 g
Amaranth Solution BP	2 mL
Compound Tartrazine Solution BP	20 mL
Chloroform Spirit BP	150 mL
Syrup BP	to 1000 mL

Dose: 5 mL.

This product would be Recently Prepared and therefore would attract a four-week discard date.

Use: Cough suppressant.

16.68 Pholcodine Linctus BPC (Linctus Pholcodinae) (BPC 1973, page 724)

Ingredients	Quantities
Strong Pholcodine Linctus BP	500 mL
Syrup BP	500 mL

Dose: 5 mL.

This product would be Recently Prepared and therefore would attract a four-week discard date.

Use: Cough suppressant.

16.69 Simple Linctus BPC (Linctus Simplex) (BPC 1973, page 724)

Ingredients	Quantities
Citric Acid BP	25 g
Concentrated Anise Water BP	10 mL
Amaranth Solution BP	15 mL
Chloroform Spirit BP	60 mL
Syrup BP	to 1000 mL

Dose: 5 mL.

This product would be Recently Prepared and therefore would attract a four-week discard date.

Use: Demulcent cough mixture.

16.70 Simple Linctus Paediatric BPC (Linctus Simplex pro Infantibus) (BPC 1973, page 725)

Ingredients	Quantities
Simple Linctus BP	250 mL
Syrup BP	to 1000 mL

Dose: Child 5–10 mL.

This product would be Recently Prepared and therefore would attract a four-week discard date.

Use: Demulcent cough mixture.

16.71 Linctus Squill Opiate BPC (also known as Gees Linctus) (Linctus Scillae Opiatus) (BPC 1973, page 725)

Ingredients	Quantities
Squill Oxymel BP	300 mL
Camphorated Opium Tincture BP	300 mL
Tolu Syrup BP	300 mL

Dose: 5 mL.

This product would be Recently Prepared and therefore would attract a four-week discard date.

Use: Cough suppressant.

16.72 Squill Linctus Opiate Paediatric BPC (Linctus Scillae Opiatus pro Infantibus) (BPC 1973, page 725)

Ingredients	Quantities
Squill Oxymel BP	60 mL
Camphorated Opium Tincture BP	60 mL
Tolu Syrup BP	60 mL
Glycerol BP	200 mL
Syrup BP	to 1000 mL

Dose: Child 5–10 mL.

This product would be Recently Prepared and therefore would attract a four-week discard date.

Use: Cough suppressant.

16.73 Compound Tolu Linctus Paediatric BPC (Linctus Tolutanus Compositus pro Infantibus) (BPC 1973, page 725)

Ingredients	Quantities
Citric Acid BP	6 g
Benzaldehyde Spirit BP	2 mL
Compound Tartrazine Solution BP	10 mL
Glycerol BP	200 mL
Invert Syrup BP	200 mL
Tolu Syrup BP	to 1000 mL

Dose: Child 5–10 mL.

This product would be Recently Prepared and therefore would attract a four-week discard date.

Use: Demulcent cough mixture.

17

Liniments, lotions and applications

17.1 Benzyl Benzoate Application BP (Benzyl Benz Applic) (BP 1988, page 621)

Ingredients	Quantities
Benzyl Benzoate BP	250 g
Emulsifying Wax BP	20 g
Freshly boiled and cooled purified water	to 1000 mL

Directions: Apply over the whole body; repeat without bathing on the following day and wash off 24 hours later. A third application may be required in some cases.

Not recommended for use in children.

Use: Used as an ascaricide in the treatment of scabies and pediculosis.

17.2 Soap Liniment BPC (Linimentum Saponis, also known as Opodeldoc) (BPC 1973, page 726)

Ingredients	Quantities
Camphor BP	40 g
Oleic Acid BP	40 g
Alcohol 90% BP	700 mL
Potassium Hydroxide Solution BP	140 mL
Rosemary Oil BP	15 mL
Freshly boiled and cooled purified water	to 1000 mL

This product should be prepared in advance, left for not less than seven days and filtered prior to dispensing.

Use: Soap Liniment is a mild counterirritant that is used in the treatment of sprains and bruises.

17.3 Calamine Lotion BP (Calam Lot) (BP 1988, page 702)

Ingredients	Quantities
Calamine BP	150 g
Zinc Oxide BP	50 g
Bentonite BP	30 g
Sodium Citrate BP	5 g
Liquified Phenol BP	5 mL
Glycerin BP	50 mL
Freshly boiled and cooled purified water	to 1000 mL

Use: Used as a protective application to the skin. Reduces itching.

17.4 Salicylic Acid Lotion BP (Lotio Acidi Salicylici) (BP 1988, page 702)

Ingredients	Quantities
Salicylic Acid BP	20 g
Castor Oil BP	10 mL
Alcohol (95%) BP	to 1000 mL

Use: Salicylic acid is a bacteriostatic and fungicide. The lotion is used to treat chronic ulcers, psoriasis, dandruff, eczema, etc.

17.5 Sulphur Lotion Compound BPC (Lotio Sulph Co) (BPC 1973, page 729)

Ingredients	Quantities
Precipitated Sulphur BP	40 g
Alcohol (95%) BP	60 mL
Glycerin BP	20 mL
Quillaia Tincture BP	5 mL
Calcium Hydroxide Solution BP	to 1000 mL

Use: This product was used to treat acne.

17.6 Copper and Zinc Sulphates Lotion BPC (Dalibour Water) (BPC 1973, page 727)

Ingredients	Quantities
Zinc Sulphate BP	15 g
Copper Sulphate BP	10 g
Concentrated Camphor Water BP	25 mL
Water	to 1000 mL

Use: Dalibour Water was used as a wet dressing to treat eczema, impetigo and intertrigo.

17.7 Zinc Sulphate Lotion BP (Lotio Rubra) (BP 1988, page 703)

Ingredients	Quantities
Zinc Sulphate BP	10 g
Amaranth Solution BP	10 mL
Water	to 1000 mL

Use: Lotio Rubra was used as an astringent lotion for indolent ulcers and to assist granulation.

17.8 Calamine Lotion Oily BP (Lotio Calamine Oleosa) (BP 1980, page 682)

Ingredients	Quantities
Calamine BP	50 g
Wool Fat BP	10 g
Arachis Oil BP	500 mL
Oleic Acid BP	5 mL
Calcium Hydroxide Solution BP	to 1000 mL

Use: Calamine Lotion Oily was used as a mild astringent to soothe irritating rashes such as prickly heat or chickenpox.

17.9 White Liniment BPC (Linimentum Album) (BPC 1973, page 726)

Ingredients	Quantities
Ammonium Chloride BP	12.5 g
Turpentine Oil BP	250 mL
Oleic Acid BP	85 mL
Dilute Ammonia Solution BP	45 mL
Water	625 mL

Use: Lin Alb was also known as White Embrocation. The turpentine acts as a rubefacient and liniments such as this were used for rheumatic pains and stiffness.

17.10 Compound Calamine Application BPC (Applicatio Calaminae Composita) (BPC 1973, page 648)

Ingredients	Quantities
Calamine BP	100 g
Zinc Oxide BP	50 g
Wool Fat BP	25 g
Zinc Stearate BP	25 g
Yellow Soft Paraffin BP	250 g
Liquid Paraffin BP	550 g

Also known as Compound Calamine Cream and Compound Calamine Liniment.

Use: Soothing application used to treat the discomfort of dermatitis and eczema.

18

Ointments and pastes

18.1 Compound Benzoic Acid Ointment BP (Whitfield's Ointment)
(BP 1988, page 705)

Ingredients	Quantities
Emulsifying Ointment BP	910 g
Benzoic Acid BP	60 g
Salicylic Acid BP	30 g

Dose: Apply twice a day.

Use: Benzoic Acid BP has antifungal and antibacterial properties and this ointment was commonly used to treat fungal infections of the skin.

18.2 Calamine Ointment BP (Unguentum Calaminae) (BP 1988, page 706)

Ingredients	Quantities
Calamine BP	150 g
White Soft Paraffin BP	850 g

Dose: Apply when required.

Use: Calamine is a soothing astringent and this preparation is used to soothe rashes and itching.

18.3 Cetomacrogol Emulsifying Ointment BP, also called Non-ionic Emulsifying Ointment BP (Unguentum Cetomacrogolis Emulsificans) (BP 1988, page 706)

Ingredients	Quantities
White Soft Paraffin BP	500 g
Cetomacrogol Emulsifying Wax BP	300 g
Liquid Paraffin BP	200 g

Dose: Apply when required. Frequency determined by any addition of active ingredient.

Use: A suitable base into which can be incorporated active ingredients. Particularly suitable when easy removal from the skin is required. Other advantages include easy miscibility with any exudates, high cosmetic acceptability and, because of the emulsifying properties, easy removal from the scalp.

Unguentum Cetrimidi Emulsificans (Cetrimide Emulsifying Ointment BP, also called Cationic Emulsifying Ointment BP) can be made by replacing Cetomacrogol Emulsifying Wax BP with Cetrimide Emulsifying Wax BP. Similarly, if the Cetomacrogol Emulsifying Wax BP is replaced by Emulsifying Wax BP, Unguentum Emulsificans (Emulsifying Ointment BP) is formed. The choice of base ointment is determined by the properties of the active ingredient to be incorporated.

18.4 Calamine and Coal Tar Ointment BP, also known as Compound Calamine Ointment BP (Unguentum Calaminae et Picis Carbonis) (BP 1988, page 706)

Ingredients	Quantities
White Soft Paraffin BP	475 g
Hydrous Wool Fat BP	250 g
Calamine BP	125 g
Zinc Oxide BP	125 g
Strong Coal Tar Solution BP	25 g

Dose: Apply once or twice daily.

Use: Used in the treatment of psoriasis and other scaly skin conditions as the coal tar in the preparation has anti-inflammatory, antipruritic and antiscaling properties.

18.5 Zinc and Salicylic Acid Paste BP (Lassar's Paste) (BP 1988, page 868)

Ingredients	Quantities
Zinc Oxide BP	240 g
Salicylic Acid BP	20 g
Starch BP	240 g
White Soft Paraffin BP	500 g

Dose: Apply twice a day.

Use: Used for hyperkeratoses.

18.6 Zinc and Coal Tar Paste BP (White's Tar Paste) (BP 1988, page 868)

Ingredients	Quantities
Yellow Soft Paraffin BP	450 g
Starch BP	380 g
Coal Tar BP	60 g
Zinc Oxide BP	60 g
Emulsifying Wax BP	50 g

Dose: Apply once or twice daily.

Use: Used to treat psoriasis and chronic atopic eczema.

18.7 Simple Ointment BP (Ung Simp) (BP 1988, page 713)

Ingredients	Quantities
Wool Fat BP	50 g
Hard Paraffin BP	50 g
Cetostearyl Alcohol BP	50 g
White/Yellow Soft Paraffin BP	850 g

Dose: Apply when required.

Use: Used as an emollient or base for other ingredients.

18.8 Sulphur Ointment BP (BP 1980, page 701)

Ingredients	Quantities
Sulphur (precipitated) BP	100 g
Simple Ointment BP (prepared with White Soft Paraffin BP)	900 g

Dose: Apply twice daily.

Use: Used to treat acne and scabies.

18.9 Methyl Salicylate Ointment BP (Unguentum Methylis Salicylatis) (BP 1988, page 712)

Ingredients	Quantities
Methyl Salicylate BP	500 g
White Beeswax BP	250 g
Hydrous Wool Fat BP	250 g

Dose: Apply two to three times a day.

Use: Used as a rubefacient to relieve pain in lumbago, sciatica and other rheumatic conditions.

18.10 Zinc Ointment BP (Ung Zinc) (BP 1988, page 715)

Ingredients	Quantities
Zinc Oxide BP	150 g
Simple Ointment BP	850 g

Use: Used to treat nappy and urinary rash and eczematous conditions.

18.11 Cetrimide Emulsifying Ointment BP (Unguentum Cetrimidi Emulsificans) (BP 1988, page 707)

Ingredients	Quantities
Cetrimide BP	30 g
Cetostearyl Alcohol BP	270 g
White Soft Paraffin BP	500 g
Liquid Paraffin BP	200 g

Use: Used as an antiseptic ointment.

18.12 Compound Zinc Paste BP (Co Zinc Paste) (BP 1988, page 868)

Ingredients	Quantities
Zinc Oxide BP	250 g
Starch BP	250 g
White Soft Paraffin BP	500 g

Use: Used to treat nappy and urinary rash and eczematous conditions. Also forms an effective sun block.

18.13 Salicylic Acid Ointment BP (Ung Acid Salicyl) (BP 1988, page 713)

Ingredients	Quantities
Salicylic Acid BP	20 g
Wool Alcohols Ointment BP	980 g

Use: Used to treat acne, ringworm and eczema.

18.14 Salicylic Acid and Sulphur Ointment BPC (Ung Acid Salicyl et Sulph) (BPC 1973, page 763)

Ingredients	Quantities
Salicylic Acid BP	30 g
Precipitated Sulphur BP	30 g
Oily Cream BP	940 g

Use: Used to treat acne.

18.15 Coal Tar Paste BPC (Pasta Picis Carbonis) (BPC 1973, page 767)

Ingredients	Quantities
Strong Coal Tar Solution BP	75 g
Compound Zinc Paste BP	925 g

Use: Used in the treatment of psoriasis.

18.16 Emulsifying Ointment BP (Ung Emulsif) (BP 1988, page 707)

Ingredients	Quantities
Emulsifying Wax BP	300 g
White Soft Paraffin BP	500 g
Liquid Paraffin BP	200 g

Used: A water-miscible ointment base, particularly useful for application to the scalp or as a soap substitute.

18.17 Ichthammol Ointment BP (Unguentum Ichthammolis) (BP 1980, page 700)

Ingredients	Quantities
Wool Fat BP	450 g
Yellow Soft Paraffin BP	450 g
Ichthammol BP	100 g

Use: Mild antibacterial and anti-inflammatory. Traditional 'drawing' ointment.

19

Powders

19.1 Effervescent Powder Compound BPC (Pulvis Effervescens Compositus, also known as Seidlitz Powder) (BPC 1973, page 776)

Ingredients	Quantities
No.1 Powder	
Sodium Potassium Tartrate Powder BP	7.5 g
Sodium Bicarbonate BP	2.5 g
No.2 Powder	
Tartaric Acid Powder BP	2.5 g

Dose: One of each powder. Dissolve powder 1 in a tumblerful of cold water. Add powder 2, stir and take while the mixture is still effervescing.

Use: Used as a saline purgative.

19.2 Compound Sodium Chloride and Dextrose Oral Powder BP (per powder) (BP 1980, page 710)

Ingredients	Quantities
Sodium Chloride BP	500 mg
Sodium Bicarbonate BP	750 mg
Potassium Chloride BP	750 mg
Dextrose BP	20 g

Use: Each powder is dissolved in 500 mL of recently boiled and cooled water to make a solution used for rehydration and electrolyte replacement in the treatment of infantile diarrhoea.

19.3 Oral Rehydration Salts Formula A BP (BP 1988, page 874)

Ingredients	Quantities
Sodium Chloride BP	1 g
Sodium Bicarbonate BP	1.5 g
Potassium Chloride BP	1.5 g
Anhydrous Glucose BP	36.4 g

This formula is sufficient to prepare 1 litre of solution.

Use: Each dose of 8.08 g is usually packed separately in an individual amber glass jar or plastic pot. Each dose of this powder is dissolved in 200 mL of recently boiled and cooled water to make a solution used for rehydration and electrolyte replacement in the treatment of diarrhoea.

19.4 Magnesium Trisilicate Powder Compound BP (Pulvis Magnesii Trisilicatis Compositus) (BP 1988, page 873)

Ingredients	Quantities
Chalk Powder BP	250 g
Heavy Magnesium Carbonate BP	250 g
Magnesium Trisilicate BP	250 g
Sodium Bicarbonate BP	250 g

Dose: 1–5 g mixed with a little water between meals.

Use: Used as an adsorbent and antacid in the treatment of dyspepsia.

20

Miscellaneous formulae

20.1 Ephedrine Nasal Drops BPC (Naristillae Ephedrinae) (BPC 1973, page 757)

Ingredients	Quantities
Ephedrine Hydrochloride BP	0.5 g
Chlorbutol BP	0.5 g
Sodium Chloride BP	0.5 g
Water	to 100 mL

Use: Used as a nasal decongestant.

20.2 Sodium Bicarbonate Ear Drops BP (Auristillae Sodii Bicarbonatis) (BP 1988, page 670)

Ingredients	Quantities
Sodium Bicarbonate BP	5 g
Glycerol BP	30 mL
Water	to 100 mL

Use: Used for the softening and removal of ear wax.

20.3 Compound Sodium Chloride Mouthwash BP (Collutorium Sodii Chloridi Compositum) (BP 1988, page 703)

Ingredients	Quantities
Sodium Chloride BP	15 g
Sodium Bicarbonate BP	10 g
Concentrated Peppermint Emulsion BP	25 mL
Double Strength Chloroform Water BP	500 mL
Water	to 1000 mL

Dose: Use approximately 15 mL diluted with an equal volume of water each morning and night.
Use: Used to cleanse and freshen the mouth.

20.4 Menthol and Eucalyptus Inhalation BP (Vapor Mentholis et Eucalypti) (BP 1980, page 577)

Ingredients	Quantities
Light Magnesium Carbonate BP	70 g
Menthol BP	20 g
Eucalyptus Oil BP	100 mL
Water	to 1000 mL

Dose: Add one teaspoonful to a pint of hot (not boiling) water and inhale the vapour.

Use: Used as a nasal decongestant.

20.5 Zinc Sulphate and Zinc Chloride Mouthwash BPC (Collutorium Zinci Sulphatis et Zinci Chloridi) (BPC 1973, page 756)

Ingredients	Quantities
Zinc Sulphate BP	20 g
Zinc Chloride BP	10 g
Dilute Hydrochloric Acid BP	10 mL
Compound Tartrazine Solution BP	10 mL
Double Strength Chloroform Water BP	500 mL
Water	To 1000 mL

Dose: This preparation should be diluted with 20 times its own volume of water before use.

Use: Used as an astringent mouthwash.

20.6 Chloroxylenol Solution BP (Liquor Chloroxylenolis) (BP 1988, page 879)

Ingredients	Quantities
Chloroxylenol BP	50.0 g
Potassium Hydroxide BP	13.6 g
Oleic Acid BP	7.5 mL
Castor Oil BP	63.0 g
Terpineol BP	100 mL
Ethanol 96% (IMS is suitable)	200 mL
Purified water freshly boiled and cooled	to 1000 mL

Use: Antiseptic for skin.

Appendix 1

Glossary of terms used in formulations

Application	A liquid or semi-liquid preparation intended for application to the skin.
Bougie (nasal)	A solid dosage form intended for insertion into the nostril.
Bougie (urethral)	A solid dosage form intended for insertion into the urethra.
Cachet	An oral preparation consisting of dry powder enclosed in a shell of rice paper.
Capsule	An oral preparation consisting of a medicament enclosed in a shell usually of gelatin basis. Soft gelatin capsules are used to enclose liquids and hard capsules to enclose solids.
Cream	A semi-solid emulsion intended for application to the skin. The emulsion may be an oil-in-water (aqueous creams) or a water-in-oil type (oily creams).
Douche	A liquid preparation intended for introduction into the vagina.
Douche (nasal)	A liquid preparation intended for introduction into the nostril.
Draught	A liquid oral preparation of fairly small volume and usually consisting of one dose.
Drops	A liquid preparation in which the quantity to be used at any one time is so small that it is measured as a number of drops (e.g. in a small pipette). Drops may comprise an oral preparation (usually paediatric), or may be intended for introduction into the nose, ear or eye; the title of the product is amended accordingly.
Dusting powder	A preparation consisting of one or more substances in fine powder intended for the application to intact skin.
Elixir	An aromatic liquid preparation including a high proportion of alcohol glycerine, propylene glycol or other solvent, and intended for the oral administration of potent or nauseous medicaments, in a small dose volume.
Emulsion	As a preparation, this term is generally restricted to an oil-in-water preparation intended for internal use.
Enema	An aqueous or oily solution or suspension intended for rectal administration.
Gargle	An aqueous solution, usually in concentrated form, intended for the treatment of the membranous lining of the throat.
Granules	A dry preparation in which each granule consists of a mixture of the ingredients in the correct proportions.
Inhalation	A preparation in which the active principle is drawn into the respiratory tract by inhalation. The active principle may be vapour when it is obtained from a liquid preparation by volatilisation, or it may be a solid when a special appliance, often an aerosol, is needed.
Injection	A preparation intended for parenteral administration which may consist of an aqueous or non-aqueous solution or suspension.
Irrigation	A solution intended for introduction into body cavities or deep wounds. Includes nasal and vaginal douches.
Linctus	A viscous liquid preparation, usually containing sucrose, which is administered in small dose volumes and which should be sipped and swallowed slowly without the addition of water.

Liniment	A liquid or semi-liquid intended for application to intact skin, usually with considerable friction produced by massaging with the hand.
Lotion	A liquid preparation intended for application to the skin without friction. Eye lotions are lotions intended for application to the eye.
Lozenge	A solid oral preparation consisting of medicaments incorporated in a flavoured base and intended to dissolve or disintegrate slowly in the mouth.
Mixture	Liquid oral preparation consisting of one or more medicaments dissolved, suspended or diffused in an aqueous vehicle.
Mouthwash	An aqueous solution, often in concentrated form, intended for local treatment of the membranous lining of the mouth and gums.
Ointment	A semi-solid preparation consisting of one or more medicaments dissolved or dispersed in a suitable base and intended for application to the skin.
Paint	A liquid preparation intended for application to the skin or mucous membranes.
Pastille	A solid oral preparation consisting of one or medicaments in an inert base and intended to dissolve slowly in the mouth.
Pessary	A solid dosage form intended for insertion into the vagina for local treatment.
Pill	A solid oral dose form consisting of one or more medicaments incorporated in a spherical or ovoid mass.
Poultice	A thick pasty preparation intended for application to the skin while hot.
Powder	A preparation consisting of one or more components in fine powder. It may be in bulk form or individually wrapped quantities and is intended for oral administration.
Spirit	An alcoholic solution of volatile medicinal substances or flavouring agents.
Suppository	A solid dosage form intended for insertion into the rectum for local or systemic treatment.
Syrup	A liquid preparation containing a high proportion of sucrose or other sweetening agent.
Tablet	A solid oral dosage form where one or more medicaments are compressed and moulded into shape.

Appendix 2

Abbreviations commonly used in pharmacy

aa.	ana	of each
a.c.	ante cibum	before food
ad/add	addendus	to be added (up to)
ad lib	ad libitum	as much as desired
alt	alternus	alternate
alt die	alterno die	every other day
amp	ampulla	ampoule
applic	applicetur	let it be applied
aq	aqua	water
aq ad	aquam ad	water up to
aur/aurist	auristillae	ear drops
BNF		British National Formulary
BP		British Pharmacopoeia
BPC		British Pharmaceutical Codex
bd/bid	bis in die	twice a day
c	cum	with
cap	capsula	capsule
cc	cum cibus	with food
collut	collutorium	mouthwash
co/comp	compositus	compound
conc	concentratus	concentrated
corp	corpori	to the body
crem	cremor	cream
d	dies	a day
dd	de die	daily
dil	dilutus	diluted
div	divide	divide
DPF		Dental Practitioners' Formulary
DT		Drug Tariff
EP		European Pharmacopoeia
et	et	and
ex aq	ex aqua	in water
ext	extractum	an extract
fort	fortis	strong
freq	frequenter	frequently
f/ft/fiat	fiat	let it be made
ft mist	fiat mistura	let a mixture be made
ft pulv	fiat pulvis	let a powder be made
garg	gargarisma	a gargle
gutt/guttae/gtt	guttae	drops
h	hora	at the hour
hs	hora somni	at the hour of sleep (bedtime)

ic	inter cibos	between meals
inf	infusum	infusion
inh		inhalation/inhaler
irrig	irrigatio	irrigation
liq	liquor	solution
lin	linimentum	liniment
lot	lotio	lotion
m/mane	mane	in the morning
md	more dicto	as directed
mdu	more dicto utendus	use as directed
mist	mistura	mixture
mitt/mitte	mitte	send (quantity to be given)
n/nocte	nocte	at night
n et m	nocte maneque	night and morning
np	nomen proprium	the proper name
narist	naristillae	nose drops
neb	nebula	spray
ocul	oculo	to (for) the eye
oculent/oc	oculentum	an eye ointment
oh	omni hora	every hour
om	omni mane	every morning
od	omni die	every day
on	omni nocte	every night
paa	parti affectae applicandus	apply to the affected part
pc	post cibum	after food
PC		prescriber contacted
po	per os	by mouth
PNC		prescriber not contacted
pr	per rectum	rectally
pv	per vaginam	vaginally
prn	pro re nata	when required
pess	pessus	pessary
pig	pigmentum	a paint
ppt	praecipitatus	precipitated
pulv	pulvis	a powder
qqh/q4h	quater quaque hora	every 4 hours
qds/qid	quater die	four times a day
qs	quantum sufficiat	sufficient
R	recipe	take
rep/rept	repetatur	let it be repeated
sos	si opus sit	when necessary
sig	signa	let it be labelled
solv	solve	dissolve
stat	statim	immediately
supp	suppositorium	suppository
syr	syrupus	syrup
tds/tid	ter in die	three times a day
tinct	tinctura	tincture
tuss urg	tussi urgente	when the cough is troublesome
ung	unguentum	ointment
ut dict/ud	ut dictum	as directed
vap	vapor	an inhalation

Appendix 3

Changing substance names from British Approved Names to recommended International Non-Proprietary Names

The MHRA (Medicines and Healthcare Products Regulatory Agency) published the following information in relation to the change of substance names from British Approved Names (BANs) to recommended International Non-Proprietary Names (rINNs). The information in A3.1 Drug names and A3.2 Radicals and groups has been taken from the MHRA website which is available at the following internet address: http://medicines.mhra.gov.uk/.

A3.1 Drug names

The following is a list of medicinal substances for which the British Approved Names (BANs) have been changed to match the corresponding recommended International Non-Proprietary Names (rINNs). These changes were published in the British Pharmacopoeia 2003, which became effective on 1 December 2003. BANs have been changed to match rINNs where the names differ to achieve consistency in the names of medicines available in the UK and to ensure compliance with EC legislation.

BAN	rINN
Changed from:	**To:**
Acepifylline	Acefylline Piperazine
Acinitrazole	Aminitrozole
Acrosoxacin	Rosoxacin
Allyloestrenol	Allylestrenol
Aloxidone	Allomethadione
Alphadolone	Alfadolone
Alphaxalone	Alfaxalone
Amethocaine	Tetracaine
Amidephrine	Amidefrine
Aminacrine	Aminoacridine
Amoxycillin	Amoxicillin
Amphetamine	Amfetamine
Amylobarbitone	Amobarbital
Amylobarbitone Sodium	Amobarbital Sodium
Angiotensin Amide	Angiotensinamide
Azetepa	Azatepa
Balipramine	Depramine
Barbitone	Barbital
Beclomethasone	Beclometasone
Benapryzine	Benaprizine

Bendrofluazide	Bendroflumethiazide
Benorylate	Benorilate
Benzathine Penicillin	Benzathine Benzylpenicillin
Benzhexol	Trihexyphenidyl
Benzphetamine	Benzfetamine
Benztropine	Benzatropine
Bethanidine	Betanidine
Bismuth Glycollylarsanilate	Glycobiarsol
Bromocyclen	Bromociclen
Bromodiphenhydramine	Bromazine
Buniodyl	Bunamiodyl
Busulphan	Busulfan
Butamyrate	Butamirate
Butethamate	Butetamate
Buthalitone Sodium	Buthalital Sodium
Butobarbitone	Butobarbital
Butoxamine	Butaxamine
Carbiphene	Carbifene
Carbolonium Bromide	Hexcarbacholine Bromide
Carbophenothion	Carbofenotion
Carphenazine	Carfenazine
Carticaine	Articaine
Cellacephate	Cellacefate
Cephamandole	Cefamandole
Cephamandole Nafate	Cefamandole Nafate
Cephoxazole	Cefoxazole
Cephradine	Cefradine
Certoparin	Certoparin Sodium
Chlophedianol	Clofedanol
Chloral Betaine	Cloral Betaine
Chloramine	Tosylchloramide Sodium
Chlorbutol	Chlorobutanol
Chlordantoin	Clodantoin
Chlorfenvinphos	Clofenvinfos
Chlorhexadol	Chloralodol
Chlormethiazole	Clomethiazole
Chlorpheniramine	Chlorphenamine
Chlorthalidone	Chlortalidone
Chlorthenoxazin	Chlorthenoxazine
Cholecalciferol	Colecalciferol
Cholestyramine	Colestyramine
Clamoxyquin	Clamoxyquine
Cloguanamile	Cloguanamil
Clomiphene	Clomifene
Clorgyline	Clorgiline
Clothiapine	Clotiapine
Co-Carboxylase	Cocarboxylase
Colistin Sulphomethate Sodium	Colistimethate Sodium
Corticotrophin	Corticotropin
Coumaphos	Coumafos

Cromoglycic Acid	Cromoglicic Acid
Crotethamide	Crotetamide
Cumetharol	Coumetarol
Cyacetazide	Cyacetacide
Cyclobarbitone Calcium	Cyclobarbital Calcium
Cycloprolol	Cicloprolol
Cysteamine	Mercaptamine
Danthron	Dantron
Deoxycortone	Desoxycortone
Desoxymethasone	Desoximetasone
Diamphenethide	Diamfenetide
Diazinon	Dimpylate
Dibromopropamidine	Dibrompropamidine
Dichlorphenamide	Diclofenamide
Dicyclomine	Dicycloverine
Dienoestrol	Dienestrol
Dimenoxadole	Dimenoxadol
Dimepropion	Metamfepramone
Dimethicone(s)	Dimeticone
Dimethindene	Dimetindene
Dimethisoquin	Quinisocaine
Dimethothiazine	Dimetotiazine
Dimethyl Sulphoxide	Dimethyl Sulfoxide
Dioxathion	Dioxation
Dipenine Bromide	Diponium Bromide
Diphenidol	Difenidol
Dothiepin	Dosulepin
Doxybetasol	Doxibetasol
Doxycycline Hydrochloride (Hemihydrate, Hemiethanolate)	Doxycycline Hyclate
Dyclocaine	Dyclonine
Eformoterol	Formoterol
Epioestriol	Epiestriol
Epithiazide	Epitizide
Etenzamide	Ethenzamide
Ethacrynic Acid	Etacrynic Acid
Ethamivan	Etamivan
Ethamsylate	Etamsylate
Ethebenecid	Etebenecid
Ethinyloestradiol	Ethinylestradiol
Ethoglucid	Etoglucid
Ethopropazine	Profenamine
Ethosalamide	Etosalamide
Ethybenztropine	Etybenzatropine
Ethyloestrenol	Ethylestrenol
Ethylphenaxemide	Pheneturide
Etifoxin	Etifoxine
Fanthridone	Fantridone
Fenchlorphos	Fenclofos
Fenethylline	Fenetylline

Fetoxylate	Fetoxilate
Flumethasone	Flumetasone
Fluopromazine	Triflupromazine
Flupenthixol	Flupentixol
Flurandrenolone	Fludroxycortide
Flurothyl	Flurotyl
Frusemide	Furosemide
Gestronol	Gestonorone
Glycalox	Glucalox
Guaiphenesin	Guaifenesin
Halethazole	Haletazole
Halopyramine	Chloropyramine
Heptabarbitone	Heptabarb
Hexachlorophane	Hexachlorophene
Hexamine Hippurate	Methenamine Hippurate
Hexobarbitone	Hexobarbital
Hydroxamethocaine	Hydroxytetracaine
Hydroxyamphetamine	Hydroxyamfetamine
Hydroxyprogesterone Hexanoate	Hydroxyprogesterone Caproate
Hydroxyurea	Hydroxycarbamide
Icomethasone Enbutate	Icometasone Enbutate
Indomethacin	Indometacin
Iodipamide	Adipiodone
Iophendylate	Iofendylate
Iothalamic Acid	Iotalamic Acid
Isobuzole	Glysobuzole
Isoetharine	Isoetarine
Isometamidium	Isometamidium Chloride
Levamphetamine	Levamfetamine
Lignocaine	Lidocaine
Lynoestrenol	Lynestrenol
Lysuride	Lisuride
Malethamer	Maletamer
Medigoxin	Metildigoxin
Meprothixol	Meprotixol
Methadyl Acetate	Acetylmethadol
Methallenoestril	Methallenestril
Methallibure	Metallibure
Methamphazone	Metamfazone
Metharbitone	Metharbital
Methenolone	Metenolone
Methetoin	Metetoin
Methicillin Sodium	Meticillin Sodium
Methimazole	Thiamazole
Methindizate	Metindizate
Methisazone	Metisazone
Methixene	Metixene
Methohexitone	Methohexital
Methoin	Mephenytoin
Methotrimeprazine	Levomepromazine

Methsuximide	Mesuximide
Methyl Cysteine	Mecysteine
Methylene Blue	Methylthioninium Chloride
Methylphenobarbitone	Methylphenobarbital
Methyprylone	Methyprylon
Metriphonate	Metrifonate
Metyzoline	Metizoline
Mitozantrone	Mitoxantrone
Monosulfiram	Sulfiram
Mustine	Chlormethine
Naphthalophos	Naftalofos
Nealbarbitone	Nealbarbital
Nicoumalone	Acenocoumarol
Nitroxynil	Nitroxinil
Norbutrine	Norbudrine
Norethynodrel	Noretynodrel
Noxiptyline	Noxiptiline
Noxythiolin	Noxytiolin
Nylestriol	Nilestriol
Octacosactrin	Tosactide
Octaphonium Chloride	Octafonium Chloride
Oestradiol	Estradiol
Oestriol	Estriol
Oestriol Sodium Succinate	Estriol Sodium Succinate
Oestriol Succinate	Estriol Succinate
Oestrone	Estrone
Oxethazaine	Oxetacaine
Oxpentifylline	Pentoxifylline
Oxyphenisatin	Oxyphenisatine
Oxypurinol	Oxipurinol
Pentaerythritol Tetranitrate	Pentaerithrityl Tetranitrate
Pentobarbitone	Pentobarbital
Pentolinium Tartrate	Pentolonium Tartrate
Phanquone	Phanquinone
Phenbenicillin	Fenbenicillin
Phenbutrazate	Fenbutrazate
Phenethicillin	Pheneticillin
Phenobarbitone	Phenobarbital
Phenoxypropazine	Fenoxypropazine
Phenyl Aminosalicylate	Fenamisal
Phenyramidol	Fenyramidol
Phthalylsulphathiazole	Phthalylsulfathiazole
Pipazethate	Pipazetate
Pipothiazine	Pipotiazine
Plasmin	Fibrinolysin (Human)
Polyhexanide	Polihexanide
Polymyxin	Polymyxin B
Polyoxyl 40 Stearate	Macrogol Ester
Potassium Clorazepate	Dipotassium Clorazepate
Pramoxine	Pramocaine

Procaine Penicillin	Procaine Benzylpenicillin
Promethoestrol	Methestrol
Promoxolan	Promoxolane
Pronethalol	Pronetalol
Proquamezine	Aminopromazine
Prothionamide	Protionamide
Psilocybin	Psilocybine
Quinalbarbitone	Secobarbital
Riboflavine	Riboflavin
Rolicypram	Rolicyprine
Salazosulphadimidine	Salazosulfadimidine
Salcatonin	Calcitonin (Salmon)
Secbutobarbitone	Secbutabarbital
Sissomicin	Sisomicin
Sodium Anoxynaphthonate	Anazolene Sodium
Sodium Calciumedetate	Sodium Calcium Edetate
Sodium Cromoglycate	Sodium Cromoglicate
Sodium Diatrizoate	Sodium Amidotrizoate
Sodium Ipodate	Sodium Iopodate
Sodium Ironedetate	Sodium Feredetate
Sodium Picosulphate	Sodium Picosulfate
Sorbitan Mono-Oleate	Sorbitan Oleate
Sorbitan Monolaurate	Sorbitan Laurate
Sorbitan Monopalmitate	Sorbitan Palmitate
Sorbitan Monostearate	Sorbitan Stearate
Stanolone	Androstanolone
Stibocaptate	Sodium Stibocaptate
Stilboestrol	Diethylstilbestrol
Streptonicozid	Streptoniazid
Succinylsulphathiazole	Succinylsulfathiazole
Sulglycotide	Sulglicotide
Sulphacetamide	Sulfacetamide
Sulphachlorpyridazine	Sulfachlorpyridazine
Sulphadiazine	Sulfadiazine
Sulphadimethoxine	Sulfadimethoxine
Sulphadimidine	Sulfadimidine
Sulphaethidole	Sulfaethidole
Sulphaguanidine	Sulfaguanidine
Sulphaloxic Acid	Sulfaloxic Acid
Sulphamethizole	Sulfamethizole
Sulphamethoxazole	Sulfamethoxazole
Sulphamethoxydiazine	Sulfametoxydiazine
Sulphamethoxypyridazine	Sulfamethoxypyridazine
Sulphamoxole	Sulfamoxole
Sulphaphenazole	Sulfaphenazole
Sulphaproxyline	Sulfaproxyline
Sulphapyridine	Sulfapyridine
Sulphasalazine	Sulfasalazine
Sulphasomidine	Sulfisomidine
Sulphasomizole	Sulfasomizole

Sulphathiazole	Sulfathiazole
Sulphathiourea	Sulfathiourea
Sulphatolamide	Sulfatolamide
Sulphaurea	Sulfacarbamide
Sulphinpyrazone	Sulfinpyrazone
Sulphomyxin Sodium	Sulfomyxin Sodium
Sulthiame	Sultiame
Tetracosactrin	Tetracosactide
Tetrahydrozoline	Tetryzoline
Thiabendazole	Tiabendazole
Thiacetazone	Thioacetazone
Thialbarbitone	Thialbarbital
Thiazesim	Tiazesim
Thiocarlide	Tiocarlide
Thioguanine	Tioguanine
Thiomesterone	Tiomesterone
Thiopentone	Thiopental
Thiothixene	Tiotixene
Thioxolone	Tioxolone
Thymoxamine	Moxisylyte
Thyroxine Sodium	Levothyroxine Sodium
Triacetyloleandomycin	Troleandomycin
Tribavirin	Ribavirin
Trimeprazine	Alimemazine
Trimustine	Trichlormethine
Troxidone	Trimethadione
Tyformin	Tiformin
Urofollitrophin	Urofollitropin
Vinbarbitone	Vinbarbital
Vinylbitone	Vinylbital
Viprynium Embonate	Pyrvinium Pamoate
Xanthinol Nicotinate	Xantinol Nicotinate
Xanthocillin	Xantocillin

A3.2 Radicals and groups

The following changes in spelling apply to names for radicals and groups.

Changed from:	To:
Besylate	Besilate
Camsylate	Camsilate
Closylate	Closilate
Cypionate	Cipionate
Edisylate	Edisilate
Enanthate	Enantate
Esylate	Esilate
Ethylsulphate	Etilsulfate
Isethionate	Isetionate

Mesylate	Mesilate
Methylsulphate	Metilsulfate
Napadisylate	Napadisilate
Napsylate	Napsilate
Theoclate	Teoclate
Tosylate	Tosilate

Bibliography

Aulton M E (ed) 1988, *Pharmaceutics – The Science of Dosage For Design*. Churchill Livingstone, Edinburgh.

British Pharmaceutical Codex 1911. Pharmaceutical Press, London.

British Pharmaceutical Codex 1934. Pharmaceutical Press, London.

British Pharmaceutical Codex 1949. Pharmaceutical Press, London.

British Pharmaceutical Codex 1954. Pharmaceutical Press, London.

British Pharmaceutical Codex 1959. Pharmaceutical Press, London.

British Pharmaceutical Codex 1963. Pharmaceutical Press, London.

British Pharmaceutical Codex 1968. Pharmaceutical Press, London.

British Pharmaceutical Codex 1973. Pharmaceutical Press, London.

British Pharmacopoeia 1885. Spottiswoode & Co, London.

British Pharmacopoeia 1914. Constable & Co, London.

British Pharmacopoeia 1932. Constable & Co, London.

British Pharmacopoeia 1948. Constable & Co, London.

British Pharmacopoeia 1953. The Pharmaceutical Press, London.

British Pharmacopoeia 1958. The Pharmaceutical Press, London.

British Pharmacopoeia 1963. The Pharmaceutical Press, London.

British Pharmacopoeia 1968. The Pharmaceutical Press, London.

British Pharmacopoeia 1973. HMSO, London.

British Pharmacopoeia 1980. HMSO, London.

British Pharmacopoeia 1988. HMSO, London.

British Pharmacopoeia 2001. TSO, London.

British Pharmacopoeia 2002. TSO, London.

British Pharmacopoeia 2004. TSO, London.

Collett D M, Aulton M E (ed) 1990, *Pharmaceutical Practice*. Churchill Livingstone, Edinburgh.

Cooper J W, Gunn C 1950, *Dispensing for Pharmaceutical Students*. Pitman, London.

Cooper J W, Gunn C 1957, *Tutorial Pharmacy*. Pitman, London.

Matthews L G 1962, *History of Pharmacy in Britain*. E & S Livingston Ltd, Edinburgh.

Medicines, Ethics and Practice – A Guide for Pharmacists. Royal Pharmaceutical Society of Great Britain, London (updated twice yearly).

Museum of the Royal Pharmaceutical Society of Great Britain. Information Sheets. Available at http://www.rpsgb. org.uk/members/museum/index.html. Last accessed July 2005.

Remington J P 1905, *The Practice of Pharmacy*. J B Lippincott, Philadelphia, USA.

The Pharmaceutical Codex (12th Edition) 1994, *Principles and Practice of Pharmaceutics*. The Pharmaceutical Press, London.

Thompson J E 1998, *A Practical Guide to Contemporary Pharmacy Practice*. Lippincott, Williams & Wilkins, Baltimore, Maryland, USA.

Trease G E 1964, *Pharmacy in History*. Baillière Tindall & Cox, London.

Wade A (ed) 1980, *The Pharmaceutical Handbook*. The Pharmaceutical Press, London.

Wade A, Weller P J (ed) 1994, *Handbook of Pharmaceutical Excipients*. The Pharmaceutical Press, London.

Winfield A J, Richards R M E (ed) 1998, *Pharmaceutical Practice*. Churchill Livingstone, Edinburgh.

Index

Page references to figures are **bold**. Page references to tables are *italic*.